Vestibular Schwannoma

Editors

ERIKA WOODSON
MATTHEW L. CARLSON

OTOLARYNGOLOGIC CLINICS OF NORTH AMERICA

www.oto.theclinics.com

Consulting Editor
SUJANA S. CHANDRASEKHAR

June 2023 • Volume 56 • Number 3

ELSEVIER

1600 John F. Kennedy Boulevard • Suite 1800 • Philadelphia, Pennsylvania, 19103-2899

http://www.oto.theclinics.com

OTOLARYNGOLOGIC CLINICS OF NORTH AMERICA Volume 56, Number 3
June 2023 ISSN 0030-6665, ISBN-13: 978-0-443-18370-6

Editor: Stacy Eastman
Developmental Editor: Diana Grace Ang

Otolaryngologic Clinics of North America (ISSN 0030-6665) is published bimonthly by Elsevier, Inc., 360 Park Avenue South, New York, NY 10010-1710. Months of issue are February, April, June, August, October, and December. Business and Editorial Offices: 1600 John F. Kennedy Blvd., Suite 1800, Philadelphia, PA 19103-2899. Customer Service Office: 6277 Sea Harbor Drive, Orlando, FL 32887-4800. Periodicals postage paid at New York, NY and additional mailing offices. Subscription prices are $468.00 per year (US individuals), $1117.00 per year (US institutions), $100.00 per year (US & Canadian student/resident), $599.00 per year (Canadian individuals), $1416.00 per year (Canadian institutions), $653.00 per year (international individuals), $1416.00 per year (international institutions), $270.00 per year (international student/resident). Foreign air speed delivery is included in all *Clinics'* subscription prices. All prices are subject to change without notice. **POSTMASTER:** Send address changes to *Otolaryngologic Clinics of North America*, Elsevier Health Sciences Division, Subscription Customer Service, 3251 Riverport Lane, Maryland Heights, MO 63043. **Telephone: 1-800-654-2452 (U.S. and Canada); 314-447-8871 (outside U.S. and Canada). Fax: 314-447-8029. E-mail: journalscustomerservice-usa@elsevier.com (for print support); journalsonlinesupport-usa@elsevier.com (for online support).**

Reprints. For copies of 100 or more of articles in this publication, please contact the Commercial Reprints Department, Elsevier Inc., 360 Park Avenue South, New York, NY 10010-1710. Tel.: 212-633-3874; Fax: 212-633-3820; E-mail: reprints@elsevier.com.

Otolaryngologic Clinics of North America is also published in Spanish by McGraw-Hill Interamericana Editores S.A., P.O. Box 5-237, 06500 Mexico D.F., Mexico.

Otolaryngologic Clinics of North America is covered in *MEDLINE/PubMed (Index Medicus), Current Contents/Clinical Medicine, Excerpta Medica, BIOSIS, Science Citation Index,* and *ISI/BIOMED.*

Contributors

CONSULTING EDITOR

SUJANA S. CHANDRASEKHAR, MD, FACS, FAAOHNS
Consulting Editor, Otolaryngologic Clinics of North America, Secretary-Treasurer,
American Otological Society, Partner, ENT & Allergy Associates, LLP, Past President,
American Academy of Otolaryngology-Head and Neck Surgery, Partner, ENT & Allergy
Associates, LLP, Clinical Professor, Department of Otolaryngology-Head and Neck
Surgery, Zucker School of Medicine at Hofstra-Northwell, Clinical Associate Professor,
Department of Otolaryngology-Head and Neck Surgery, Icahn School of Medicine at
Mount Sinai, New York, New York, USA

EDITORS

ERIKA WOODSON, MD, FACS
Associate Physician, Head and Neck Surgery, Kaiser Permanente—Southern California,
San Diego, San Diego, California, USA

MATTHEW L. CARLSON, MD
Professor of Otolaryngology and Neurologic Surgery, Division Chair, Otology and
Neurotology, Program Director, Neurotology and Lateral Skull Base Surgery Fellowship,
Medical Director, Cochlear Implant Program, Department of Otolaryngology, Mayo Clinic,
Rochester, Minnesota, USA

AUTHORS

MEREDITH E. ADAMS, MD, MS
Associate Professor, Department of Otolaryngology–Head and Neck Surgery, Center for
Skull Base and Pituitary Surgery, University of Minnesota, Minneapolis, Minneapolis, USA

SEILESH C. BABU, MD
Otology, Neurotology and Skull Base Surgery, President, Michigan Ear Institute,
Farmington Hills, Michigan, USA

SAMUEL BARNETT, MD
Professor, Departments of Neurological Surgery and Otolaryngology, The University of
Texas Southwestern Medical Center, Dallas, Texas, USA

KAITLYN A. BROOKS, MD
Department of Otolaryngology–Head and Neck Surgery, Emory University, Atlanta, Georgia,
USA

MATTHEW L. CARLSON, MD
Professor of Otolaryngology and Neurologic Surgery, Division Chair, Otology and
Neurotology, Program Director, Neurotology and Lateral Skull Base Surgery Fellowship,
Medical Director, Cochlear Implant Program, Department of Otolaryngology, Mayo Clinic,
Rochester, Minnesota, USA

JANET S. CHOI, MD, MPH
Neurotology Fellow, Department of Otolaryngology–Head and Neck Surgery, University of Minnesota, Minneapolis, Minnesota, USA

PETER J. CIOLEK, MD
Facial Plastic and Reconstructive Surgery, Head and Neck Institute, Cleveland Clinic, Cleveland, Ohio, USA

ALEXANDER D. CLAUSSEN, MD
Department of Otolaryngology–Head and Neck Surgery, University of Iowa Hospitals and Clinics, University of Iowa, Iowa City, Iowa, USA

MAURA K. COSETTI, MD
Associate Professor, Department of Otolaryngology–Head and Neck Surgery, Icahn School of Medicine at Mount Sinai, New York, New York, USA

CHRISTINE T. DINH, MD
Associate Professor of Otolaryngology, Otology, Neurotology, & Lateral Skull Base Surgery, Director of Schwannoma Laboratory, Co-Director of Auditory Brainstem Implant Program, Department of Otolaryngology, University of Miami Miller School of Medicine, Miami, Florida, USA

ALLISON R. DURHAM, MD
Department of Otolaryngology, University of Utah Health, Salt Lake City, Utah, USA

CALEB J. FAN, MD
Otology, Neurotology and Skull Base Surgery, Michigan Ear Institute, Farmington Hills, Michigan, USA

SIMON FREEMAN, MB, ChB, BSc (Hons), MPhil, FRCS (ORL-HNS)
Consultant ENT and Skull Base Surgeon, Salford Royal Hospital and Manchester University NHS Trust, Manchester, United Kingdom

RICK A. FRIEDMAN MD, PhD
Professor of Otolaryngology and Neurosurgery, Co-Director of the UCSD Acoustic Neuroma Center, Division of Otolaryngology–Head and Neck Surgery, Department of Neurosurgery, University of California San Diego School of Medicine, San Diego, California, USA

ARIEL S. FROST, MD
Facial Plastic and Reconstructive Surgery, Head and Neck Institute, Cleveland Clinic, Cleveland, Ohio, USA

BRUCE J. GANTZ, MD
Department of Otolaryngology–Head and Neck Surgery, University of Iowa Hospitals and Clinics, University of Iowa, Iowa City, Iowa, USA

RICHARD K. GURGEL, MD, MSCI
Department of Otolaryngology, University of Utah Health, Salt Lake City, Utah, USA

MARLAN R. HANSEN, MD
Department of Otolaryngology–Head and Neck Surgery, University of Iowa Hospitals and Clinics, University of Iowa, Iowa City, Iowa, USA

JACOB B. HUNTER, MD
Associate Professor of Otolaryngology, The University of Texas Southwestern Medical Center, Dallas Texas, USA

BRANDON ISAACSON, MD
Professor, Departments of Otolaryngology and Neurological Surgery, The University of Texas Southwestern Medical Center, Dallas, Texas, USA

JEFFREY T. JACOB, MD
Neurosurgery, Michigan Head and Spine Institute, Southfield, Michigan, USA

PAWINA JIRAMONGKOLCHAI, MD, MSCI
Division of Otolaryngology–Head and Neck Surgery, University of California San Diego School of Medicine, San Diego, California, USA

RUSTIN G. KASHANI, MD
Department of Otolaryngology–Head and Neck Surgery, University of Iowa Hospitals and Clinics, University of Iowa, Iowa City, Iowa, USA

EMILY KAY-RIVEST, MD, MSc
Assistant Professor, Division of Otology and Neurotology, Department of Otolaryngology–Head and Neck Surgery, McGill University, Montreal, Quebec, Canada; Division of Otology and Neurotology, Department of Otolaryngology–Head and Neck Surgery, New York University, New York, New York, USA

ARMINE KOCHARYAN, MD
Department of Otolaryngology–Head and Neck Surgery, University of Iowa Hospitals and Clinics, University of Iowa, Iowa City, Iowa, USA

JOE WALTER KUTZ Jr, MD
Professor, Departments of Otolaryngology and Neurological Surgery, The University of Texas Southwestern Medical Center, Dallas, Texas, USA

MICHAEL J. LINK, MD
Departments of Otolaryngology–Head and Neck Surgery, and Neurologic Surgery, Mayo Clinic, Rochester, Minnesota, USA

SIMON LLOYD, MBBS, BSc (Hons), MPhil(Oxon), FRCS(ORL-HNS)
Professor, Consultant ENT and Skull Base Surgeon, Salford Royal Hospital and Manchester University NHS Trust, Manchester, United Kingdom

CHRISTINE M. LOHSE, MS
Department of Quantitative Health Sciences, Mayo Clinic, Rochester, Minnesota, USA

JACOB C. LUCAS, MD
Otology, Neurotology and Skull Base Surgery, Michigan Ear Institute, Farmington Hills, Michigan, USA

JOHN P. MARINELLI, MD
Department of Otolaryngology–Head and Neck Surgery, Mayo Clinic, Rochester, Minnesota, USA; Department of Otolaryngology–Head and Neck Surgery, San Antonio Uniformed Services Health Education Consortium, JBSA, Texas, USA

FIONA MCCLENAGHAN, MBBS, BSc, (Hons), FRCS (ORL-HNS)
Skull Base Fellow, Salford Royal Hospital and Manchester University NHS Trust, Manchester, United Kingdom

LINDSAY SCOTT MOORE, MD
Tahbazof Clinical and Research Fellow, Clinician Scientist Training Program, Department of Otolaryngology–Head and Neck Surgery, Stanford University School of Medicine, Stanford, California, USA

AIDA NOURBAKHSH, MD, PhD
T32 Resident, Department of Otolaryngology, University of Miami Miller School of Medicine, Miami, Florida, USA

NEIL S. PATEL, MD
Department of Otolaryngology, University of Utah Health, Salt Lake City, Utah, USA

JOHN THOMAS ROLAND Jr, MD
Professor and Chair, Division of Otology and Neurotology, Department of Otolaryngology–Head and Neck Surgery, New York University, New York, New York, USA

ZACHARY G. SCHWAM, MD
Neurotology Fellow, Department of Otolaryngology–Head and Neck Surgery, Icahn School of Medicine at Mount Sinai, New York, New York, USA

MARC S. SCHWARTZ, MD
Department of Neurosurgery, University of California San Diego School of Medicine, San Diego, California, USA

VUSALA SNYDER, MD
Department of Otolaryngology, University of Pittsburgh, Pittsburgh, Pennsylvania, USA

KONSTANTINA M. STANKOVIC, MD, PhD
Bertarelli Foundation Professor and Chair, Departments of Otolaryngology–Head and Neck Surgery, and Neurosurgery, Stanford University School of Medicine, Stanford, California, USA

EMMA STAPLETON, MB, ChB, FRCS (ORL-HNS)
Consultant ENT and Auditory Implant Surgeon, Manchester University NHS Trust, Manchester, United Kingdom

DONALD TAN, MD
The University of Texas Southwestern Medical Center, Dallas Texas, USA

EVAN L. TOOKER, MS
Department of Otolaryngology, University of Utah Health, Salt Lake City, Utah, USA

ANDREW S. VENTEICHER, MD, PhD
Assistant Professor, Department of Neurosurgery, Center for Skull Base and Pituitary Surgery, University of Minnesota, Minneapolis, Minneapolis, USA

ESTHER X. VIVAS, MD
Professor, Department of Otolaryngology–Head and Neck Surgery, Emory University, Atlanta, Georgia, USA

GEORGE B. WANNA, MD
Professor, Department of Otolaryngology–Head and Neck Surgery, Icahn School of Medicine at Mount Sinai, New York, New York, USA

D. BRADLEY WELLING, MD, PhD
Walter Augustus Lecompte Distinguished Professor, Harvard Department of Otolaryngology–Head and Neck Surgery, Massachusetts Eye and Ear Infirmary, Massachusetts General Hospital, Boston, Massachusetts, USA

CAMERON C. WICK, MD
Associate Professor, Department of Otolaryngology–Head and Neck Surgery, Washington University, St Louis, Missouri, USA

ERIKA WOODSON, MD, FACS
Associate Physician, Head and Neck Surgery, Kaiser Permanente—Southern California, San Diego, San Diego, California, USA

KEVIN Y. ZHAN, MD
Department of Otolaryngology–Head and Neck Surgery, Washington University, St Louis, Missouri, USA

Contents

> Vestibular schwannomas (VSs) are benign, slow-growing tumors of the eighth cranial nerve. Sporadic unilateral VSs constitute approximately 95% of all newly diagnosed tumors. There is little known about risk factors for developing sporadic unilateral VS. Potential risk factors that have been reported are familial or genetic risk, noise exposure, cell phone use, and ionizing radiation, whereas protective factors may include smoking and aspirin use. More research is needed to elucidate the risk factors for development of these rare tumors.

> Vestibular schwannomas (VSs) are benign tumors that develop after biallelic inactivation of the NF2 gene that encodes the tumor suppressor merlin. Merlin inactivation leads to cell proliferation by dysregulation of receptor tyrosine kinase signaling and other intracellular pathways. In VS without NF2 mutations, dysregulation of non-NF2 genes can promote pathways favoring cell proliferation and tumorigenesis. Furthermore, the tumor microenvironment of VS consists of multiple cell types that influence VS tumor biology through complex intercellular networking and communications.

> Hearing loss is the most common and earliest symptom of sporadic vestibular schwannoma (VS). The most common pattern of hearing loss is asymmetric sensorineural hearing loss. Throughout its natural history, patients with serviceable hearing (SH) maintain SH at 94% to 95% after 1 year, 73% to 77% after 2 years, 56% to 66% after 5 years, and 32% to 44% after 10 years. For patients newly diagnosed with VS, it is likely their hearing will worsen despite small initial tumor size or lack of tumor growth.

The advent of MRI has led to more sporadic vestibular schwannomas diagnosed today than ever before. Despite the average patient being diagnosed in their sixth decade of life with a small tumor and minimal symptoms, population-based data demonstrate that more tumors per capita are treated today than ever before. Emerging natural history data justify either an upfront treatment approach or the "Size Threshold Surveillance" approach. Specifically, if the patient elects to pursue observation, then existing data support the tolerance of some growth during observation in appropriately selected patients up until a specific size threshold range (about 15 mm of CPA extension). The current article discusses the rationale behind a shift in the existing observation management approach, where initial detection of growth typically begets treatment, and outlines the application of a more flexible and nuanced approach based on existing evidence.

Decision-making in management of sporadic vestibular schwannoma aims to identify the most appropriate options based on tumor characteristics, symptoms, health, and goals for each patient. Advances in knowledge of tumor natural history, improvements in radiation techniques, and achievements in neurologic preservation with microsurgery have shifted emphasis toward maximizing quality of life using a personalized approach. To empower patients to make informed decisions, we present a framework to help match patient values and priorities with reasonable expectations from modern management options. Introduced herein are practical examples of communication strategies and decision aids to support shared decision-making in modern practice.

Monitoring the cochlear nerve during vestibular schwannoma (VS) microsurgery depends on the hearing status and surgical approach. Traditional hearing preservation VS microsurgery relies on acoustically driven auditory brainstem response (ABR) and cochlear nerve action potential. Both modalities have advantages and disadvantages that need to be understood for proper implementation. When hearing is lost or the approach violates the otic capsule, electrically evoked monitoring methods may be used. Evoked ABR (eABR) is feasible and safe but may be limited by artifact. Combining eABR with near-field measures such as electrocochleography or neural telemetry shows promise.

Herein we briefly describe the translabyrinthine approach to vestibular schwannoma resection as well as a focused literature review as to the best candidates, technical recommendations, and key outcomes with respect to other approaches.

Rustin G. Kashani, Armine Kocharyan, Alexander D. Claussen, Bruce J. Gantz, and Marlan R. Hansen

The middle fossa approach is an excellent technique for removing appropriate vestibular schwannomas in patients with serviceable hearing. Knowledge of the intricate middle fossa anatomy is essential for optimal outcomes. Gross total removal can be achieved with preservation of hearing and facial nerve function, both in the immediate and long-term periods. This article provides an overview of the background and indications for the procedure, a description of the operative protocol, and a summary of the literature on postoperative hearing outcomes.

Jacob C. Lucas, Caleb J. Fan, Jeffrey T. Jacob, and Seilesh C. Babu

The retrosigmoid corridor provides the most broadly applied approach for resection of sporadic vestibular schwannoma. It may be utilized for any size tumor and for patients with intact hearing with the intention of hearing preservation. For larger tumors, the skull base surgeon must weigh the benefits the retrosigmoid approach against those of the translabyrinthine route. For smaller tumors where hearing preservation is a goal, the retrosigmoid approach is contrasted to the middle fossa route. Hearing preservation is most likely for patients with small and medially located intracanalicular tumors with minimal extension into the cerebellopontine angle, and excellent preoperative hearing.

Erika Woodson

Stereotactic radiosurgery (SRS) is a valid option for most patients undergoing treatment of small- and medium-sized vestibular schwannoma. Predictors of hearing preservation are the same for observation or surgery: when pretreatment hearing is normal, the tumor is smaller, and when a cerebrospinal fluid fundal cap exists. Hearing outcomes are poor when hearing loss exists pre-treatment. Rates of facial and trigeminal neuropathy are higher post-treatment after fractionated plans than single-fraction SRS. Subtotal resection and adjuvant radiation appears to offer patients with large tumors optimal outcomes for hearing, tumor control, and cranial nerve function versus gross total resection.

Pawina Jiramongkolchai, Marc S. Schwartz, and Rick A. Friedman

Neurofibromatosis type 2 (NF2) is an autosomal dominant syndrome caused by a mutation in the NF2 suppressor gene and is characterized by the development of multiple benign tumors throughout the central nervous system. Bilateral vestibular schwannomas (VSs) are pathogno-monic for NF2 and are associated with progressive hearing loss and even-tual deafness in most patients. This review presents current management options for NF-2-associated VSs.

D. Bradley Welling

Vestibular schwannomas continue to cause hearing loss, facial nerve pa-ralysis, imbalance, and tinnitus. These symptoms are compounded by germline neurofibromatosis type 2 (NF2) gene loss and multiple intracranial and spinal cord tumors associated with NF2-related schwannomatosis. The current treatments of observation, microsurgical resection, or stereo-tactic radiation may prevent catastrophic brainstem compression but are all associated with the loss of cranial nerve function, particularly hearing loss. Novel targeted treatment options to stop tumor progression include small molecule inhibitors, immunotherapy, anti-inflammatory drugs, radio-sensitizing and sclerosing agents, and gene therapy.

Emily Kay-Rivest and John Thomas Roland Jr

The current management of vestibular schwannomas (VS) includes obser-vation, microsurgery (MS), and stereotactic radiosurgery (SRS) or radio-therapy, and treatment failures may occur with any primary modality. SRS is most often used for microsurgical failures, as it carries a low risk of adverse events. Salvage MS following previous MS is reserved for spe-cific cases and can present certain surgical challenges. Irradiation failures can be managed with both salvage MS and repeat SRS. This article is in-tended to review an approach to the failure of primary interventions for VS, with a focus on the time interval between modalities, rates of tumor con-trol, functional outcomes, and possible complications.

Joe Walter Kutz Jr, Donald Tan, Jacob B. Hunter, Samuel Barnett, and Brandon Isaacson

Microsurgical removal of acoustic neuroma has advanced tremendously; however, complications still occur. Facial nerve injury is the most common detrimental complication and should take precedence over gross tumor removal in cases where there is an unfavorable tumor-facial nerve interface. Cerebrospinal fluid leakage can occur even with meticulous closure tech-niques and is generally treatable with either lumbar-subarachnoid drainage or revision wound closure. Meningitis is a serious complication that requires a high index of suspicion in the postoperative period. Other less common complications include intraoperative and postoperative vascular injuries. Early identification and treatment can prevent devastating outcomes.

John P. Marinelli, Christine M. Lohse, Michael J. Link, and Matthew L. Carlson

The focus of management in sporadic vestibular schwannoma has dramatically evolved over the last 100 years. The centrality of quality of life (QoL) is being underscored by an ongoing epidemiologic shift toward an older patient demographic that is being diagnosed with smaller tumors and often with few associated symptoms. Two disease-specific QoL instruments have been developed for sporadic vestibular schwannoma: the Penn Acoustic Neuroma Quality of Life Scale in 2010, and more recently, the Mayo Clinic Vestibular Schwannoma Quality of Life Index in 2022. The current article examines disease-specific quality-of-life outocmes in the management of ssporadic vestibular schwannoma.

Cochlear implantation offers significantly better hearing outcomes than auditory brainstem implantation in patients with vestibular schwannoma. Neither the primary treatment modality nor the cause of the tumor (neurofibromatosis type 2 related or sporadic) seems to have a significant effect on hearing outcome with cochlear implantation. Some uncertainty remains regarding long-term hearing outcomes; however, cochlear implantation in vestibular schwannoma serves to offer patients, with a functioning cochlear nerve, the probability of open set speech discrimination with a consequent positive impact on quality of life.

Facial nerve paralysis is a debilitating clinical entity that presents as a complete or incomplete loss of facial nerve function. The etiology of facial nerve palsy and sequelae varies tremendously. The most common cause of facial paralysis is Bell's palsy, followed by malignant or benign tumors, iatrogenic insults, trauma, virus-associated paralysis, and congenital etiologies.

The future of the management of both sporadic and neurofibromatosis type 2-asscoiated vestibular schwannomas (VSs) will be shaped by cutting-edge technologic and biomedical advances to enable personalized, precision medicine. This scoping review envisions the future by highlighting the most promising developments published, ongoing, planned, or potential that are relevant for VS, including integrated omics approaches, artificial intelligence algorithms, biomarkers, liquid biopsy of the inner ear, digital medicine, inner ear endomicroscopy, targeted molecular imaging, patient-specific stem cell-derived models, ultra-high dose rate radiotherapy, optical imaging-guided microsurgery, high-throughput development of targeted therapeutics, novel immunotherapeutic strategies, tumor vaccines, and gene therapy.

OTOLARYNGOLOGIC CLINICS OF NORTH AMERICA

SERIES OF RELATED INTEREST

Facial Plastic Surgery Clinics
Available at: https://www.facialplastic.theclinics.com/

THE CLINICS ARE AVAILABLE ONLINE!
Access your subscription at:
www.theclinics.com

Foreword

Vestibular Schwannoma: The Current Knowledge

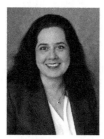

Sujana S. Chandrasekhar, MD, FACS
Consulting Editor

Vestibular schwannoma (VS) is a rare tumor. The incidence of VS in the United States is somewhere between 1.2 and 2.6 cases per 100,000 per year, with a median age at diagnosis of 55 years. Eighty-nine percent of all nerve sheath tumors are schwannomas, and 60% of benign schwannomas are VSs. The incidence of VS diagnosis is increasing as brain MRI scans are done for various reasons, with VS often being found incidentally. When they are symptomatic, they often present with asymmetric or sudden hearing loss, often with tinnitus, due to pressure on the adjacent cochlear nerve in the internal auditory canal. When presenting early, these tumors lend themselves to significant shared decision making between patient/family and physician. In the United States, it is less likely that we encounter a large or giant VS these days; unfortunately, the same cannot be said about other countries, where life-saving measures are often the first intervention for these benign but space-occupying lesions.

When I first learned about VS, the tumor was mis-called Acoustic Neuroma (AN). It is neither Acoustic, as it arises from the Vestibular portion of the eighth cranial nerve, nor is it a Neuroma, as its cell of origin is the Schwann cell surrounding the nerve. By the time the nomenclature changed officially, both VS and AN were used interchangeably, and the distinction seemed somewhat semantic, as the tumors could not be dissected off of intact vestibular nerves. But, of course, better understanding of tumor anatomy and biology, as well as interchange of ideas and approaches between neurotologists, neurosurgeons, radiation oncologists, physicists, and medical oncologists and immunologists, can only make patient outcomes better.

Sporadic VS behaves quite differently from the often bilateral and aggressive VS seen in Neurofibromatosis 2 (NF2). The three options for sporadic VS: observation, microsurgery, and radiation, may not be appropriate for patients with NF2. Many of the advances in medical interventions, in particular, for VS, have been made because

Otolaryngol Clin N Am 56 (2023) xv–xvi
https://doi.org/10.1016/j.otc.2023.03.002
0030-6665/23/

of the different tumor biology and significant quality-of-life impact of NF2. And, of course, we cannot forget the fourth traveler in the internal auditory canal and cerebellopontine angle, the facial nerve, as well as other cranial nerves in the vicinity.

The Guest Editors of this issue of *Otolaryngologic Clinics of North America*, Drs Erika Woodson and Matthew Carlson, have lent their clinical and research perspectives to designing an issue that explores all aspects of care for patients with VS. Even though this is a rare tumor, it remains in the minds of otolaryngologists, as we are usually the ones making the initial diagnosis and discussing the possible treatment plan, even in broad strokes. I think that all clinicians who interact with patients who may have this tumor will benefit from reading this issue of *Otolaryngologic Clinics of North America* on Vestibular Schwannoma, as the resources found within are outstanding.

Sujana S. Chandrasekhar, MD, FACS
Consulting Editor
Otolaryngologic Clinics of North America
Past President
American Academy of Otolaryngology–
Head and Neck Surgery
Secretary-Treasurer
American Otological Society
Partner
ENT & Allergy Associates, LLP
18 East 48th Street, 2nd Floor
New York, NY 10017, USA

Clinical Professor
Department of Otolaryngology–
Head and Neck Surgery
Zucker School of Medicine at Hofstra–Northwell
Hempstead, NY, USA

Clinical Associate Professor
Department of Otolaryngology–
Head and Neck Surgery
Icahn School of Medicine at Mount Sinai
New York, NY, USA

E-mail address:
ssc@nyotology.com

Preface

Welcome to the *Otolaryngologic Clinics of North America*, Vestibular Schwannoma Issue

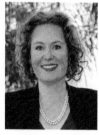
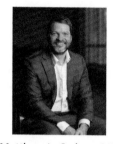

Erika Woodson, MD, FACS   Matthew L. Carlson, MD

Editors

Despite vestibular schwannoma being relatively uncommon, otolaryngologists and neurosurgeons have maintained an enduring fascination with the management of sporadic and NF2-associated vestibular schwannoma. Within the last 100 years, vestibular schwannomas characteristically defined the subspecialties of neurotology and neurologic skull base surgery—supporting refinements in middle and posterior fossa skull base approaches, driving innovation, such as intraoperative cranial nerve monitoring and early adoption of the operating microscope, and fostering the multidisciplinary collaboration that exists today.

Though substantial investments in clinical and basic science research have occurred, the management of vestibular schwannoma remains challenging and controversial. Management trends continue to evolve for tumors of all sizes. Patient-centered decision making is now an appropriate focus of the counseling process. The initial management of small tumors with the goal of function preservation is complex and nuanced, and this issue explores multiple viewpoints. Considerations regarding extent of resection, adjuvant radiosurgery, and salvage management of sporadic large vestibular schwannoma are a few of many topics debated here with updated data and more patient-centered perspective. Novel perspectives on management of NF2 disease, tumor modulating clinical trials, and cochlear implantation all await the reader.

Our primary objective in this issue was to provide an update on timely topics related to the management of this disease. Each article covers fundamental considerations directed toward residents, fellows, and early attending physicians as well as more complex concepts that will appeal to experienced surgeons and clinicians who treat patients with vestibular schwannoma. Indeed, we hope that this issue provides

Otolaryngol Clin N Am 56 (2023) xvii–xviii
https://doi.org/10.1016/j.otc.2023.03.001
0030-6665/23/© 2023 Published by Elsevier Inc.

guidance to improve the care of patients with vestibular schwannoma now, and optimism for innovation in managing this challenging disease in years to come.

Sincerely yours,

Erika Woodson, MD, FACS
Head and Neck Surgery
Kaiser Permanente
San Diego, CA 92111, USA

Matthew L. Carlson, MD
Department of Otolaryngology
Mayo Clinic
Rochester, MN 55905, USA

E-mail addresses:
ewoodsonmd@gmail.com (E. Woodson)
Carlson.matthew@mayo.edu (M.L. Carlson)

Epidemiology and Risk Factors for Development of Sporadic Vestibular Schwannoma

Allison R. Durham, MD, Evan L. Tooker, MS, Neil S. Patel, MD,
Richard K. Gurgel, MD, MSCI*

KEYWORDS

- Vestibular schwannoma • Acoustic neuroma • Risk factors • Incidence
- Epidemiology • Familial risk • Noise exposure • Smoking

KEY POINTS

- The incidence of vestibular schwannoma ranges from 3 to 5 per 100,000.
- Familial risk may be a factor in the development of unilateral vestibular schwannoma.
- Cell phone use remains a controversial risk factor for vestibular schwannoma.
- Noise exposure has been identified as a potential risk factor; leisure noise seems to incur greater risk than occupational noise exposure.
- There is a decreased incidence of vestibular schwannoma among current smokers.

INTRODUCTION AND EPIDEMIOLOGY

Vestibular schwannomas (VSs), also historically referred to as acoustic neuromas, arise from Schwann cells ensheathing the vestibular portion of the vestibulocochlear nerve. These benign tumors typically exhibit indolent growth within the internal auditory canal with the potential to extend into the cerebellopontine angle and compress the cerebellum, brainstem, and cranial nerves V, VII, and VIII. Sporadic VSs are unilateral tumors that account for 94% to 96% of cases, whereas the other 5% develop in individuals with the autosomal dominant genetic condition neurofibromatosis type II (NF2), characterized by bilateral VS or other central nervous system (CNS) tumors.[1,2]

A recent systemic review by Marinelli and colleagues[3] suggests the incidence rate of sporadic VS is much higher than the historically quoted rate of one per 100,000 person-years.[4-6] Among international population-based studies published between 2010 and 2022 in Denmark, the Netherlands, Taiwan, and the United States, incidence rates ranged between 3.0 and 5.2 per 100,000 person-years with a median age of 60 years

Department of Otolaryngology, University of Utah Health, 50 North Medical Drive, SOM 3C120, Salt Lake City, UT 84132, USA
* Corresponding author.
E-mail address: richard.gurgel@hsc.utah.edu

Otolaryngol Clin N Am 56 (2023) 413–420
https://doi.org/10.1016/j.otc.2023.02.003
0030-6665/23/Published by Elsevier Inc.

at diagnosis.[3,7–11] All four cohorts reported no difference in incidence rates between female and male sex.

Collectively, an incidence rate of threefold to fivefold greater than previously reported represents a much higher prevalence of sporadic VS that more closely aligns with historical temporal bone studies that cite a lifetime prevalence of up to one in 100 persons.[12,13] Considering the increase in incidence rates of 3 to 5 per 100,000 person-years, the lifetime chance of developing a sporadic VS that is diagnosed in the clinical setting by MRI is greater than one in 500 people.[11] The rising incidence of VS is largely attributed to the increased sensitivity of MRI technology, established criteria for asymmetric sensorineural hearing loss, and increased access to health care screening in the post-MRI era, though few studies have tested this theory. Between 2004 and 2016, the incidence of head MRI in Olmsted County, Minnesota, remained stable, whereas the incidence rates of incidentally diagnosed VS continued to increase in the study population.[14] These findings suggest that etiologies other than increased MRI screening and utilization may be contributing to the rising incidence of sporadic VS. Are there other known risk factors for developing VS? This article explores the evidence regarding a number of potential genetic and environmental risk factors for unilateral, sporadic VS.

FAMILIAL RISK

There is evidence in the literature for a genetic or familial link between sporadic VS cases, occurring in patients who do not meet criteria for NF2.[15] Bikhazi and colleagues reported on a case series of nine families with sporadic unilateral VS. In this series, there were five first-degree relative relationships (four parent-offspring and one sibling) and four second-degree relative relationships (three first-degree cousins' relationships and one aunt-nephew relationship). No family had a diagnosis or evidence of NF2. The observed frequency of unilateral VS occurrence was much higher than the expected frequency based on available epidemiologic incidence data.[15] Interestingly, 50% of the patients in the series presented with tumors larger than 3 cm.[15]

In a more recent 2022 study, Gurgel and colleagues[16] reported similar findings in an analysis of two large, independent genealogical databases: the Veterans Health Administration Genealogy Resource and the Utah Population Database. In this study, the investigators analyzed familial clustering of individuals with unilateral VS and found that the relatedness of unilateral VS cases exceeded the expected relatedness of cases in the Veterans Health Administration database. **Fig. 1** shows a high-risk

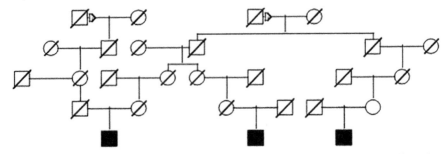

Fig. 1. High-risk pedigree for unilateral VS from the Utah Population Database. Affected individuals are shaded. Females are circles, and males are squares. Deceased individuals have a slash. (*From* Gurgel RK, Couldwell WT, Patel NS, Cannon-Albright LA. Is There an Inherited Contribution to Risk for Sporadic Unilateral Vestibular Schwannoma? Evidence of Familial Clustering. Otol Neurotol. 2022, with permission.)

pedigree that was identified in the Utah Population Database.[16] This study demonstrated a significantly elevated risk for unilateral VS in more distant cousins of cases in both databases: there was a relative risk of 60.83 to third-degree relatives and a relative risk of 2.3 to 11.88 in fifth-degree relatives.[16] Taken together, these findings provide strong evidence for an underlying heritable risk factor present in these families, which has been confirmed by different authors using independent databases.

CELL PHONE USE

Currently, there is no consensus linking cellular telephone use with an increased risk of cancer, but most of the literatures suggest that there is no correlation.[17–20] Starting with the introduction of cellular telephones in the mid-1980s, there was a concern for a risk of brain tumors given the proximity of the brain to the radiofrequency radiation emitted by cellular antennas. Exposure to moderate-to-high doses of ionizing radiation among atomic bomb survivors and dental x-rays are the only two established environmental risks for brain and CNS tumors.[21–24] However, ionizing radiation in the clinical setting, which includes diagnostic radiation (5–50 EHz) and therapeutic radiation (500–5,000 EHz), is a 10^6 magnitude greater than the 39 GHz emitted by 5G cellular antennas and far below the human exposure limits specified by the International Commission on Non-Ionizing Radiation Protection (ICNIRP).[25,26]

Early epidemiologic studies by the National Cancer Institute (NCI) between 1994 and 1998 found no relationship between cell phone use and risk of VS in adults.[27,28] One of the largest animal studies by the US National Toxicology Program investigating 2G and 3G frequencies in rats and mice observed smalls amounts of cancerous cardiac Schwann cells in male rats but not in female rats or mice.[28,29] Given the similarities between cardiac and vestibular Schwann cells, there was concern about the potential risk for VS. However, these findings were not found in similar mouse[30] and rat[31] animal models, raising questions about inconsistency. The ICNIRP has largely discredited conclusions about the increased risk of cancer associated with radiofrequency exposure in subsequent animal studies.[32]

The Million Women study and the Danish Cohort, two of the largest epidemiologic reviews to date, collectively concluded that there is no evidence linking cell phone use with an increased risk of sporadic VS.[20,33–35] The Million Women Study, a prospective cohort of more than 790,000 women in the United Kingdom, analyzed data of self-reported cell phone questionnaires and rates of VS. The initial outcomes reported higher rates of VS among participants with greater than 10 years of cell phone use but was not reported in follow-up studies.[20] Researchers acknowledged limitations in the interpretation of the increased risk of VS and noted that rates in the United Kingdom did not increase over the same period of increased mobile phone use. The most comprehensive study, the Danish Cohort Study, compared subscriber information from more than 358,000 cell phones with the Danish Cancer Registry brain tumor incidence data and found no association between cell phone use and the incidence of VS, even among subscribers with 13 or more years of cell phone use.[33]

As of 2011, the International Agency for Research on Cancer classifies radiofrequency electromagnetic fields as a Group 2B (possibly carcinogenic to humans) based on the limited evidence of an increased risk for glioma (not VS).[36] The Food and Drug Administration, NCI and the Center for Disease Control collectively state that there is no scientific evidence that definitively links cell phone use and cancer.[25,37,38] Although long-term studies are ongoing, to date there is no convincing evidence linking cell phone use to an increased risk of sporadic VS.[17–20]

NOISE EXPOSURE

There have been a number of studies reporting on a link between noise exposure and the development of VS with varying results. A large population-based case-control study in Europe reported increased odds ratio (OR) of developing VS in individuals with leisure-based noise exposure (1.9) and occupational noise exposure (1.7).[39] A separate meta-analysis of eight studies reported similar findings of increased risk for both occupational and leisure noise exposure, with a higher OR for leisure noise exposure (4.9 vs 2.2).[40] However, other studies have reported no increased risk of VS with occupational noise exposure.[41–43] It has been hypothesized that the increased risk observed with leisure noise exposure may be due to different noise type or that individuals are less likely to use ear protection when exposed to leisure noise compared with occupational noise.[40] The presence of a true causal relationship between noise exposure and the development of VS is unknown as most of these studies are subject to recall bias.

SMOKING

Cigarette smoking may be a protective factor in the risk of developing VS.[41,44–46] A large international case-based control study demonstrated a decreased OR of developing VS in ever smokers (0.7), which was lower in current smokers (0.5).[45] A decreased incidence of VS in current smokers was also reported in a prospective study of women in the United Kingdom.[44] It is unclear why smoking may be a protective factor in the development of VS; some investigators have proposed that female sex hormones may play a role, which are modulated by smoking.[44,45] It should also be stated that VS are significantly more rare than other tumors known to be associated with smoking, so the potential protective benefits for VS do not outweigh the other known risks of smoking for cancer development and other associated health problems.

ASPIRIN

Certain medications may be protective against the development of VS and could therefore be considered negative risk factors for VS. Pharmacologic treatment of sporadic VS with aspirin (ASA) has been proposed as an alternative to surgical resection and stereotactic radiotherapy and thus may also have potential protective benefits against developing sporadic VS. ASAs potential to slow VS growth via inhibition of the cyclooxygenase-2 enzyme has been documented with limited results.[47,48] In 2018, the Congress of Neurological Surgeons recommended that ASA may be considered for use in patients undergoing observation of their VS.[49] However, the recent meta-analysis on the efficacy of ASA on sporadic VS by Ignacio and colleagues[50] found no significant difference in tumor growth between VS patients with ASA intake and those without. Among the four cohorts in the retrospective study, no significant difference in the OR between linear tumor growth (1.2), volumetric tumor growth (1.4) and both combined (1.0) was found. Currently, there is a phase II, prospective, double-blind, multicenter longitudinal study examining the effect of ASA on growth of VS. Although there is insufficient evidence to recommend ASA as a therapy for patients with VS at this time, there may be a potential protective benefit against developing sporadic VS.

SUMMARY

In summary, the incidence rates of sporadic VS increased over the last two decades—ranging between 3.0 and 5.2 per 100,000 person-years. Increased incidence rates are largely attributed to greater access to medical care and MRI, particularly regarding incidentally diagnosed tumors. However, there may be additional etiologies contributing to the increase in the incidence of VS beyond detection alone. Among potential risk factors, there is strong evidence for an underlying heritable risk factor in a subset of patients. Although cell phone use and noise exposure are proposed risk factors, the connection remains controversial due to limited evidence and study design bias. Smoking has been identified as a negative (ie, protective) risk factor in multiple studies; however, it has limited benefit due to a much higher risk of developing cancers and other serious medical problems. ASA may be a negative risk factor; however, the results of its effect on VS growth are mixed and it has not been shown to significantly reduce tumor growth. Future studies with additional large, independent genealogical databases as well as an ongoing randomized clinical trial on the effect of ASA show promise in further characterizing the risk factors for sporadic VS.

CLINICS CARE POINTS

- In order of prevalence, the most common presenting symptoms include ipsilateral sensorineural hearing loss, imbalance, tinnitus, and ear fullness.
- There is limited data to support an association between tumor size and severity of symptoms.
- Tumor growth is not strongly correlated with new or worsening symptoms.
- Thin-sliced, gadolinium contrast enhanced MRI of the head is the standard method for diagnosis without confirmatory biopsy.
- Current treatment options include active tumor surveillance with MRI, microsurgical resection, and radiosurgery.
- The choice of treatment is based on patient preference, clinical presentation, tumor size, and institutional expertise.
- For the treatment of small tumors, there is a paradigm shift towards active tumor surveillance with MRI instead of traditional up-front microsurgical resection.

DISCLOSURE

R.K. Gurgel serves on the surgical advisory board for MedEl and receives institutional research support from Cochlear, Australia and Advanced Bionics. No disclosures for other authors.

REFERENCES

1. Evans DG, Moran A, King A, et al. Incidence of vestibular schwannoma and neurofibromatosis 2 in the North West of England over a 10-year period: higher incidence than previously thought. Otol Neurotol 2005;26(1):93–7.
2. Evans DG, Huson SM, Donnai D, et al. A clinical study of type 2 neurofibromatosis. Q J Med 1992;84(304):603–18.
3. Marinelli JP, Beeler CJ, Carlson ML, et al. Global incidence of sporadic vestibular schwannoma: a systematic review. Otolaryngol Head Neck Surg 2022;167(2):209–14.
4. Cleveland Clinic Health Library-Acoustic Neuroma. Cleveland Clinic Health Library. 2022. Available at: https://my.clevelandclinic.org/health/diseases/16400-acoustic-neuroma. Accessed October 1, 2022.

5. National Institute on Deafness and Other Communication Disorders. Vestibular Schwannoma (Acoustic Neuroma) and Neurofibromatosis. Available at: https://www.nidcd.nih.gov/health/vestibular-schwannoma-acoustic-neuroma-and-neurofibromatosis. Accessed October 1, 2022.

6. Bangiyev JN, Gurgel R, Vanderhooft SL, et al. Reversible profound sensorineural hearing loss due to propranolol sensitive hemangioma in an infant with PHACE syndrome. Int J Pediatr Otorhinolaryngol 2017;103:55–7.

7. Kleijwegt M, Ho V, Visser O, et al. Real incidence of vestibular schwannoma? estimations from a national registry. Otol Neurotol 2016;37(9):1411–7.

8. Reznitsky M, Petersen MMBS, West N, et al. Epidemiology Of Vestibular Schwannomas – Prospective 40-Year Data From An Unselected National Cohort</p&gt. Clin Epidemiol 2019;11:981–6.

9. Koo M, Lai JT, Yang EY, et al. Incidence of vestibular schwannoma in Taiwan from 2001 to 2012: a population-based national health insurance study. Ann Otol Rhinol Laryngol 2018;127(10):694–7.

10. Marinelli JP, Lohse CM, Carlson ML. Incidence of vestibular schwannoma over the past half-century: a population-based study of Olmsted County, Minnesota. Otolaryngol Head Neck Surg 2018;159(4):717–23.

11. Marinelli JP, Grossardt BR, Lohse CM, et al. Prevalence of sporadic vestibular schwannoma: reconciling temporal bone, radiologic, and population-based Studies. Otol Neurotol 2019;40(3):384–90.

12. Stewart TJ, Liland J, Schuknecht HF. Occult schwannomas of the vestibular nerve. Arch Otolaryngol Head Neck Surg 1975;101(2):91–5.

13. Leonard JR, Talbot ML. Asymptomatic acoustic neurilemoma. Arch Otolaryngol Head Neck Surg 1970;91(2):117–24.

14. Marinelli JP, Lohse CM, Grossardt BR, et al. Rising incidence of sporadic vestibular schwannoma: true biological shift versus simply greater detection. Otol Neurotol 2020;41(6):813–47.

15. Bikhazi NB, Slattery WH 3rd, Lalwani AK, et al. Familial occurrence of unilateral vestibular schwannoma. Laryngoscope 1997;107(9):1176–80.

16. Gurgel RK, Couldwell WT, Patel NS, et al. Is there an inherited contribution to risk for sporadic unilateral vestibular schwannoma? Evidence of familial clustering. Otol Neurotol 2022;43(10):e1157–63.

17. Schüz J, Pirie K, Reeves GK, et al. Cellular telephone use and the risk of brain tumors: update of the UK million women study. JNCI: J Natl Cancer Inst 2022; 114(5):704–11.

18. Corona AP, Oliveira JC, Souza FP, et al. Risk factors associated with vestibulocochlear nerve schwannoma: systematic review. Braz J Otorhinolaryngol 2009; 75(4):593–615.

19. Pettersson D, Mathiesen T, Prochazka M, et al. Long-term mobile phone use and acoustic neuroma risk. Epidemiology 2014;25(2):233–41.

20. Benson VS, Pirie K, Schuz J, et al. Authors' response to: the case of acoustic neuroma: comment on mobile phone use and risk of brain neoplasms and other cancers. Int J Epidemiol 2014;43(1):275.

21. Braganza MZ, Kitahara CM, Berrington de Gonzalez A, et al. Ionizing radiation and the risk of brain and central nervous system tumors: a systematic review. Neuro Oncol 2012;14(11):1316–24.

22. Bondy ML, Scheurer ME, Malmer B, et al. Brain tumor epidemiology: consensus from the Brain Tumor Epidemiology Consortium. Cancer 2008;113(S7):1953–68.

23. Yonehara S, Brenner AV, Kishikawa M, et al. Clinical and epidemiologic characteristics of first primary tumors of the central nervous system and related organs

among atomic bomb survivors in Hiroshima and Nagasaki, 1958-1995. Cancer 2004;101(7):1644–54.

24. Corona AP, Ferrite S, Lopes Mda S, et al. Risk factors associated with vestibular nerve schwannomas. Otol Neurotol 2012;33(3):459–65.

25. Santa Maria PL, Shi Y, Gurgel RK, et al. Long-term hearing outcomes following stereotactic radiosurgery in vestibular schwannoma patients-a retrospective cohort study. Neurosurgery 2019;85(4):550–9.

26. Karipidis K, Mate R, Urban D, et al. 5G mobile networks and health—a state-of-the-science review of the research into low-level RF fields above 6 GHz. J Expo Sci Environ Epidemiol 2021;31(4):585–605.

27. Inskip PD, Tarone RE, Hatch EE, et al. Cellular-telephone use and brain tumors. N Engl J Med 2001;344(2):79–86.

28. Capstick MH, Kuehn S, Berdinas-Torres V, et al. A radio frequency radiation exposure system for rodents based on reverberation chambers. IEEE Trans Electromagn C 2017;59(4):1041–52.

29. Gong Y, Capstick MH, Kuehn S, et al. Life-time dosimetric assessment for mice and rats exposed in reverberation chambers for the two-year NTP cancer bioassay study on cell phone radiation. IEEE Trans Electromagn C 2017;59(6): 1798–808.

30. Oberto G, Rolfo K, Yu P, et al. Carcinogenicity study of 217 Hz pulsed 900 MHz electromagnetic fields in Pim1 transgenic mice. Radiat Res 2007;168(3):316–26.

31. Zook BC, Simmens SJ. The effects of pulsed 860 MHz radiofrequency radiation on the promotion of neurogenic tumors in rats. Radiat Res 2006;165(5):608–15.

32. ICNIRP note: critical evaluation of two radiofrequency electromagnetic field animal carcinogenicity studies published in 2018. Health Phys 2020;118(5):525–32.

33. Schuz J, Steding-Jessen M, Hansen S, et al. Long-term mobile phone use and the risk of vestibular schwannoma: a Danish nationwide cohort study. Am J Epidemiol 2011;174(4):416–22.

34. Benson VS, Pirie K, Schuz J, et al. Mobile phone use and risk of brain neoplasms and other cancers: prospective study. Int J Epidemiol 2013;42(3):792–802.

35. Moon IS, Kim BG, Kim J, et al. Association between vestibular schwannomas and mobile phone use. Tumor Biol 2014;35(1):581–7.

36. IARC classifies radiofrequency electromagnetic fields as possibly carcinogenic to humans. International Agency for Research on Cancer 2011. Available at: https://www.iarc.who.int/wp-content/uploads/2018/07/pr208_E.pdf. Accessed September 24, 2022.

37. Shuren J. National toxicology program draft report on radiofrequency energy exposure. United states food and drug administration. 2018. Available at: https://www.fda.gov/news-events/press-announcements/statement-jeffrey-shuren-md-jd-director-fdas-center-devices-and-radiological-health-recent-national. Accessed September 25, 2022.

38. Cell Phones and Your Health. Centers for Disease Control and Prevention. 2022. Available at: https://www.cdc.gov/nceh/radiation/cell_phones._FAQ.html. Accessed September 25, 2022.

39. Deltour I, Schlehofer B, Massardier-Pilonchery A, et al. Exposure to loud noise and risk of vestibular schwannoma: results from the INTERPHONE international casecontrol study. Scand J Work Environ Health 2019;45(2):183–93.

40. Cao Z, Zhao F, Mulugeta H. Noise exposure as a risk factor for acoustic neuroma: a systematic review and meta-analysis. Int J Audiol 2019;58(9):525–32.

41. Chen M, Fan Z, Zheng X, et al. Risk factors of acoustic neuroma: systematic review and meta-analysis. Yonsei Med J 2016;57(3):776–83.

42. Aarhus L, Kjaerheim K, Heikkinen S, et al. Occupational noise exposure and vestibular schwannoma: a case-control study in Sweden. Am J Epidemiol 2020;189(11):1342–7.

43. Fisher JL, Pettersson D, Palmisano S, et al. Loud noise exposure and acoustic neuroma. Am J Epidemiol 2014;180(1):58–67.

44. Benson VS, Green J, Pirie K, et al. Cigarette smoking and risk of acoustic neuromas and pituitary tumours in the Million Women Study. Br J Cancer 2010; 102(11):1654–6.

45. Schoemaker MJ, Swerdlow AJ, Auvinen A, et al. Medical history, cigarette smoking and risk of acoustic neuroma: an international case-control study. Int J Cancer 2007;120(1):103–10.

46. Berkowitz O, Iyer AK, Kano H, et al. Epidemiology and environmental risk factors associated with vestibular schwannoma. World Neurosurg 2015;84(6):1674–80.

47. Dilwali S, Kao SY, Fujita T, et al. Nonsteroidal anti-inflammatory medications are cytostatic against human vestibular schwannomas. Transl Res 2015;166(1):1–11.

48. Kandathil CK, Dilwali S, Wu CC, et al. Aspirin intake correlates with halted growth of sporadic vestibular schwannoma in vivo. Otol Neurotol 2014;35(2):353–7.

49. Van Gompel JJ, Agazzi S, Carlson ML, et al. Congress of neurological surgeons systematic review and evidence-based guidelines on emerging therapies for the treatment of patients with vestibular schwannomas. Neurosurgery 2018;82(2): E52–4.

50. Ignacio KHD, Espiritu AI, Diestro JDB, et al. Efficacy of aspirin for sporadic vestibular schwannoma: a meta-analysis. Neurol Sci 2021;42(12):5101–6.

Updates on Tumor Biology in Vestibular Schwannoma

Aida Nourbakhsh, MD, PhD[a,b], Christine T. Dinh, MD[a,b],*

KEYWORDS

• Tumor biology • Vestibular schwannoma • Tumor microenvironment • Merlin • NF2

KEY POINTS

• Vestibular schwannomas (VSs) arise from biallelic inactivation of the neurofibromatosis type 2 (*NF2*) gene that encodes tumor suppressor merlin.
• Merlin inactivation causes cell proliferation by dysregulation of receptor- and non-receptor-mediated pathways.
• In VS without *NF2* mutations, dysregulation of non-*NF2* genes promotes cell proliferation and tumorigenesis.
• The VS tumor microenvironment is dynamic with multiple cell types engaging in intercellular communications that act in conjunction with VS intracellular signaling to modulate tumor progression and hearing loss.

OVERVIEW OF VESTIBULAR SCHWANNNOMA

Vestibular schwannomas (VSs) are benign intracranial tumors that arise from the Schwann cells of the vestibulocochlear nerve. They occur sporadically as unilateral tumors or exist bilaterally as part of an autosomal dominant tumor disposition syndrome called neurofibromatosis type 2 (NF2). VS can cause hearing loss, tinnitus, and dizziness, among other neurologic complications.[1] In this review, the authors summarize the key pathways in VS tumor biology and the regulation of its microenvironment that contribute to tumorigenesis, tumor progression, and hearing loss.

Tumor Biology of Vestibular Schwannoma

Biallelic NF2 inactivation

The *NF2* gene is located on chromosome 22q11 and encodes the tumor suppressor merlin.[2] In NF2-associated VS, one *NF2* allele is inactivated through a germline mutation.[1] Tumorigenesis occurs when the other *NF2* allele is lost, acquires a somatic mutation, or silenced by other means. In sporadic VS, however, a Schwann cell acquires

a Department of Otolaryngology, University of Miami Miller School of Medicine, 1120 Northwest 14th Street, Suite 579, Miami, FL 33136, USA; b Sylvester Comprehensive Cancer Center, 1475 Northwest 12th Avenue, Miami, FL 33136, USA
* Corresponding author.
E-mail address: ctdinh@med.miami.edu

Otolaryngol Clin N Am 56 (2023) 421–434
https://doi.org/10.1016/j.otc.2023.02.004
0030-6665/23/© 2023 Elsevier Inc. All rights reserved.

oto.theclinics.com

Abbreviations	
GTP	guanosine triphosphate
Ras	rat sarcoma
Akt	protein kinase B
c-MET	mesenchymal epithelial transition factor
ERBB	epidermal growth factor
LIM	LIN-11, Isl-1 and MEC-3
PIKE-L	phosphoinositide 3-kinase enhancer – L isoform
Rac1	Rac Family Small GTPase 1
CRL4[DCAF]	cullin4A-RING E3 ubiquitin ligase[DDB1-and CUL4-associated factors]
NF-kB	nuclear factor kappa B
IkBa	nuclear factor kappa B inhibitor alpha
IL	interleukin
TNFa	tumor necrosis factor alpha
TGFb1	transforming growth factor beta 1
CpG	5′—C—phosphate—G—3′
MiRNA	MicroRNA
mRNA	messenger ribonucleic acid

de novo, somatic inactivation of both NF2 alleles to initiate tumorigenesis.[3] Following biallelic *NF2* inactivation, merlin is truncated and dysfunctional or expressed at lower levels with minimal effect on intrinsic function.[4,5] Truncating mutations are associated with worse disease severity in NF2 patients.[6]

Merlin function

Merlin is a scaffold protein that links membrane receptors and intracellular effectors to regulate signaling pathways that control cell proliferation and survival.[2] Merlin activity is modulated through conformational changes that are complex.[7] In general, unphosphorylated merlin remains in its closed conformation and acts as a tumor suppressor. When merlin is phosphorylated, it transitions to an open configuration and acts as a scaffolding protein that facilitates cell proliferation through receptor-mediated and intracellular pathways.[2]

Receptor tyrosine kinases

Receptor tyrosine kinases (RTKs) are plasma membrane proteins that regulate cell proliferation in VS. VS have increased expression of multiple RTKs, including (1) hepatocyte growth factor receptor, also known as c-MET, (2) the ERBB family of RTKs, including epidermal growth factor receptor (EGFR, also known as ErbB1/HER1), ErbB2 (HER2), and ErbB3 (HER3), (3) the platelet-derived growth factor receptor (PDGFR) family including PDGFR-α and PDGFR-β, and (4) the vascular endothelial growth factor receptor (VEGFR) family.[8–13]

When unphosphorylated, merlin co-localizes with RTKs and CD44 (cell surface adhesion receptor) at the plasma membrane, blocking the assembly of Ras (GTP-binding protein) complex and inhibiting downstream signaling through PI3K/Akt/JNK (phosphatidylinositol-3-kinase/Akt/c-Jun N-terminal kinase) and Raf/MEK/ERK (Raf/mitogen-activated protein kinase kinase/extracellular signal-regulated kinase) pathways (**Fig. 1**).[2] Merlin can also inhibit Src tyrosine kinase-mediated activation of Raf/MEK/ERK signaling and focal adhesion kinase (FAK) signaling, promoting cell proliferation by p53 degradation through ubiquitination (see **Fig. 1**).[14,15]

Merlin can interact with c-MET and inactivate Rac1, resulting in p21-activated kinase (PAK) inhibition.[16,17] In turn, PAK inhibition downregulates Raf/MEK/ERK signaling to block cell proliferation.[18] In addition, PAK inhibition downregulates

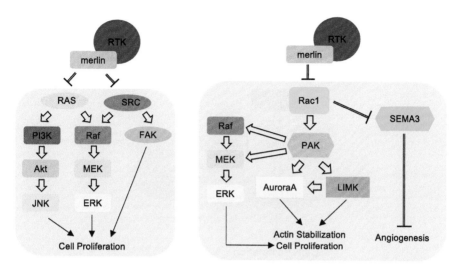

Fig. 1. Receptor tyrosine kinase signaling. Merlin co-localizes with RTKs and inhibits downstream Ras, SRC, and Rac1 signaling to suppress cell proliferation.

AuroraA and LIM domain kinases, which lead to actin stabilization and blockage of cell proliferation (see **Fig. 1**).[2]

VEGF binds VEGFR RTKs to promote tumor angiogenesis, supporting a microenvironment rich in nutrients and oxygen to sustain growth. VEGF expression has been correlated positively to VS tumor volume and growth.[19] Hypoxic VS cells can express hypoxia-inducible factor 1α, stimulating VEGF expression and angiogenesis.[20] Semaphorin 3 F (SEMA3F) is a secreted protein that regulates angiogenesis. In schwannoma, merlin deficiency activates Rac1, downregulating SEMA3F and increasing angiogenesis through VEGF signaling (see **Fig. 1**).[21]

Merlin can regulate cell survival and proliferation by inhibiting PIKE-L, a GTPase responsible for PI3K/Akt activation and downstream mammalian target of rapamycin (mTOR) signaling (**Fig. 2**).

Histone deacetylases

Histone deacetylases (HDAC) are enzymes that remove the acetyl groups from the lysine residues of histones and nonhistone substrates. HDACs regulate tumorigenesis by repressing expression of tumor suppressor genes or regulating oncogenic signaling. HDAC can bypass merlin suppression of PIKE-L and activate Akt by interacting with PP1 phosphatase and releasing PP1 inhibition of Akt (see **Fig. 2**).[2,22] In turn, Akt activates mTORC1 and downstream effects to promote cell proliferation and survival.

Hippo pathway

Merlin is also an upstream regulator of the Hippo pathway. When merlin binds large tumor suppressor kinases (LATS1/2), mammalian Ste20-like kinases (MST1/2) can phosphorylate the LATS1/2 complex, facilitating cytoplasmic retention and degradation of the transcriptional coactivator Yes-associated protein (YAP) and its homolog TAZ. By preventing YAP/TAZ nuclear localization, TEA domain transcription is halted, thus blocking cell proliferation and survival.[2] Merlin also regulates YAP cytoplasmic localization by interacting with angiomotin (AMOT), which binds YAP and regulates Rac1 signaling.[2] In addition, merlin inhibits E3 ubiquitin ligase CRL4[DCAF1],

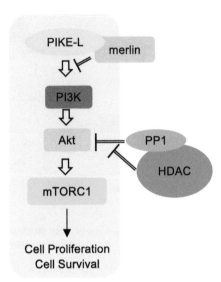

Fig. 2. PI3K/Akt/mTOR signaling. Merlin regulates cell proliferation by suppressing PI3K/Akt/mTOR signaling. HDAC bypasses merlin suppression by releasing PP1 inhibition on Akt.

resulting in LATS1/2 activation, YAP downregulation, and reduced cell proliferation (**Fig. 3**).[2] RTKs interact extensively with the Hippo pathway, with investigations demonstrating YAP/TAZ as downstream effectors of RTK/RAS-mediated signaling through PI3K/Akt and Raf/MEK pathways. Furthermore, YAP promotes transcription of multiple genes, including amphiregulin, an EGFR ligand.[23] VS have demonstrated aberrant YAP/TAZ expression, with TAZ correlating positively to tumor growth. Increased nuclear YAP correlated positively with high Ki-67 proliferative index and low merlin expression.[24]

NF-κB signaling
Merlin also inhibits degradation of IκBα (a member of the IκB kinase family of proteins), which in turn, reduces NF-κB-dependent transcription (**Fig. 4**). Thus, merlin inactivation promotes NF-κB, a transcription factor that regulates inflammation and cell death genes. Aberrant NF-κB signaling is a critical event in VS tumorigenesis.[25]

Thus, merlin inactivation can lead to cell proliferation and tumor progression by dysregulation of several pathways: RTKs including VEGF-VEGFR, Ras-mediated PI3K/Akt/JNK and Raf/MEK/ERK, SRC-mediated Raf/MEK/ERK and FAK, PI3K/Akt/mTOR, Rac1/PAK, HDAC/Akt, YAP/TAZ, and NF-κB signaling pathways (**Fig. 5**).

Tumor Microenvironment

Considerable progress has been made in understanding merlin signaling; however, less is known about the tumor microenvironment (TME) of VS. The TME is a dynamic entity, consisting of complex intercellular networks where communications between multiple cell types regulate intracellular signaling in VS (**Fig. 6**). Yidian and colleagues performed single-cell sequencing on three sporadic VS and found the TME to consist of 6-cell clusters: Schwann cells, myeloid cells, T cells, B cells, endothelial cells, and fibroblasts.[26] Schwann cells and myeloid cells were the predominant cells. Schwann cells were heterogenous, demonstrating varying degrees of differentiation, proliferation, and immune cell chemotaxis. Myeloid cells were composed of monocytes and

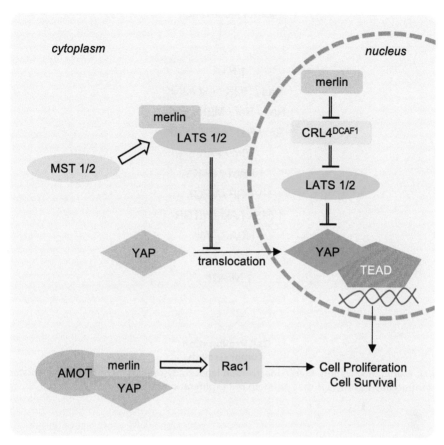

Fig. 3. Mammalian Hippo pathway. Merlin regulates LATS kinases and AMOT to prevent YAP nuclear localization and transcription of cell proliferation genes.

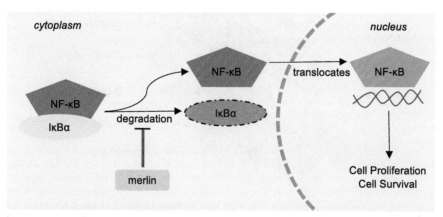

Fig. 4. NF-κB pathway. Merlin inhibits NF-κB signaling by preventing degradation of IκBα.

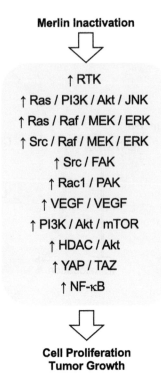

Merlin Inactivation

↑ RTK

↑ Ras / PI3K / Akt / JNK

↑ Ras / Raf / MEK / ERK

↑ Src / Raf / MEK / ERK

↑ Src / FAK

↑ Rac1 / PAK

↑ VEGF / VEGF

↑ PI3K / Akt / mTOR

↑ HDAC / Akt

↑ YAP / TAZ

↑ NF-κB

**Cell Proliferation
Tumor Growth**

Fig. 5. Merlin inactivation. Merlin inactivation leads to dysregulation of receptor-mediated and intracellular pathways that promote cell proliferation.

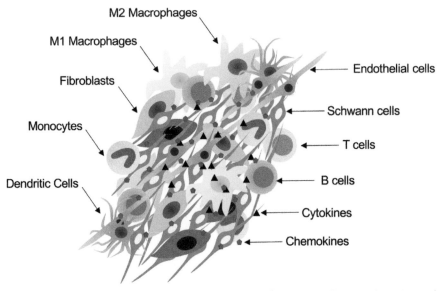

Fig. 6. VS tumor microenvironment. The TME consists of multiple cell types whose intercellular communications occur through cell-to-cell and paracrine signaling.

dendritic cells, of which intermediate monocytes could be further differentiated into M1 and M2 phenotypic macrophages. Expression analysis also showed that myeloid cells have prominent roles in chemotaxis and cytokine–cytokine receptor signaling. Furthermore, they identified significant interactions between fibroblasts and immune cells through the chemokine CXCL (C-X-C motif ligand) pathway.[26]

Tumor-associated macrophages

More recent studies in VS have focused on understanding the role of tumor-associated macrophages (TAMs) on tumor growth and hearing loss.[27] Although TAMs exist functionally along a spectrum, they are commonly classified into two broad types that can be differentiated by their surface glycoproteins and the cytokines they secrete.[28] M1 macrophages are pro-inflammatory, classically activated macrophages that secrete cytokines, such as TNFα. M2 macrophages are protumorigenic, alternatively activated macrophages that secrete cytokines that promote angiogenesis and facilitate tumor growth.[28] VS tumor growth has been associated with macrophage infiltration.[29] Increased CD163 expression (M2 macrophage marker) correlated positively to volumetric tumor growth and microvessel density, supporting the role of M2 macrophages in angiogenesis and tumor progression.[30,31] CD163 was also associated with poor hearing outcomes.[32]

Secretome

The secretome plays an important role in the development of the TME, tumor progression, and hearing loss in VS. Myeloid cells contribute largely to chemotaxis and cytokine signaling.[26] VS can upregulate multiple cytokines and chemokines, including the CXC family (eg, CXCL12 and CXCL16), IL-1β, IL-6, IL-34, macrophage colony stimulating factor, macrophage inflammatory protein-1alpha, TNFα, and TGFβ1.[31,33–36] These proteins are involved in the polarization of macrophages or can facilitate the inflammatory activities of TAMs critical in tumor formation and progression.[37] In ex vivo investigations using cultured VS, Dilwali and colleagues identified fibroblast growth factor 2 to be otoprotective and TNFα to be ototoxic cytokines that modulate hearing in VS patients.[38,39]

Furthermore, VS expresses other pro-inflammatory proteins, including cyclooxygenase-2 (COX-2) and the NLRP3 (NOD-, LRR- and pyrin domain-containing protein 3) inflammasome.[40,41] COX-2 is an enzyme important in arachidonic acid metabolism and biosynthesis of prostaglandin E2 (PGE2). PGE2 can modulate macrophage activity, including the production of other inflammatory cytokines.[42] COX-2 was aberrantly expressed in VS, and PGE2 expression correlated with cell proliferation rates in cultured VS.[40] VS also increases VEGF by upregulating COX-2 through Hippo signaling.[43] The NLRP3 inflammasome is a large cytosolic protein complex that initiates an inflammatory immune response by cleavage of the inflammatory protease procaspase-1 into its activated form, caspase-1. This process will lead to cleavage of pro-IL-1β and pro-IL-18 into their active forms. VS also upregulates NLRP3-associated genes along with macrophage infiltration, further suggesting the role of TAMs in facilitating the inflammatory response.[41]

Matrix metalloproteinases

Matrix metalloproteinases (MMPs) are proteases that are secreted into the extracellular space or anchored on the plasma membrane. They function to degrade extracellular matrix components and are secreted by many cell types, but particularly macrophages.[44] MMP-2 was found in the cyst fluid and wall of cystic VS and may be involved in cyst formation, growth, and adhesion to surrounding structures.[45] Upregulation of MMP-9 has been linked to tumor growth in VS.[46] Plasma MMP-14 correlated positively to the degree of hearing loss and extent of surgical resection.[47] MMP-14 may also enhance VEGF activity, contribute to collagen degradation in Antoni B areas, and promote cyst formation in VS.[48]

Non-neurofibromatosis Type 2 Pathways

Although NF2 gene inactivation and merlin deficiency are critical events, not all VS have identifiable *NF2* mutations. Approximately 15% to 84% of sporadic VS harbor at least one *NF2* mutation on genetic testing.[49] In addition, not all cells in the VS tumor harbor *NF2* mutations, as suggested by a variant allelic fraction ranging from 8% to 69% for the *NF2* gene. This suggests that cellular heterogeneity (eg, infiltration by fibroblasts and immune cells) or clonal evolution may contribute to the genetic complexity.[26] As such, recent investigations have focused on integrative analyses to broadly assess the cellular composition, genome, epigenome, transcriptome, proteome, and secretome of VS, in an effort to better understand the TME and pathways involved in tumorigenesis, tumor progression, and hearing loss (**Fig. 7**).[50–52]

Non-neurofibromatosis type 2 mutations

Scientific advances with next-generation sequencing have revealed non-*NF2* mutations in VS, suggesting alternative or secondary mechanisms responsible for tumorigenesis. In an investigation by Havik and colleagues, 46 VS and matched blood samples were analyzed using whole-exome sequencing (WES).[50] Excluding one tumor, 716 mutations affecting 692 genes were identified, with a median of 14 genes per tumor sample. The most common mutation was *NF2* (78%), followed by cell division cycle protein 27 (*CDC27*; 11%) and ubiquitin-specific peptidase 8 (*USP8*; 7%). CDC27 has tumor suppressor functions, whereas USP8 can inhibit RTK degradation.[53,54] Pathway analysis showed clustering of mutations in the axonal guidance canonical pathway, providing insight on potential non-*NF2* mechanisms of tumorigenesis. [50] Mutations also linked to pathways upstream and downstream of merlin, including Rac1, CD44, mTOR, and mitogen-activated protein kinase signaling.

Agnohitri and colleagues performed WES on 13 cranial and 13 spinal schwannomas and found 441 somatic single-nucleotide variants. *NF2* mutations were most common (77%). Of the 13 VS, other mutations were identified including mutations of *LTZR1* (leucine zipper like transcription regulator 1), *ARID1A* (SWI-SNF chromatin-

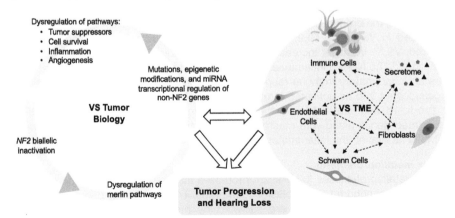

Fig. 7. Biological factors affecting tumor progression and hearing loss in VS. *NF2* inactivation and dysregulated non-*NF2* genes lead to tumorigenesis and evolution of the TME to facilitate tumor progression and hearing loss in VS.

remodeling complex), and *TSC1* (tuberous sclerosis protein 1), among others. LTZR1 and ARID1A encode proteins with tumor suppressor activity.[55,56] The *TSC* genes encodes hamartin, a protein that inhibits mTOR signal transduction.[57] Pathway analysis identified enrichment of MEK, mTOR, NFκB, ErbB2, TNFα, and inflammatory signaling. Furthermore, they identified and characterized a common event occurring in several VS tumors, that is, an in-frame fusion involving SH3PXD2A and HTRA1, arising through a balanced translocation on chromosome 10q. The authors postulate that SH3PXD2A-HTRA1 fusion causes upregulation of phosphorylated MEK to promote tumorigenesis.[51]

DNA methylation

Hypermethylation of the CpG islands in the promoter regions can lead to gene silencing and is an important epigenetic mechanism causing tumor suppressor inactivation. Conversely, hypomethylation can cause upregulation of gene products. Up to 61% of VS demonstrate aberrant methylation of the NF2 gene, suggesting an alternate pathway of *NF2* inactivation.[58–60] Using methylation profiling, Agnihotri and colleagues identified loss of 22q as the only recurrent chromosomal aberration, found in 61% of 125 schwannomas. However, there was aberrant methylation of several non-*NF2* genes, with pathway analysis demonstrating enrichment in Ras signaling, among other pathways.[51] Other VS studies have found aberrant methylation of genes that encode tumor suppressors, DNA repair enzymes, apoptosis initiators, MMP suppressors, and angiogenesis mediators. Some tumor suppressor genes expressing aberrant methylation were *RASSF1* (Ras association domain family member 1) and *PTEN* (phosphatase and tensin homolog).[59,61] Torres-Martin and colleagues found a trend toward hypomethylation in VS, with upregulation of gene products confirmed for multiple hypomethylated genes, including *MET* proto-oncogene that encodes c-MET.[62]

MicroRNA

MiRNAs are small non-coding RNAs that are complementary to target mRNAs. They function by binding mRNA and inhibiting translation into their respective proteins. VS tumors demonstrate aberrant expression of several miRNAs, some associated with rapid tumor growth.[52,63,64] In a study by Torres-Martin and colleagues, 174 deregulated miRNAs were identified, among which global upregulation of a miRNA cluster in the chromosomal region of 14q32 indicate a potential role in VS tumorigenesis.[52] Increased expression of miR-19, miR-21, and miR-221 were common findings, whose expression can decrease tumor suppressor PTEN in various cell types.[63,65,66] Targeting miRNAs is a novel therapeutic approach to VS tumor control, and Torres-Martin and colleagues demonstrated that miR-21 downregulation reduced cell proliferation and induced apoptosis and autophagy in VS cells.[52]

Transcriptome

The culmination of these mutations, epigenetic modifications, and miRNA-associated transcriptional changes of *NF2* and non-*NF2* genes ultimately impacts the VS transcriptome. Transcriptome analysis can provide insight into dysregulated signaling pathways that lead to tumorigenesis. In brief, transcriptional analyses of VS demonstrated increased expression of (1) several tumor suppressor genes including *CAV1* and *PTEN*, (2) RTKs and their associated ligands, (3) downstream effectors involved with merlin (eg, PI3K, Akt1), and (4) angiogenesis mediators, such as *VEGF*.[8,9,25,51,67–71] The osteopontin gene (*SPP1*), which is involved in merlin protein degradation, was also upregulated.[8] Pathway analysis of dysregulated genes link to merlin-associated signaling, including EGFR, VEGFR, mTOR, and FAK, among others.[25,51,71]

SUMMARY

In summary, the mechanisms involved in VS tumorigenesis and progression are complex and involve thorough understanding of *NF2* and non-*NF2* signaling pathways and the dynamic interplay of cell types and secreted proteins in the TME. Understanding these molecular and cellular events will provide important insight into potential therapies for tumor control and hearing protection in VS.

CLINICS CARE POINTS

- Vestibular schwannoma (VS) tumorigenesis occurs following biallelic neurofibromatosis type 2 (*NF2*) inactivation.
- In VS without *NF2* mutations, dysregulation of non-NF2 genes can promote tumorigenesis.
- Tumor progression and hearing loss in VS are governed by VS tumor biology and the tumor microenvironment.

DISCLOSURE

The authors do not have any conflicts of interest. A Nourbakhsh is funded by the Alpha Omega Alpha Postgraduate Award and the American Neurotology Society Research Grant. C Dinh is funded by NIH/NIDCD K08DC017508, NIH/NIDCD R01DC017264, and NIH/NCI Sylvester K-supplement/NF2 Program Grants.

REFERENCES

1. Dinh CT, Nisenbaum E, Chyou D, et al. Genomics, Epigenetics, and Hearing Loss in Neurofibromatosis Type 2. Otol Neurotol 2020;41(5):e529–37.
2. Petrilli AM, Fernandez-Valle C. Role of Merlin/NF2 inactivation in tumor biology. Oncogene 2016;35(5):537–48.
3. Irving RM, Moffat DA, Hardy DG, et al. Somatic NF2 gene mutations in familial and non-familial vestibular schwannoma. Hum Mol Genet 1994;3(2):347–50.
4. Yang C, Asthagiri AR, Iyer RR, et al. Missense mutations in the NF2 gene result in the quantitative loss of merlin protein and minimally affect protein intrinsic function. Proc Natl Acad Sci U S A 2011;108(12):4980–5.
5. Welling DB, Guida M, Goll F, et al. Mutational spectrum in the neurofibromatosis type 2 gene in sporadic and familial schwannomas. Hum Genet 1996;98(2):189–93.
6. Halliday D, Emmanouil B, Pretorius P, et al. Genetic Severity Score predicts clinical phenotype in NF2. J Med Genet 2017;54(10):657–64.
7. Sher I, Hanemann CO, Karplus PA, et al. The tumor suppressor merlin controls growth in its open state, and phosphorylation converts it to a less-active more-closed state. Dev Cell 2012;22(4):703–5.
8. Torres-Martin M, Lassaletta L, San-Roman-Montero J, et al. Microarray analysis of gene expression in vestibular schwannomas reveals SPP1/MET signaling pathway and androgen receptor deregulation. Int J Oncol 2013;42(3):848–62.
9. Dilwali S, Roberts D, Stankovic KM. Interplay between VEGF-A and cMET signaling in human vestibular schwannomas and schwann cells. Cancer Biol Ther 2015;16(1):170–5.
10. Ammoun S, Cunliffe CH, Allen JC, et al. ErbB/HER receptor activation and preclinical efficacy of lapatinib in vestibular schwannoma. Neuro Oncol 2010;12(8):834–43.

11. Bush ML, Burns SS, Oblinger J, et al. Treatment of vestibular schwannoma cells with ErbB inhibitors. Otol Neurotol 2012;33(2):244–57.

12. Petrilli AM, Garcia J, Bott M, et al. Ponatinib promotes a G1 cell-cycle arrest of merlin/NF2-deficient human schwann cells. Oncotarget 2017;8(19):31666–81.

13. Caye-Thomasen P, Werther K, Nalla A, et al. VEGF and VEGF receptor-1 concentration in vestibular schwannoma homogenates correlates to tumor growth rate. Otol Neurotol 2005;26(1):98–101.

14. Fuse MA, Plati SK, Burns SS, et al. Combination Therapy with c-Met and Src Inhibitors Induces Caspase-Dependent Apoptosis of Merlin-Deficient Schwann Cells and Suppresses Growth of Schwannoma Cells. Mol Cancer Therapeut 2017;16(11):2387–98.

15. Troutman S, Moleirinho S, Kota S, et al. Crizotinib inhibits NF2-associated schwannoma through inhibition of focal adhesion kinase 1. Oncotarget 2016; 7(34):54515–25.

16. Wang Y, Wang B, Li P, et al. Reduced RAC1 activity inhibits cell proliferation and induces apoptosis in neurofibromatosis type 2(NF2)-associated schwannoma. Neurol Res 2017;39(12):1086–93.

17. Singleton PA, Salgia R, Moreno-Vinasco L, et al. CD44 regulates hepatocyte growth factor-mediated vascular integrity. Role of c-Met, Tiam1/Rac1, dynamin 2, and cortactin. J Biol Chem 2007;282(42):30643–57.

18. Flaiz C, Chernoff J, Ammoun S, et al. PAK kinase regulates Rac GTPase and is a potential target in human schwannomas. Exp Neurol 2009;218(1):137–44.

19. Koutsimpelas D, Stripf T, Heinrich UR, et al. Expression of vascular endothelial growth factor and basic fibroblast growth factor in sporadic vestibular schwannomas correlates to growth characteristics. Otol Neurotol 2007;28(8):1094–9.

20. Kim JY, Song JJ, Kwon BM, et al. Tanshinone IIA exerts antitumor activity against vestibular schwannoma cells by inhibiting the expression of hypoxia-inducible factor-1alpha. Mol Med Rep 2015;12(3):4604–9.

21. Wong HK, Shimizu A, Kirkpatrick ND, et al. Merlin/NF2 regulates angiogenesis in schwannomas through a Rac1/semaphorin 3F-dependent mechanism. Neoplasia 2012;14(2):84–94.

22. Jacob A, Oblinger J, Bush ML, et al. Preclinical validation of AR42, a novel histone deacetylase inhibitor, as treatment for vestibular schwannomas. Laryngoscope 2012;122(1):174–89.

23. Guerrant W, Kota S, Troutman S, et al. YAP Mediates Tumorigenesis in Neurofibromatosis Type 2 by Promoting Cell Survival and Proliferation through a COX-2-EGFR Signaling Axis. Cancer Res 2016;76(12):3507–19.

24. Zhao F, Yang Z, Chen Y, et al. Deregulation of the Hippo Pathway Promotes Tumor Cell Proliferation Through YAP Activity in Human Sporadic Vestibular Schwannoma. World Neurosurg 2018;117:e269–79.

25. Dilwali S, Briet MC, Kao SY, et al. Preclinical validation of anti-nuclear factor-kappa B therapy to inhibit human vestibular schwannoma growth. Mol Oncol 2015;9(7):1359–70.

26. Yidian C, Chen L, Hongxia D, et al. Single-cell sequencing reveals the cell map and transcriptional network of sporadic vestibular schwannoma. Front Mol Neurosci 2022;15:984529.

27. Wang S, Liechty B, Patel S, et al. Programmed death ligand 1 expression and tumor infiltrating lymphocytes in neurofibromatosis type 1 and 2 associated tumors. J Neuro Oncol 2018;138(1):183–90.

28. Orecchioni M, Ghosheh Y, Pramod AB, et al. Macrophage Polarization: Different Gene Signatures in M1(LPS+) vs. Classically and M2(LPS-) vs. Alternatively Activated Macrophages. Front Immunol 2019;10:1084.
29. Perry A, Graffeo CS, Carlstrom LP, et al. Predominance of M1 subtype among tumor-associated macrophages in phenotypically aggressive sporadic vestibular schwannoma. J Neurosurg 2019;1–9.
30. de Vries M, Briaire-de Bruijn I, Malessy MJ, et al. Tumor-associated macrophages are related to volumetric growth of vestibular schwannomas. Otol Neurotol 2013; 34(2):347–52.
31. de Vries WM, Briaire-de Bruijn IH, van Benthem PPG, et al. M-CSF and IL-34 expression as indicators for growth in sporadic vestibular schwannoma. Virchows Arch 2019;474(3):375–81.
32. Nisenbaum E, Misztal C, Szczupak M, et al. Tumor-Associated Macrophages in Vestibular Schwannoma and Relationship to Hearing. OTO Open 2021;5(4). 2473974X211059111.
33. Breun M, Schwerdtfeger A, Martellotta DD, et al. CXCR4: A new player in vestibular schwannoma pathogenesis. Oncotarget 2018;9(11):9940–50.
34. Taurone S, Bianchi E, Attanasio G, et al. Immunohistochemical profile of cytokines and growth factors expressed in vestibular schwannoma and in normal vestibular nerve tissue. Mol Med Rep 2015;12(1):737–45.
35. Held-Feindt J, Rehmke B, Mentlein R, et al. Overexpression of CXCL16 and its receptor CXCR6/Bonzo promotes growth of human schwannomas. Glia 2008; 56(7):764–74.
36. Mori K, Chano T, Yamamoto K, et al. Expression of macrophage inflammatory protein-1alpha in Schwann cell tumors. Neuropathology 2004;24(2):131–5.
37. Boutilier AJ, Elsawa SF. Macrophage Polarization States in the Tumor Microenvironment. Int J Mol Sci 2021;22(13).
38. Dilwali S, Lysaght A, Roberts D, et al. Sporadic vestibular schwannomas associated with good hearing secrete higher levels of fibroblast growth factor 2 than those associated with poor hearing irrespective of tumor size. Otol Neurotol 2013;34(4):748–54.
39. Dilwali S, Landegger LD, Soares VY, et al. Secreted Factors from Human Vestibular Schwannomas Can Cause Cochlear Damage. Sci Rep 2015;5:18599.
40. Dilwali S, Kao SY, Fujita T, et al. Nonsteroidal anti-inflammatory medications are cytostatic against human vestibular schwannomas. Transl Res 2015;166(1):1–11.
41. Sagers JE, Sahin MI, Moon I, et al. NLRP3 inflammasome activation in human vestibular schwannoma: Implications for tumor-induced hearing loss. Hear Res 2019;381:107770.
42. Tang T, Scambler TE, Smallie T, et al. Macrophage responses to lipopolysaccharide are modulated by a feedback loop involving prostaglandin E2, dual specificity phosphatase 1 and tristetraprolin. Sci Rep 2017;7(1):4350.
43. Gately S. The contributions of cyclooxygenase-2 to tumor angiogenesis. Cancer Metastasis Rev 2000;19(1–2):19–27.
44. Elkington PT, Green JA, Friedland JS. Analysis of matrix metalloproteinase secretion by macrophages. Methods Mol Biol 2009;531:253–65.
45. Moon KS, Jung S, Seo SK, et al. Cystic vestibular schwannomas: a possible role of matrix metalloproteinase-2 in cyst development and unfavorable surgical outcome. J Neurosurg 2007;106(5):866–71.
46. Moller MN, Werther K, Nalla A, et al. Angiogenesis in vestibular schwannomas: expression of extracellular matrix factors MMP-2, MMP-9, and TIMP-1. Laryngoscope 2010;120(4):657–62.

47. Ren Y, Hyakusoku H, Sagers JE, et al. MMP-14 (MT1-MMP) Is a Biomarker of Surgical Outcome and a Potential Mediator of Hearing Loss in Patients With Vestibular Schwannomas. Front Cell Neurosci 2020;14:191.

48. Xia L, Yang S, Wang C, et al. Immunohistochemical Profiles of Matrix Metalloproteinases and Vascular Endothelial Growth Factor Overexpression in the Antoni B Area of Vestibular Schwannomas. World Neurosurg 2020;144:e72–9.

49. de Vries M, van der Mey AG, Hogendoorn PC. Tumor Biology of Vestibular Schwannoma: A Review of Experimental Data on the Determinants of Tumor Genesis and Growth Characteristics. Otol Neurotol 2015;36(7):1128–36.

50. Havik AL, Bruland O, Myrseth E, et al. Genetic landscape of sporadic vestibular schwannoma. J Neurosurg 2018;128(3):911–22.

51. Agnihotri S, Jalali S, Wilson MR, et al. The genomic landscape of schwannoma. Nat Genet 2016;48(11):1339–48.

52. Torres-Martin M, Lassaletta L, de Campos JM, et al. Global profiling in vestibular schwannomas shows critical deregulation of microRNAs and upregulation in those included in chromosomal region 14q32. PLoS One 2013;8(6):e65868.

53. Row PE, Prior IA, McCullough J, et al. The ubiquitin isopeptidase UBPY regulates endosomal ubiquitin dynamics and is essential for receptor down-regulation. J Biol Chem 2006;281(18):12618–24.

54. Reincke M, Sbiera S, Hayakawa A, et al. Mutations in the deubiquitinase gene USP8 cause Cushing's disease. Nat Genet 2015;47(1):31–8.

55. Smith MJ, Isidor B, Beetz C, et al. Mutations in LZTR1 add to the complex heterogeneity of schwannomatosis. Neurology 2015;84(2):141–7.

56. Wu JN, Roberts CW. ARID1A mutations in cancer: another epigenetic tumor suppressor? Cancer Discov 2013;3(1):35–43.

57. James MF, Han S, Polizzano C, et al. NF2/merlin is a novel negative regulator of mTOR complex 1, and activation of mTORC1 is associated with meningioma and schwannoma growth. Mol Cell Biol 2009;29(15):4250–61.

58. Kino T, Takeshima H, Nakao M, et al. Identification of the cis-acting region in the NF2 gene promoter as a potential target for mutation and methylation-dependent silencing in schwannoma. Gene Cell 2001;6(5):441–54.

59. Gonzalez-Gomez P, Bello MJ, Alonso ME, et al. CpG island methylation in sporadic and neurofibromatis type 2-associated schwannomas. Clin Cancer Res 2003;9(15):5601–6.

60. Kullar PJ, Pearson DM, Malley DS, et al. CpG island hypermethylation of the neurofibromatosis type 2 (NF2) gene is rare in sporadic vestibular schwannomas. Neuropathol Appl Neurobiol 2010;36(6):505–14.

61. Lassaletta L, Bello MJ, Del Rio L, et al. DNA methylation of multiple genes in vestibular schwannoma: Relationship with clinical and radiological findings. Otol Neurotol 2006;27(8):1180–5.

62. Torres-Martin M, Lassaletta L, de Campos JM, et al. Genome-wide methylation analysis in vestibular schwannomas shows putative mechanisms of gene expression modulation and global hypomethylation at the HOX gene cluster. Genes Chromosomes Cancer 2015;54(4):197–209.

63. Cioffi JA, Yue WY, Mendolia-Loffredo S, et al. MicroRNA-21 overexpression contributes to vestibular schwannoma cell proliferation and survival. Otol Neurotol 2010;31(9):1455–62.

64. Sass HCR, Hansen M, Borup R, et al. Tumor miRNA expression profile is related to vestibular schwannoma growth rate. Acta Neurochir 2020;162(5):1187–95.

65. Poenitzsch Strong AM, Setaluri V, Spiegelman VS. MicroRNA-340 as a modulator of RAS-RAF-MAPK signaling in melanoma. Arch Biochem Biophys 2014;563: 118–24.
66. Ghafouri-Fard S, Abak A, Shoorei H, et al. Regulatory role of microRNAs on PTEN signaling. Biomed Pharmacother 2021;133:110986.
67. Caye-Thomasen P, Borup R, Stangerup SE, et al. Deregulated genes in sporadic vestibular schwannomas. Otol Neurotol 2010;31(2):256–66.
68. Jacob A, Lee TX, Neff BA, et al. Phosphatidylinositol 3-kinase/AKT pathway activation in human vestibular schwannoma. Otol Neurotol 2008;29(1):58–68.
69. Stonecypher MS, Chaudhury AR, Byer SJ, et al. Neuregulin growth factors and their ErbB receptors form a potential signaling network for schwannoma tumorigenesis. J Neuropathol Exp Neurol 2006;65(2):162–75.
70. Aarhus M, Bruland O, Saetran HA, et al. Global gene expression profiling and tissue microarray reveal novel candidate genes and down-regulation of the tumor suppressor gene CAV1 in sporadic vestibular schwannomas. Neurosurgery 2010;67(4):998–1019 [discussion: 1019].
71. Sass HC, Borup R, Alanin M, et al. Gene expression, signal transduction pathways and functional networks associated with growth of sporadic vestibular schwannomas. J Neuro Oncol 2017;131(2):283–92.

Natural History of Hearing Loss in Sporadic Vestibular Schwannoma

Kaitlyn A. Brooks, MD[a], Esther X. Vivas, MD[a],*

KEYWORDS

- Sporadic vestibular schwannoma • Natural history • Hearing loss
- Asymmetric hearing • Sudden hearing loss

KEY POINTS

- Hearing loss due to untreated sporadic vestibular schwannoma (VS) commonly presents as an asymmetric sensorineural loss on audiogram.
- Hearing loss typically progresses slowly with incremental shifts in pure-tone audiometry (PTA) and speech discrimination testing.
- Better hearing (PTA < 30 dB and word recognition score (WRS) > 70%) at the time of diagnosis is correlated with the preservation of serviceable hearing (SH).
- At 5 and 10 years after diagnosis, roughly 60% and 40% of patients who had SH at time of VS diagnosis will maintain SH, respectively.
- The mechanism behind hearing loss in VS patients is currently controversial and the correlation between tumor growth or size and the progression of hearing loss specifically is not well understood.
- All patients with VS should be counseled on the natural progression of disease and inevitable evolution of hearing loss, regardless of tumor growth or initial size.

BACKGROUND

The start of the twenty-first century has seen a revolution in terms of vestibular schwannoma (VS) management because posttreatment morbidity, particularly associated hearing loss, has been less tolerated.[1] Patients and physicians have opted for less-invasive treatment modalities, with an increasing number of patients undergoing a period of observation rather than therapeutic intervention.[1,2] Various factors can be attributed to the de-escalation in treatment. For example, recent trends show greater age, smaller tumor size, and less severe symptomatology at time of VS diagnosis,[1,3,4]

a Department of Otolaryngology- Head and Neck Surgery, Emory University Hospital Midtown, 11th Floor, Suite 1135, Medical Office Tower, 550 Peachtree Street NE, Atlanta, GA 30308, USA
* Corresponding author. Emory University Hospital Midtown, 11th Floor, Suite 1135, Medical Office Tower, 550 Peachtree Street NE, Atlanta, GA 30308, USA.
E-mail address: evivas@emory.edu

Otolaryngol Clin N Am 56 (2023) 435–444
https://doi.org/10.1016/j.otc.2023.02.005

in addition to a shift in prioritizing functional outcomes versus total disease clearance.[5,6] VS observation is done with a "wait-and-scan" approach where the goal is to monitor change in tumor size on serial imaging and change in symptomatology to determine when intervention is warranted.[7] With growing popularity of an observational period for sporadic VS, the natural history of hearing loss is an important point to understand in order to fully counsel patients on their treatment options.

Definitions

At the time of diagnosis, patients are typically categorized by the severity of hearing loss, which can be done using several methods including American Academy of Otolaryngology- Head and Neck Surgery (AAO-HNS) Hearing Classification and Gardner- Robertson hearing classification. Hearing loss can be further categorized into those with serviceable hearing (SH) and nonserviceable hearing (NSH). SH can be defined as AAO-HNS Hearing Classification A or B and Gardner-Robertson hearing classification I or II. These hearing classification scales are shown below in **Tables 1 and 2.**

EVALUATION

All patients with VS or complaint of hearing loss should undergo audiologic testing consisting of pure-tone audiometry (PTA) and speech discrimination testing (SDS). The vast majority of patients (95%) with sporadic VS will present with hearing loss[8]; hearing loss is both the most common and earliest VS symptom.[9] Roughly half of patients at the time of diagnosis have SH,[5,10] with one-fifth to one-third of patients presenting with AAO Class A hearing ($\leq$30 dB PTA and SDS $\geq$ 70%).[4,10]

The most common hearing loss pattern at time of presentation is an asymmetric sensorineural hearing loss (SNHL), defined as 10-dB (dB) difference or greater in hearing between the 2 ears at 2 or more contiguous frequencies or greater than 15-dB difference at 1 frequency as seen below in **Fig. 1.**[11] A 15-dB difference or greater interaural difference at 3000 Hz specifically has the highest positive predictive value. Asymmetric tinnitus can also be a presenting symptom but only yields a diagnosis of a new VS in 1% of instances.[11]

About 5% to 15% of patients with VS may present with a sudden sensorineural hearing loss (SSNHL).[11] It is suggested that more than half of patients experiencing their first VS-associated SSNHL episode will have complete recovery.[12] With each subsequent SSNHL episode in patients with sporadic VS, rates of hearing recovery decrease.

Quality of life (QOL) at the time of presentation is often affected by VS-associated hearing loss in multiple ways, including inability to use the telephone with the affected ear, difficulty with personal relationships, and difficulty with conversations.[10] All of these QOL outcomes are more strongly associated with decreased SDS when compared with increased PTA; patients experience significant change in QOL

Table 1			
AAO-HNS hearing classification system			
Classification	**PTA (dB)**	**SDS (%)**	**Serviceable vs Nonserviceable**
Class A	<30	70–100	Serviceable
Class B	31–50	50–69	Serviceable
Class C	>50	50–69	Nonserviceable
Class D	Any PTA	<50	Nonserviceable

Table 2			
Gardner-Robertson hearing grading scale for vestibular schwannoma			
Grade	PTA (dB)	SDS (%)	Hearing
I	0–30	70–100	Good
II	31–50	50–69	Serviceable
III	51–90	5–49	Nonserviceable
IV	>91	1–4	Poor
V	Cannot test	0	Deaf

depending on presentation as AAO-HNS Class A hearing versus AAO-HNS Class B hearing, despite both indicating SH.[10]

Auditory brainstem response (ABR) has been used historically for evaluation; its role, however, has been lost due to the advent of MRI as the gold standard for VS diagnosis. ABR changes seen in sporadic VS include dissynchrony with reduced amplitude of ABR peaks or absent ABR peaks altogether.[13] Meta-analysis showed a sensitivity of 93% and specificity of 82% of ABR for suspected VS but the data were widely skewed.[14]

PROGRESSION

Hearing loss for sporadic VS is typically slow and progressive at a rate of 3.5 dB increase per year.[5] Poorer baseline hearing at time of diagnosis portends hearing deterioration from SH to NSH[6]; every 10-dB increase in PTA and 10% decrease in SDS at the time of diagnosis increase the risk of progression to NSH.[15,16] Patients with AAO-HNS Class B hearing are more at risk for progressive hearing loss than those with Class A hearing.[6,15] The pattern in which SDS worsens is roughly linear for patients who start with SDS at 100% because these patients typically lose 2% to 4% of SDS annually; for patients with initial SDS between 70% and 99%, the pattern of SDS deterioration is inversely logarithmic as SDS decreases at rates of 13%, 8%, and 6% in the first, second, and third years after diagnosis, respectively.[4] Patterns

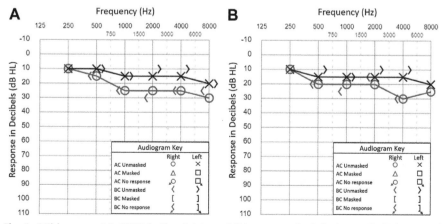

Fig. 1. Mild asymmetric SNHL in the right ear. (*A*) Image on the left shows 10-dB interaural difference among 3 contiguous frequencies and (*B*) Image on the right shows 15-dB interaural difference at one frequency.

of SDS deterioration are shown below in **Fig. 2** for patients with initial SDS of 100% and initial SDS between 70% and 99%.

Patients with 100% speech discrimination at diagnosis have a 75% chance of preserving good hearing after 10 years.[4] The overall probability of maintaining SH at the 5-year and 10-year postdiagnosis mark range from 50% to 70% and 30% to 50%, respectively, for tumors less than 1.5 cm in greatest dimension.[6] Rates of progression to NSH among patients who have SH at time of VS diagnosis are shown below in **Table 3**.[4,5] For patients that have NSH loss at time of VS diagnosis, hearing may continue to worsen but does not significantly change or improve, regardless of tumor progression or nonprogression.[17]

PATHOGENESIS

The available literature has presented conflicting results regarding the pathophysiology behind the slow deterioration of hearing in sporadic VSs. One-dimensional tumor size is likely not correlated to hearing loss but there is positive correlation with 3-dimensional tumor volume and severity of hearing loss[18]; increased tumor volume is associated with increased PTA and decreased SDS at the time of diagnosis.[16] **Figs. 3** and **4** show a patient with a 2.1 cm × 1.3 cm × 1.5 cm right VS who presented with subtle subjective hearing loss. Despite the large size of this tumor, audiograms at diagnosis and 6-month follow-up show no SNHL and mild asymmetric SNHL, respectively. This patient had 100% SDS on both evaluations. A second patient is shown with a large 2.1 cm × 2.6 cm × 1.8 cm right VS in **Fig. 5**; this patient presented with complaints of severe subjective hearing loss, which was confirmed on audiogram with SDS 12% (**Fig. 6**).

It has been hypothesized that an increased growth rate in a VS highlights aggressive features and the ability to disrupt cochlear nerve function.[19] Increased tumor size and growth effect on hearing is hypothesized to be due to compression on neighboring

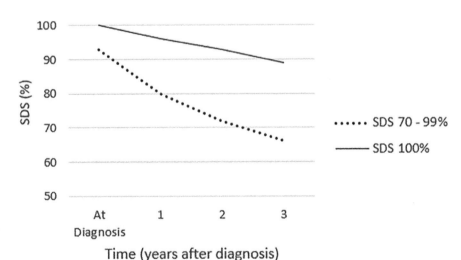

Fig. 2. Linear SDS loss for patients with initial SDS 100% versus inversely logarithmic SDS loss for patients with initial SDS 70% to 99%, data used from ref.[4]

Table 3
Maintenance of serviceable hearing over natural history of sporadic vestibular schwannoma

Years after Diagnosis (year)	Percent of Patients with Serviceable Hearing (%)
1	94–95
3	73–77
5	56–66
10	32–44

Data from from Stangerup SE, Thomsen J, Tos M, Caye-Thomasen P. Long-term hearing preservation in vestibular schwannoma. Otol Neurotol. Feb 2010;31(2):271 to 5. doi:10.1097/MAO.0-b013e3181c34bda; Khandalavala KR, Saba ES, Kocharyan A, et al. Hearing Preservation in Observed Sporadic Vestibular Schwannoma: A Systematic Review. Otol Neurotol. Jul 1 2022;43(6):604 to 610. https://doi.org/10.1097/MAO.0000000000003520

neurovascular structures leading to ischemic changes.[16] Just under half of patients with VS will have growth in their tumor during observation; the remaining patients will see no growth or regression in size.[20] The average growth rate for patients who experience tumor growth was 1.9 mm per year.[20] Tumor growth, however, has been both proven and disproven to be correlated with hearing loss.[6,18,19] Cystic tumors in particular have been correlated with tumor growth but an association between cystic nature of tumor and worsened hearing loss has not been described.[21]

Pathologic changes have been explored as to the mechanism behind hearing loss, which includes changes at the cellular layer of the cochlea involving degeneration of spiral ganglion cells, inner and outer hair cells, and the stria vascularis.[22,23] Changes in chemical composition of endolymph and perilymph have also been described in addition to cochlear hydrops as a factor in hearing loss due to sporadic VS.[23] Finally, factors secreted from VS tumors were proposed as the mechanism behind changes on the cellular level in the cochlea with the proposition that elevated intracochlear levels of TNF-α were correlated with hearing loss and that elevated intracochlear levels of fibroblast growth factor 2 (FGF-2) were otoprotective.[24]

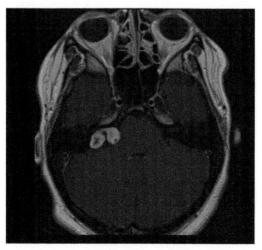

Fig. 3. Axial postcontrast T1-sequence MRI showing large right VS measuring 2.1 cm × 1.3 cm × 1.5 cm (corresponding audiograms in **Fig. 4**).

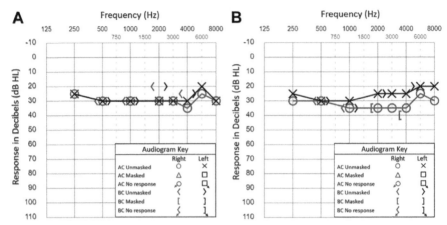

Fig. 4. Corresponding audiograms to patient with large VS in **Fig. 3**. (*A*) Image on the left shows no asymmetric SNHL at the time of diagnosis, and (*B*) image on the right shows a mild asymmetric SNHL at 6-month follow-up.

Therapeutic Options

Auditory rehabilitation can be done with numerous options, including traditional amplification with hearing aids. Hearing aids can significantly improve both objective hearing outcomes in terms of PTA and SDS and subjective QOL for these patients, even if treatment is not pursued for the VS.[25] A cross-sectional study demonstrated that 32% of patients with unilateral VS use a hearing-assistive device; for patients with NSH in the VS ear, a contralateral routing of signals (CROS) hearing aid can feed sonic input to the better hearing ear. Bone-anchored hearing devices are a good alternative to CROS devices when the patient does not wish to wear a receiver in the better hearing ear.

When a VS is present in the only hearing ear, the contralateral ear can be implanted with a cochlear implant.[17,26] There have been recent reports of implanting patients ipsilateral to their tumor.[27] The role of implantable hearing technologies in patients with VS will be discussed in detail in another article of this issue.

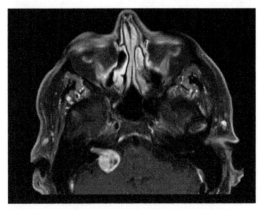

Fig. 5. Axial postcontrast T1-sequence MRI showing 2.1 cm × 2.6 cm × 1.8 cm right VS (corresponding audiogram in **Fig. 6**).

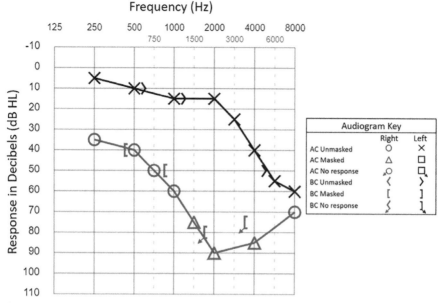

Fig. 6. Corresponding audiogram for patient with large VS in **Fig. 5** at the time of diagnosis, showing a severe asymmetric sloping SNHL.

DISCUSSION

With smaller tumor size and older patient age at the time of VS diagnosis, a significant number of patients with sporadic VS are embarking on observation periods as the initial management. It is more important than ever to understand how hearing changes during the natural history of VS to fully counsel patients in their management choices, especially given that the majority of patients with VS who undergo observation will see progression in their hearing loss ipsilateral to the tumor.[4–6] Rates of hearing loss progression during the natural history of the tumor can be compared with rates of hearing loss with microsurgical tumor resection and stereotactic radiosurgery so physicians can help patients make an informed decision. A point to highlight is that higher SDS and lower PTA at time of diagnosis are protective against hearing loss. Seventy-five percent of patients with 100% SDS initially are able to maintain a similar level of hearing at the 10-year mark,[4] which is much higher than the quoted 30% to 50% rate of maintaining SH at the 10-year timepoint for all patients with SH.[6] Atypical patterns of hearing loss can also be seen in patients with VS; SSNHL can affect 5% to 15% of patients, and patients can experience multiple episodes. Recovery of hearing is more probable with earlier episodes of SSNHL versus later episodes.[12]

The proposed mechanisms behind progressive hearing loss from VS, however, are controversial. Multiple studies have suggested that tumor size and tumor growth are correlated to progression of hearing loss; multiple other studies, however, suggest that tumor growth and initial tumor size are not correlated to progression of hearing loss.[6,18,19] We show 2 examples of patients with large VSs and extremely varied severity of hearing loss. Conflicting conclusions in the currently available evidence weaken the hypothesis that direct compression of neurovascular structures from the tumor is solely responsible for the progressive hearing loss seen in VS. Three-dimensional volumetric tumor sizing, however, has been correlated with hearing loss in multiple studies.[18] Data has also shown that 75% of intrameatal tumors and 60% of extrameatal tumors do not grow after 10 years of observation,[3] which is a higher rate of nongrowth than expected if progression of hearing loss was due simply to tumor growth or size. The exact mechanism behind VS-related hearing loss is currently unclear but compression and changes in intracochlear biochemical signaling have both been explored.

SUMMARY

Hearing loss is the most common and earliest symptom of VS at diagnosis. The most common pattern of hearing loss is asymmetric SNHL. Roughly half of the patients at time of diagnosis have SH in the affected ear. Throughout its natural history, patients with SH maintain SH at 94% to 95% after 1 year, 73% to 77% after 2 years, 56% to 66% after 5 years, and 32% to 44% after 10 years. Better hearing at the time of diagnosis in terms of higher SDS and lower PTA is otoprotective because these patients maintain good hearing for a longer period of time. For patients newly diagnosed with VS, it is likely their hearing will continue to deteriorate during a 10-year observational period despite small initial tumor size or lack of tumor growth. The mechanism responsible for progressive hearing loss in sporadic VS is still under investigation.

CLINICS CARE POINTS

- Hearing loss due to untreated VS commonly presents as an asymmetric sensorineural loss on audiogram.
- Hearing loss typically progresses slowly in small annual increments of increasing PTA and decreasing SDS.
- Better hearing (PTA < 30 dB and WRS > 70%) at time of diagnosis is correlated with the preservation of SH.
- Roughly 60% and 40% of patients who started with SH at the time of VS diagnosis will have SH at 5 and 10 years after diagnosis, respectively.
- The mechanism behind hearing loss in patients with VS is currently controversial, including the role of tumor growth and size and their implication on hearing loss.

DECLARATION OF INTERESTS

The authors testify no financial relationships to disclose or conflicts of interest pertaining to this study.

REFERENCES

1. Carlson ML, Habermann EB, Wagie AE, et al. The Changing Landscape of Vestibular Schwannoma Management in the United States–A Shift Toward Conservatism. Otolaryngol Head Neck Surg 2015;153(3):440–6.
2. Pena I, Chew EY, Landau BP, et al. Diagnostic Criteria for Detection of Vestibular Schwannomas in the VA Population. Otol Neurotol 2016;37(10):1510–5.
3. Reznitsky M, Petersen M, West N, et al. Epidemiology Of Vestibular Schwannomas - Prospective 40-Year Data From An Unselected National Cohort. Clin Epidemiol 2019;11:981–6.
4. Stangerup SE, Thomsen J, Tos M, et al. Long-term hearing preservation in vestibular schwannoma. Otol Neurotol. Feb 2010;31(2):271–5.

5. Khandalavala KR, Saba ES, Kocharyan A, et al. Hearing Preservation in Observed Sporadic Vestibular Schwannoma: A Systematic Review. Otol Neurotol 2022;43(6):604–10.
6. Carlson ML, Link MJ, Driscoll CLW, et al. Working Toward Consensus on Sporadic Vestibular Schwannoma Care: A Modified Delphi Study. Otol Neurotol 2020; 41(10):e1360–71.
7. Solares CA, Panizza B. Vestibular schwannoma: an understanding of growth should influence management decisions. Otol Neurotol 2008;29(6):829–34.
8. Matthies C, Samii M. Management of 1000 vestibular schwannomas (acoustic neuromas): clinical presentation. Neurosurgery 1997;40(1):1–9 [discussion: 9-10].
9. Selesnick SH, Jackler RK. Atypical hearing loss in acoustic neuroma patients. Laryngoscope. Apr 1993;103(4 Pt 1):437–41.
10. Peris-Celda M, Graffeo CS, Perry A, et al. Beyond the ABCs: Hearing Loss and Quality of Life in Vestibular Schwannoma. Mayo Clin Proc 2020;95(11):2420–8.
11. Sweeney AD, Carlson ML, Shepard NT, et al. Congress of Neurological Surgeons Systematic Review and Evidence-Based Guidelines on Otologic and Audiologic Screening for Patients With Vestibular Schwannomas. Neurosurgery 2018;82(2): E29–31.
12. Wasano K, Oishi N, Noguchi M, et al. Sudden sensorineural hearing loss in patients with vestibular schwannoma. Sci Rep 2021;11(1):1624.
13. Eggermont JJ. Auditory brainstem response. Handb Clin Neurol 2019;160: 451–64.
14. Koors PD, Thacker LR, Coelho DH. ABR in the diagnosis of vestibular schwannomas: a meta-analysis. Am J Otolaryngol 2013;34(3):195–204.
15. Hunter JB, Dowling EM, Lohse CM, et al. Hearing Outcomes in Conservatively Managed Vestibular Schwannoma Patients With Serviceable Hearing. Otol Neurotol 2018;39(8):e704–11.
16. Patel NS, Huang AE, Dowling EM, et al. The Influence of Vestibular Schwannoma Tumor Volume and Growth on Hearing Loss. Otolaryngol Head Neck Surg 2020; 162(4):530–7.
17. Jia H, Nguyen Y, De Seta D, et al. Management of sporadic vestibular schwannoma with contralateral nonserviceable hearing. Laryngoscope 2020;130(6): E407–15.
18. Gan J, Zhang Y, Wu J, et al. Current Understanding of Hearing Loss in Sporadic Vestibular Schwannomas: A Systematic Review. Front Oncol 2021;11:687201.
19. Sughrue ME, Yang I, Aranda D, et al. The natural history of untreated sporadic vestibular schwannomas: a comprehensive review of hearing outcomes. J Neurosurg 2010;112(1):163–7.
20. Smouha EE, Yoo M, Mohr K, et al. Conservative management of acoustic neuroma: a meta-analysis and proposed treatment algorithm. Laryngoscope 2005; 115(3):450–4.
21. Paldor I, Chen AS, Kaye AH. Growth rate of vestibular schwannoma. J Clin Neurosci 2016;32:1–8.
22. Mahmud MR, Khan AM, Nadol JB Jr. Histopathology of the inner ear in unoperated acoustic neuroma. Ann Otol Rhinol Laryngol 2003;112(11):979–86.
23. Roosli C, Linthicum FH Jr, Cureoglu S, et al. Dysfunction of the cochlea contributing to hearing loss in acoustic neuromas: an underappreciated entity. Otol Neurotol 2012;33(3):473–80.
24. Dilwali S, Landegger LD, Soares VY, et al. Secreted Factors from Human Vestibular Schwannomas Can Cause Cochlear Damage. Sci Rep 2015;5:18599.

25. Reffet K, Lescanne E, Bobillier C, et al. Hearing aids in patients with vestibular schwannoma: Interest of the auditory brainstem responses. Clin Otolaryngol 2018;43(4):1057–64.
26. Di Lella F, Merkus P, Di Trapani G, et al. Vestibular schwannoma in the only hearing ear: role of cochlear implants. Ann Otol Rhinol Laryngol 2013;122(2):91–9.
27. Borsetto D, Hammond-Kenny A, Tysome JR, et al. Hearing rehabilitation outcomes in cochlear implant recipients with vestibular schwannoma in observation or radiotherapy groups: A systematic review. Cochlear Implants Int 2020; 21(1):9–17.

Introducing an Evidence-Based Approach to Wait-And-Scan Management of Sporadic Vestibular Schwannoma
Size Threshold Surveillance

John P. Marinelli, MD[a,b], Christine M. Lohse, MS[c],
Matthew L. Carlson, MD[a,d],*

KEYWORDS

- Size threshold surveillance • Acoustic neuroma • Observation
- Threshold observation • Wait-and-scan • Conservative management • Treatment

KEY POINTS

- Greater disease detection has resulted in a shift toward smaller tumors diagnosed in older patients, often with fewer symptoms.
- The detection rate of new tumors has outpaced the transition to increasingly conservative management, with more vestibular schwannomas treated today than ever before.
- Emerging natural history data demonstrate that most tumors grow during observation, justifying either an upfront treatment approach or a "size threshold surveillance" approach.
- Existing data support the tolerance of some growth during observation in appropriately selected patients up until a size threshold range (approximately 15 mm of cerebellopontine angle extension) whereby further tumor growth would predispose the patient to a disproportionately elevated risk of poor posttreatment outcomes.

MOTIVATION FOR A PARADIGM SHIFT IN OBSERVATION MANAGEMENT
Major Epidemiological Shifts in the Post-Magnetic Resonance Imaging Era

Foreshadowed by publications from the early-2000s that revealed increasing diagnosis rates of incidental brain tumors with the widespread adoption of MRI,[1,2] the incidence of sporadic vestibular schwannoma has increased significantly in the post-MRI era.[3,4]

[a] Department of Otolaryngology–Head and Neck Surgery, Mayo Clinic, 200 1st St Southwest, Rochester, MN 55905, USA; [b] Department of Otolaryngology–Head and Neck Surgery, San Antonio Uniformed Services Health Education Consortium, 3551 Roger Brooke Drive, JBSA, TX 78234, USA; [c] Department of Quantitative Health Sciences, Mayo Clinic, Rochester, MN, USA; [d] Department of Neurologic Surgery, Mayo Clinic, Rochester, MN, USA
* Corresponding author.
E-mail address: carlson.matthew@mayo.edu

Otolaryngol Clin N Am 56 (2023) 445–457
https://doi.org/10.1016/j.otc.2023.02.006
0030-6665/23/© 2023 Elsevier Inc. All rights reserved.

Combined with the influence of screening protocols for asymmetrical sensorineural hearing loss, the incidence of sporadic tumors has risen to 3 to 5 per 100,000 person-years across global population-based studies since 2010 and exceeds 20 per 100,000 person-years among people aged older than 70 years.[5] In fact, the clinically detectable lifetime prevalence of sporadic vestibular schwannoma now exceeds 1 in 500 persons, rendering it no longer a rare disease state in the United States.[6,7]

In this way, more vestibular schwannomas are diagnosed today than ever before. Importantly, evidence suggests that the majority of this increase in incidence rates is accounted for by improved disease detection through the combined effects of MRI and routine screening of asymmetrical sensorineural hearing loss rather than being attributable to an underlying biological shift from environmental exposures such as cell phone use or loud noise.[8–11] Underscoring the improved detection explanation behind increasing incidence rates is the epidemiological evolution toward an older patient demographic with increasingly smaller tumors at diagnosis. To this end, population-based studies demonstrate that the typical patient diagnosed with sporadic vestibular schwannoma in the modern era is minimally symptomatic, older than 60 years of age, and has a tumor that is entirely confined to the internal auditory canal or minimal cerebellopontine angle extension.[3,4]

Concern for Ongoing Overtreatment

Following an improved understanding of the natural history of sporadic vestibular schwannoma, reports surfaced in the early-2000s introducing the observation management approach.[12–14] Since then, there has been an increasing global transition toward observation for the initial management of sporadic vestibular schwannoma,[15] with international population-based studies demonstrating that most newly diagnosed patients undergo at least an initial period of observation before receiving definitive treatment with either radiosurgery or microsurgery.[3,4] Of note, although some studies from the United States suggest that observation is not the most common initial management approach,[16] it is important to recognize the tertiary referral center bias associated with these studies—a topic discussed at-length elsewhere.[17,18]

Nevertheless, despite most newly diagnosed patients undergoing observation, population-based data also suggest that the treatment incidence of sporadic vestibular schwannoma (ie, the number of people treated with radiosurgery or microsurgery per person-years) has actually increased.[19] More specifically, the incidence rates of microsurgery in the population have remained essentially stable since 1960, whereas the rates of radiosurgery have significantly increased over time.[19] As discussed above, the number of people who develop sporadic vestibular schwannoma is thought to be relatively stable during the last 50 years, and increasing incidence rates are attributable to improved detection capabilities. Therefore, the increasing incidence of treated tumors over time suggests that the rate at which newly diagnosed patients are being allocated to observation management is being outpaced by the rate at which they are being detected and treated with either radiosurgery or microsurgery (**Fig. 1**). Patients who 30 years ago would have lived their whole lives never knowing they had a small vestibular schwannoma are now being increasingly diagnosed and treated over time. These observations indicate some degree of overtreatment is likely occurring among patients with sporadic vestibular schwannoma.

All Vestibular Schwannomas Grow: The Paradox of the Existing Observation Management Paradigm

Within the existing observation management paradigm, treatment is generally recommended as soon as "true growth" (ie, ≥ 2 mm linear diameter) is detected on serial

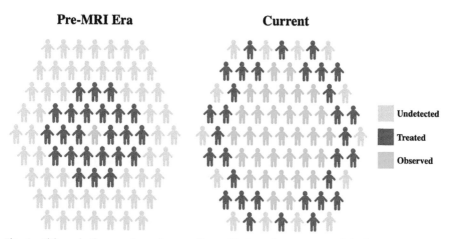

Fig. 1. Although the number of sporadic vestibular schwannomas globally is thought to have remained essentially stable for the past several decades, there has been a significant increase in the detection rate of new tumors in the post-MRI era. Although more vestibular schwannomas undergo observation today than ever before, more tumors also receive treatment than ever before. (*From* Carlson ML, Link MJ. Vestibular Schwannomas. *NEJM.* 2021 Apr 8;384(14):1335-1348.)

MRI. A 2018 survey of the North American Skull Base Society showed that 91% of providers would observe a small (<15 mm) vestibular schwannoma until growth was detected, at which time treatment with either radiosurgery or microsurgery would then be recommended.[20]

Yet, as a logical extension of the *sporadic* development of these tumors, all vestibular schwannomas necessarily grew to the size detected at diagnosis. In this sense, all patients with sporadic vestibular schwannomas have "growing" tumors at some point and would thus warrant treatment in the existing observation management paradigm. Moreover, a recent multi-institutional investigation of almost 1000 sporadic vestibular schwannomas undergoing observation, using sensitive slice-by-slice volumetric tumor measurements, demonstrated that 80% of patients had continued tumor growth within 5 years of diagnosis.[21] When patients continued observation despite earlier tumor growth, the trend continued with another approximately 80% experiencing tumor growth within 5 years following the first episode of tumor growth; moreover, another 80% had a third episode of tumor growth within 5 years following the second episode of tumor growth when observation was still continued (**Fig. 2**A).[21] These natural history data match anecdotal provider perceptions of growth during observation, with almost 75% of respondents in a 2018 North American Skull Base Society survey indicating that they estimate the likelihood of tumor growth within the first 5 years of observation to be between 50% and 90%.[20]

These findings not only underscore the notion that "all sporadic vestibular schwannomas grow" but also illustrate that there is nothing unique about the time of diagnosis or the first episode of documented growth in terms of future proclivity of growth or acute need for treatment. Instead, sporadic vestibular schwannomas seem to display an overall propensity toward growth over time. The arbitrary timepoint of diagnosis is underscored by the observation that many patients have a long-standing history of attributable symptoms before diagnosis, even multiple episodes of sudden hearing loss in some cases, while conversely, up to 25% of newly diagnosed patients since

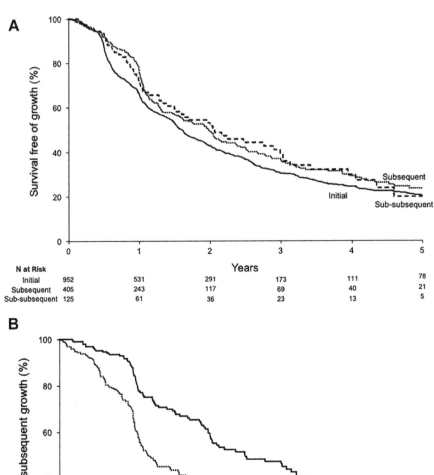

Fig. 2. Natural history of sporadic vestibular schwannoma from 952 patients undergoing observation. (*A*) The steady propensity toward growth among observed tumors, with growth patterns after diagnosis paralleling subsequent growth patterns (ie, there is nothing unique about the time of diagnosis in terms of long-term growth behavior); (*B*) The predictable nature of future growth, with tumors that have elevated growth rates (faster time to growth, larger interval size changes) being significantly more likely to continue growing; those that grew ≥50% per year displayed a hazard ratio for subsequent growth of 1.7 (95% CI 1.3–2.3; *P* < .001). (*From* Marinelli et al. Long-term natural history and patterns of sporadic vestibular schwannoma growth: A multi-institutional volumetric analysis of 952 patients. *Neuro Oncol.* 2022 Aug 1;24(8):1298-1306.)

2015 in population-based studies are diagnosed incidentally (**Fig. 3**).[5] Finally, it is worth noting that for most tumors, interval growth is small, and tumors that demonstrate growth may ultimately burnout and stop growing or even regress.[21,22]

Considered together, it should be appreciated that all *sporadic* vestibular schwannomas necessarily grow at some point during a patient's lifetime before diagnosis, and some degree of tumor growth following diagnosis will occur in most people during observation. These tumors' growth potential and behavior must fundamentally frame the way in which the observation management paradigm is conceptualized.

CLINICALLY MEANINGFUL SIZE THRESHOLDS TO GUIDE TIMING OF TREATMENT
Detectable Growth on Magnetic Resonance Imaging Does Not Necessarily Equal Clinically Meaningful Growth

Most lateral skull base surgeons would intuitively agree that growth of an intracanalicular vestibular schwannoma from 4 mm to 6 mm is unlikely to change post-treatment outcomes. Yet, this 2-mm difference represents the most widely adopted arbiter designating a tumor as a growing tumor, and as discussed previously, growing tumors in the existing observation management paradigm are typically recommended to be treated.[20]

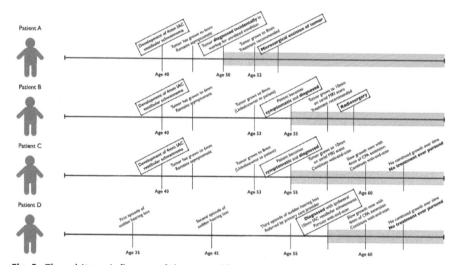

Fig. 3. The arbitrary influence of the natural history of vestibular schwannoma on the time-point at which patients undergo treatment in the existing observation management paradigm. Patients A, B, and C develop the same tumor at the same point in their lives and are otherwise identical clinically. Patient A is incidentally diagnosed, one growth episode is documented, and treatment is pursued. Patients B and C experience the same tumor growth without their knowledge because they have yet to be diagnosed. Eventually becoming symptomatic, both Patients B and C are diagnosed and undergo observation. Tumor growth is detected: Patient B undergoes radiosurgery while Patient C decides to continue observation. Slow continued growth is documented for Patient C but they decide to pursue continued observation still. Eventually, the tumor stops growing and no treatment is ever necessary. Patient D highlights how delays in diagnosis influence the progression toward treatment. In other words, the time at which a tumor comes to clinical attention is not always directly related to its natural history and prior growth episodes. (*From* Marinelli et al. Spontaneous Volumetric Tumor Regression During Wait-and-Scan Management of 952 Sporadic Vestibular Schwannomas. *Otol Neurotol.* 2022 Oct 1;43(9):e1034-e1038.)

It is critical to first recognize that the 2-mm litmus used to represent true interval tumor size change on serial MRI scans extends from scan-to-scan variability that arises from the limitations of MRI—the 2-mm litmus distinctly does not extend from posttreatment patient outcomes.[23,24] In fact, discussion of a clinically significant tumor growth threshold whereby meaningful clinical outcomes appreciably decrease has received surprisingly little attention to date. Although numerous studies have demonstrated that tumor size represents the most important factor influencing postoperative facial nerve function, most studies examining these outcomes investigate postoperative House-Brackmann (HB) grade III or greater facial nerve paresis. However, for a patient with an 8-mm intracanalicular tumor who presented with HB grade I facial nerve function and underwent 3 years of observation, anything less than maintaining normal facial nerve function and achieving durable tumor control after treatment would be considered a poor outcome.

Published Clinically Meaningful Size Thresholds for Treatment During Observation

In 2021, Macielak and colleagues[25] defined a clinically meaningful tumor size threshold range where further periods of observation beyond this tumor size threshold range disproportionately increase the likelihood of poor postoperative microsurgical outcomes should the tumor continue to grow. Chronicling more than 600 patients who underwent microsurgery at Mayo Clinic, the investigation found that tumor extension by 14–20 mm into the cerebellopontine angle represented a critical threshold range whereby foregoing preoperative HB grade I facial nerve function, gross total resection, and serviceable hearing became more likely.[25] Tumors of 13 mm or less within the cerebellopontine angle—and notably all intracanalicular tumors—demonstrated more favorable likelihoods of preserving preoperative HB grade I function, achieving gross total resection, and maintaining serviceable hearing.[25] These findings corroborate prior studies that examine tumor size and risk of HB III or greater facial nerve function and report thresholds of 16 mm of cerebellopontine angle extension.[26,27] Considered together, these data suggest that, when considering microsurgery for a patient with a growing tumor during observation—considering all factors including patient symptoms, preferences, and goals—continuing to observe tumor growth to approximately 15 mm in the cerebellopontine angle would not significantly compromise clinically meaningful postoperative outcomes.

Similar size threshold ranges whereby further tumor growth during observation would lead to deleterious posttreatment outcomes following radiosurgery have been minimally investigated to date. Forty-four percent of respondents from a 2018 North American Skull Base Society survey indicated that 25 mm represented the size cutoff where radiation becomes a poor treatment option in an otherwise healthy patient.[20] A total of 91% of respondents thought that this cutoff lies between 20 and 30 mm.[20] Published outcome data suggest that a tumor size of 25 mm or less within the cerebellopontine angle is favorable for avoiding significant brainstem edema and achieving good long-term tumor control.[28] Not considered in these estimates is the approximate 5% to 10% risk of treatment failure and subsequent need for salvage treatment. In most cases, "radiation failure" in the context of vestibular schwannoma management constitutes continued growth on serial MRI. Allowing for an initial transient postradiosurgery tumor swell (ie, pseudoprogression), tumors are often notably larger by the time radiation failure is declared. Furthermore, most studies indicate that tumor resection following earlier radiation treatment is more challenging with an increased risk of facial nerve paralysis or incomplete resection. A specific investigation into a size threshold less than this 25-mm cutoff for patients who initially underwent observation has not been investigated to date and is a current focus of research at the authors' center.

QUALITY OF LIFE DATA AND IMPLICATIONS FOR SMALL TUMORS

When assessing patient reported quality of life metrics, several large international prospective and cross-sectional assessments show there is no global advantage to active treatment over observation.[29,30] What is more, an initial period of observation (6 months or greater) seems to improve long-term quality of life regardless of the ultimate modality chosen, a finding likely explained by patients having more time to make a decision that they think is best and reconcile with their new diagnosis.[31] Prospective study of symptom evolution among 244 patients treated with either observation, radiosurgery, or microsurgery showed patients' tinnitus, dizziness or imbalance, and headaches were not significantly modified by treatment modality, suggesting that, in general, patient symptoms should not direct therapy—the exception being potentially reversible symptoms attributable to mass effect (eg, tumor-associated trigeminal neuralgia).[32]

A recent study of the Acoustic Neuroma Association and Mayo Clinic among 346 patients with small vestibular schwannomas showed that 96% of patients undergoing observation were satisfied with their treatment, and 88% of patients who initially underwent observation followed by definitive treatment with either radiosurgery or microsurgery were satisfied with their treatment.[33] This significantly contrasted with those who underwent upfront treatment with either radiosurgery or microsurgery, where 81% reported being satisfied with their choice. The reported difference across all 3 management groups was statistically significant ($P = .001$).[33]

PUTTING IT ALL TOGETHER: SIZE THRESHOLD SURVEILLANCE
Upfront Treatment Versus Size Threshold Surveillance

First, it is imperative to emphasize that the preceding discussion surrounding the rationale for a paradigm shift toward a more evidence-based approach during observation of small sporadic vestibular schwannomas must not be taken to mean that we advocate for every newly diagnosed small tumor to undergo observation. Rather, this information affords clinicians and patients a flexible approach that more accurately accounts for the nature of tumor growth and is only one of many aspects that should be considered within the greater context of patient care and shared decision-making. Especially in light of the overall propensity toward growth for these tumors,[21] if a well-informed patient desires to pursue upfront treatment, we think it is reasonable to pursue upfront radiosurgery or microsurgery at the time when the tumor is likely the smallest it will ever be and the patient is least symptomatic. Nevertheless, when initial observation is chosen, rather than reflexively treating a small tumor at first detection of linear growth, we think the evidence supports a more flexible approach that acknowledges at the outset that most tumors will show some growth during observation but continued observation in the setting of limited growth is a reasonable consideration if the patient desires, so long as follow-up can be assured (**Figs. 4** and **5**). This approach carries particular relevance for people with small tumors (eg, tumors confined to the internal auditory canal), elderly patients, patients with a vestibular schwannoma in an only-hearing ear, and those with multiple medical comorbidities.

We should recognize that it is nonsensical to counsel a patient with an 8-mm intracanalicular tumor that we can observe their tumor and they may be one of the lucky patients who has a tumor that never grows. Counseling often continues, if growth is detected, the tumor should be treated. However, because the patient did not go to bed one night without a vestibular schwannoma and wake up the next morning with an 8-mm tumor, such counseling neglects the obvious reality that all sporadic vestibular schwannomas necessarily grew before diagnosis. An approach that includes

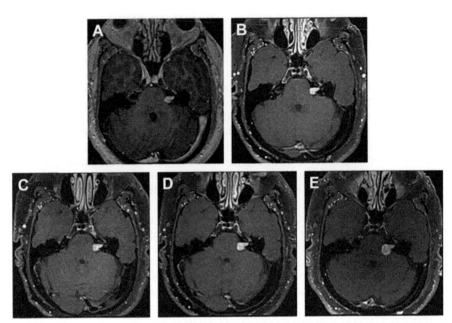

Fig. 4. A 51-year-old right-handed male patient who presented with asymmetrical sensori-neural hearing loss (pure-tone average at 0.5, 1, 2, and 3 kHz of 35 dB hearing loss; word recognition score of 88%) and was diagnosed with a left-sided sporadic vestibular schwannoma with 5 mm of cerebellopontine angle extension (*A*). He had a prior brain MRI in 2003 for an unrelated indication that did not demonstrate the presence of a tumor at that time; thus, it grew to the size detected on image A at some point during that interval. During the following 6 years, he experienced slow (1–2 mm per year) but persistent growth of his tumor (*B–E*) and elected continued observation. Six years following diagnosis, he underwent Gamma Knife radiosurgery at an eventual tumor size of 11 mm of cerebellopontine angle extension with an uncomplicated treatment course and no evidence of growth to date.

willingness to tolerate some growth during observation, particularly for slowly growing tumors, provides the opportunity for a more flexible strategy to optimize care based on individualized patient goals. In light of the existing quality of life data,[33] health-care cost-effectiveness data,[34–36] and the broader context of ongoing overtreatment of sporadic vestibular schwannoma,[19] it is likely that continued observation for many patients with small, slowly growing vestibular schwannomas is an advantageous consideration. Finally, it is worth appreciating that some groups, including our center, have intuitively already been practicing a similar approach—the "size threshold surveillance" (STS) paradigm simply provides the evidence framework to support the overarching practice,[4] with data to support strong consideration for treatment at a threshold of about 15 mm of cerebellopontine angle extension based on current evidence,[25] particularly if microsurgery is to be pursued in the setting of persistent growth.

Illustrative Patient Scenarios and Practical Considerations

Two examples at different age boundaries may help illustrate the practical application of the STS approach. Consider a 35-year-old patient who elects initial observation with a vestibular schwannoma that grows from 8 to 11 mm in cerebellopontine angle dimension during a 1-year period. Within this clinical context, treatment would often

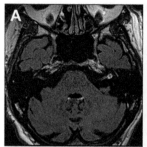 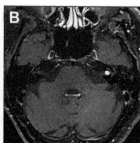 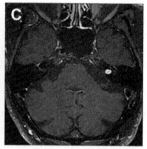

Fig. 5. A 74-year-old right-handed male patient who was diagnosed with a 4 mm intracanalicular left-sided sporadic vestibular schwannoma after presenting with asymmetrical sensorineural hearing loss (*A*). During the course of 3 years of observation (*B, C*), he experienced slow (1–2 mm per year) but persistent growth of his tumor, now 8 mm in maximal diameter in the internal auditory canal (*C*). He desires to pursue continued observation and will return in 1 year for interval imaging with plans for Gamma Knife radiosurgery if he experiences further growth.

still be recommended as the likelihood of future growth during this younger patient's lifetime is high, and the tumor size is already approximating the 15-mm threshold range. However, consider a 75-year-old patient diagnosed with a 5-mm intracanalicular tumor that grows to 9 mm by the third year of observation. This patient could justifiably consider continued observation. If the tumor grows to 11 mm 2 years later, it would still be justifiable to consider continued observation. For smaller tumors, numerous factors—chiefly of which being patient preference—must drive these decisions, and the STS paradigm allows for sufficient flexibility to continue observation in the setting of limited growth. Based on recent data, the *limited growth* motif of these scenarios warrants emphasis, as patients who have significant or more rapid size changes between interval MRI scans are significantly more likely to experience continued growth (**Fig. 2**B).[21,37,38]

One practical objection to the STS approach may surround the concern that, if further growth is tolerated, the patient may incur unnecessary additional risk. For example, one could reasonably argue that a certain poor outcome was preventable to some degree had earlier treatment been pursued. For example, consider a middle-aged patient who elected to observe an 8-mm intracanalicular tumor for 10 years until it grows to 10 mm of cerebellopontine angle extension. They then undergo resection of their tumor through a retrosigmoid approach. There is injury to the facial nerve during surgery, and they ultimately have HB grade III facial nerve function at 1 year postoperatively. Although this outcome is uncommon, it is estimated that HB II or greater facial nerve function occurs in approximately 3% to 5% of cases with 10 mm or greater of cerebellopontine angle extension at high-volume centers.[25] However, take the same patient with an 8-mm intracanalicular tumor who undergoes upfront treatment with microsurgery through a middle fossa approach. They also end up with HB III facial nerve function at 1 year—a risk estimated within the literature to occur between 3% and 16% for hearing preservation cases.[39–42] Therefore, in either approach—upfront treatment or continued observation—there is inevitable low risk of adverse events. Furthermore, from a standpoint of patient satisfaction and decisional regret, it is conceivable that patients' acceptance of a complication may be higher if they thought the treatment was truly necessary. If a relatively asymptomatic patient with a small tumor elects upfront surgery and develops nonserviceable hearing, facial nerve paralysis, or new onset debilitating headache or tinnitus, the risk for decisional regret is high because the patient could have also observed their tumor for many more years. Conversely, if a patient undertakes treatment after documented progressive growth, they may be more apt to accept such an outcome. The crucial conceptual element to the STS approach is that the risk of poor posttreatment outcomes may not substantially change up until the threshold of approximately 15 mm of cerebellopontine angle extension, particularly for microsurgery.[25]

SUMMARY

Because of the advent of MRI and widespread adoption of screening protocols for asymmetrical sensorineural hearing loss, more sporadic vestibular schwannomas are diagnosed today than ever before. Although an increasing number of patients are being allocated to observation for initial management, the detection rate of new tumors has outpaced the transition to increasingly conservative management. As a result, more sporadic vestibular schwannomas are also treated today than ever before. Emerging natural history data demonstrate that most tumors grow during observation. These findings justify either an upfront treatment approach or, what we have termed, a "Size Threshold Surveillance" approach. Specifically, if the patient elects to pursue observation, then existing data support the tolerance of some growth during observation in appropriately selected patients up until a size threshold range (approximately 15 mm of cerebellopontine angle extension) whereby further tumor growth would predispose the patient to a disproportionately elevated risk of poor posttreatment outcomes.

CLINICS CARE POINTS

- Most vestibular schwannomas will show some growth during observation.
- Reflexively recommending treatment at first indication of growth does not adequately account for natural history data as well as overarching concern for overtreatment of vestibular schwannoma.
- Tolerating some growth during observation (i.e., considering to continue observing growing tumors) allows for greater flexibility for patient-centered decision-making if the patient desires continued observation.

FUNDING

No external funding sources.

ACKNOWLEDGMENTS

The views expressed herein are those of the authors and do not reflect the official policy or position of Brooke Army Medical Center, the U.S. Army Medical Department, the U.S. Army Office of the Surgeon General, the Department of the Army, the Department of the Air Force, or the Department of Defense or the U.S. Government.

CONFLICTS OF INTEREST

No authors have relevant conflicts of interest to disclose.

REFERENCES

1. Lin D, Hegarty JL, Fischbein NJ, et al. The prevalence of "incidental" acoustic neuroma. Arch Otolaryngol Head Neck Surg 2005;131:241–4.

2. Vernooij MW, Ikram MA, Tanghe HL, et al. Incidental findings on brain MRI in the general population. N Engl J Med 2007;357:1821–8.
3. Marinelli JP, Lohse CM, Carlson ML. Incidence of vestibular schwannoma over the past half-century: a population-based study of Olmsted County, Minnesota. Otolaryngol Head Neck Surg 2018;159:717–23.
4. Reznitsky M, Petersen M, West N, et al. Epidemiology of vestibular schwannomas - prospective 40-year data from an unselected national cohort. Clin Epidemiol 2019;11:981–6.
5. Marinelli JP, Beeler CJ, Carlson ML, et al. Global incidence of sporadic vestibular schwannoma: a systematic review. Otolaryngol Head Neck Surg 2022;167(2):209–14.
6. Marinelli JP, Grossardt BR, Lohse CM, et al. Prevalence of sporadic vestibular schwannoma: reconciling temporal bone, radiologic, and population-based studies. Otol Neurotol 2019;40:384–90.
7. Zanoletti E, Mazzoni A, Martini A, et al. Surgery of the lateral skull base: a 50-year endeavour. Acta Otorhinolaryngol Ital 2019;39:S1–146.
8. Mornet E, Kania R, Sauvaget E, et al. Vestibular schwannoma and cell-phones. Results, limits and perspectives of clinical studies. Eur Ann Otorhinolaryngol Head Neck Dis 2013;130:275–82.
9. Roswall N, Stangerup SE, Caye-Thomasen P, et al. Residential traffic noise exposure and vestibular schwannoma - a Danish case-control study. Acta Oncol 2017;56:1310–6.
10. Deltour I, Schlehofer B, Massardier-Pilonchery A, et al. Exposure to loud noise and risk of vestibular schwannoma: results from the INTERPHONE international casecontrol study. Scand J Work Environ Health 2019;45:183–93.
11. Marinelli JP, Lohse CM, Grossardt BR, et al. Rising incidence of sporadic vestibular schwannoma: true biological shift versus simply greater detection. Otol Neurotol 2020;41:813–47.
12. Shin YJ, Fraysse B, Cognard C, et al. Effectiveness of conservative management of acoustic neuromas. Am J Otol 2000;21:857–62.
13. Tschudi DC, Linder TE, Fisch U. Conservative management of unilateral acoustic neuromas. Am J Otol 2000;21:722–8.
14. Raut VV, Walsh RM, Bath AP, et al. Conservative management of vestibular schwannomas - second review of a prospective longitudinal study. Clin Otolaryngol Allied Sci 2004;29:505–14.
15. Carlson ML, Habermann EB, Wagie AE, et al. the changing landscape of vestibular schwannoma management in the United States–A shift toward conservatism. Otolaryngol Head Neck Surg 2015;153:440–6.
16. Leon J, Trifiletti DM, Waddle MR, et al. Trends in the initial management of vestibular schwannoma in the United States. J Clin Neurosci 2019;68:174–8.
17. Marinelli JP, Nassiri AM, Habermann EB, et al. Underreporting of vestibular schwannoma incidence within national brain tumor and cancer registries in the United States. Otol Neurotol 2021;42:e758–63.
18. Saba ES, Marinelli JP, Lohse CM, et al. Quantifying tertiary referral center bias in vestibular schwannoma research. Otol Neurotol 2020;41:258–64.
19. Marinelli JP, Grossardt BR, Lohse CM, et al. Is Improved detection of vestibular schwannoma leading to overtreatment of the disease? Otol Neurotol 2019;40:847–50.
20. Carlson ML, Van Gompel JJ, Wiet RM, et al. A cross-sectional survey of the North American skull base society: current practice patterns of vestibular schwannoma

evaluation and management in North America. J Neurol Surg B Skull Base 2018; 79:289–96.

21. Marinelli JP, Schnurman Z, Killeen DE, et al. Long-term natural history and patterns of sporadic vestibular schwannoma growth: a multi-institutional volumetric analysis of 952 patients. Neuro Oncol 2022;24(8):1298–306.

22. Marinelli JP, Killeen DE, Schnurman Z, et al. Spontaneous volumetric tumor regression during wait-and-scan management of 952 sporadic vestibular schwannomas. Otol Neurotol 2022;43(9):e1034–8.

23. Kanzaki J, Tos M, Sanna M, et al. New and modified reporting systems from the consensus meeting on systems for reporting results in vestibular schwannoma. Otol Neurotol 2003;24:642–8 [discussion: 648-649].

24. Slattery WH 3rd, Fisher LM, Yoon G, et al. Magnetic resonance imaging scanner reliability for measuring changes in vestibular schwannoma size. Otol Neurotol 2003;24:666–70 [discussion: 670-661].

25. Macielak RJ, Wallerius KP, Lawlor SK, et al. Defining clinically significant tumor size in vestibular schwannoma to inform timing of microsurgery during wait-and-scan management: moving beyond minimum detectable growth. J Neurosurg 2021;1–9. https://doi.org/10.3171/2021.4.JNS21465.

26. Torres R, Nguyen Y, Vanier A, et al. Multivariate analysis of factors influencing facial nerve outcome following microsurgical resection of vestibular schwannoma. Otolaryngol Head Neck Surg 2017;156:525–33.

27. Ren Y, MacDonald BV, Tawfik KO, et al. Clinical predictors of facial nerve outcomes after surgical resection of vestibular schwannoma. Otolaryngol Head Neck Surg 2021;164:1085–93.

28. Carlson ML, Link MJ. Vestibular schwannomas. N Engl J Med 2021;384:1335–48.

29. Carlson ML, Tveiten OV, Driscoll CL, et al. Long-term quality of life in patients with vestibular schwannoma: an international multicenter cross-sectional study comparing microsurgery, stereotactic radiosurgery, observation, and nontumor controls. J Neurosurg 2015;122:833–42.

30. Carlson ML, Barnes JH, Nassiri AM, et al. Prospective study of disease-specific quality-of-life in sporadic vestibular schwannoma comparing observation, radiosurgery, and microsurgery. Otol Neurotol 2021;42:e199–208.

31. Carlson ML, Tombers NM, Kerezoudis P, et al. Quality of life within the first 6 months of vestibular schwannoma diagnosis with implications for patient counseling. Otol Neurotol 2018;39:e1129–36.

32. Barnes JH, Patel NS, Lohse CM, et al. Impact of treatment on vestibular schwannoma-associated symptoms: a prospective study comparing treatment modalities. Otolaryngol Head Neck Surg 2021;165:458–64.

33. Nassiri AM, Lohse CM, Tombers NM, et al. Comparing patient satisfaction after upfront treatment versus wait-and-scan for small sporadic vestibular schwannoma. Otol Neurotol 2023;44(1):e42–7.

34. Macielak RJ, Thao V, Borah BJ, et al. Lifetime cost and quality-adjusted life-years across management options for small- and medium-sized sporadic vestibular schwannoma. Otol Neurotol 2021;42(9):e1369–75.

35. Verma S, Anthony R, Tsai V, et al. Evaluation of cost effectiveness for conservative and active management strategies for acoustic neuroma. Clin Otolaryngol 2009; 34:438–46.

36. Gait C, Frew EJ, Martin TP, et al. Conservative management, surgery and radiosurgery for treatment of vestibular schwannomas: a model-based approach to cost-effectiveness. Clin Otolaryngol 2014;39:22–31.

37. Marinelli JP, Lees KA, Lohse CM, et al. Natural history of growing sporadic vestibular schwannomas: an argument for continued observation despite documented growth in select cases. Otol Neurotol 2020;41:e1149–53.
38. Marinelli JP, Carlson ML, Hunter JB, et al. Natural history of growing sporadic vestibular schwannomas during observation: an international multi-institutional study. Otol Neurotol 2021;42(8):e1118–24.
39. Raheja A, Bowers CA, MacDonald JD, et al. Middle fossa approach for vestibular schwannoma: good hearing and facial nerve outcomes with low morbidity. World Neurosurg 2016;92:37–46.
40. Meyer TA, Canty PA, Wilkinson EP, et al. Small acoustic neuromas: surgical outcomes versus observation or radiation. Otol Neurotol 2006;27:380–92.
41. Hillman T, Chen DA, Arriaga MA, et al. Facial nerve function and hearing preservation acoustic tumor surgery: does the approach matter? Otolaryngol Head Neck Surg 2010;142:115–9.
42. Ginzkey C, Scheich M, Harnisch W, et al. Outcome on hearing and facial nerve function in microsurgical treatment of small vestibular schwannoma via the middle cranial fossa approach. Eur Arch Oto-Rhino-Laryngol 2013;270:1209–16.

Guiding Patients Through Decision-Making in Management of Sporadic Vestibular Schwannoma

Janet S. Choi, MD, MPH[a], Andrew S. Venteicher, MD, PhD[b,c],
Meredith E. Adams, MD, MS[a,c,*]

KEYWORDS

- Vestibular schwannoma • Shared decision-making • Management strategies
- Management options • Counseling • Equipoise

KEY POINTS

- Contemporary management options for vestibular schwannoma (VS) have evolved, as focus has shifted to minimizing functional deficits and maximizing quality of life.
- Shared decision-making, in which clinicians and patients jointly engage in reaching decisions while prioritizing patient values and preferences, is a key concept in VS management.
- A broad range of criteria (tumor, patient, symptom-related, and contextual factors) affecting risk-benefit profiles of management options should be discussed in the context of patients' personal values and priorities.
- Various communication strategies and decision aids are available that support patients with VS and promote inclusion of patients with disability and diverse backgrounds in the decision-making process.

INTRODUCTION

Shared decision-making is a process in which clinicians and patients share the best available evidence and jointly engage in reaching a decision while prioritizing the patient's values and preferences.[1] The value of shared medical decision-making is strongest when there is more than one reasonable management option available; this is

[a] Department of Otolaryngology–Head and Neck Surgery, University of Minnesota, 420 Delaware Street Southeast, MMC 396, Minneapolis, MN 55455, USA; [b] Department of Neurosurgery, University of Minnesota, 420 Delaware Street Southeast, MMC 96, Minneapolis, MN 55455, USA; [c] Center for Skull Base and Pituitary Surgery, University of Minnesota, Minneapolis, MN 55455, USA
* Corresponding author. Department of Otolaryngology–Head and Neck Surgery, University of Minnesota, 420 Delaware Street Southeast, MMC 396, Minneapolis, MN 55455.
E-mail address: meadams@umn.edu

Otolaryngol Clin N Am 56 (2023) 459–469
https://doi.org/10.1016/j.otc.2023.02.019

increasingly true for most patients with vestibular schwannoma (VS). In the modern era, there exist multiple valid management strategies involving observation, radiation, and microsurgery with different risk-benefit profiles unique to each patient. This article outlines a framework to achieve shared decision-making for patients with sporadic VS and presents potential challenges to anticipate through the process.

MANAGEMENT OPTIONS FOR SPORADIC VESTIBULAR SCHWANNOMA

Management options for sporadic VS, largely categorized into observation, radiation, and microsurgery, have substantially evolved over recent decades (**Fig. 1**). Microsurgery was considered the predominant strategy in the 1990s with its low perioperative morbidity and mortality. Surgical objectives shifted from total resection to long-term neurologic functional preservation,[2] reflected in current discussions of goals of care that center on quality of life over "cure." Expansion of multidisciplinary surgical teams and application of various microsurgical approaches provided improvement in tumor control and facial nerve preservation. Scenarios favorable for microsurgery generally include young patients and/or large tumors. Stereotactic radiation use steadily increased in the 2000s and has been established as a similarly valid management option. The advantages of being an outpatient procedure with a low-risk profile have contributed to growth in use. Scenarios favorable for stereotactic radiation include small but growing tumors or patients with comorbidities that increase surgical risk. Observation is also increasingly used as an active management option, fueled by better understanding of VS natural history. Patients with small tumors or those who are risk adverse with respect to an intervention strategy may particularly find this option attractive. Discussion regarding timing of surveillance imaging and "trigger points"—developments warranting alternative management—are necessary components of this management strategy that can be tailored for each patient.

Although these options can seem mutually exclusive, many patients will pursue multiple paths depending on details of each clinical scenario. Relative risks and benefits are constantly weighed for each patient. Overall, contemporary management options for VS have become considerably more complex with new understanding of the disease and advancement in technologies.

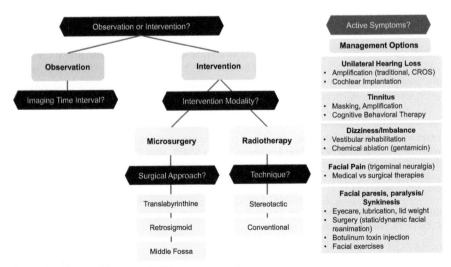

Fig. 1. Decision-making tree in VS management.

Current Trends in Vestibular Schwannoma Management

There has been a paradigm shift toward conservatism in management of VS concurrent with decreasing size of tumors at the time of diagnosis. Studies on US national cancer registry and population-based cohorts document increased rates of observation over stereotactic radiation and microsurgery.[3,4] A period of observation presents minimal risk to patients with small- to medium-sized schwannoma without brainstem compression. Prior research suggests observation as the best approach to retaining serviceable hearing, and surgical outcomes are not affected by a delay in treatment after observation.[5] When presenting observation as an option, it is important to consider its unique risk-benefit profile for each patient. For younger patients, observation is a noninvasive option that may allow retention of serviceable hearing for many years until active intervention is indicated. For older patients, life expectancy from other comorbidities may negate any benefit from intervention for a benign tumor.

Clinical Equipoise in Vestibular Schwannoma Management

Throughout the decision-making process, it is important to acknowledge that most patients with VS have multiple valid options. In some scenarios, one option may stand out as clearly "best," such as a large tumor in a young patient who would be best treated with microsurgery. However, in many cases, especially for small- to medium-sized tumors, there is *clinical equipoise* in which more than one option can be reasonably considered. Both overall and disease-specific quality-of-life outcome measures have been compared across management options, but no clearly superior strategy has emerged.[6,7] A notable exception was in the anxiety domain, for which significant improvement was observed among patients who underwent microsurgery but not those who selected observation or stereotactic radiation.[8] When surveyed, 93% of patients were satisfied with their original treatment choice and greater than 80% reported not feeling regret over their choice.[9,10] Long-term hindsight satisfaction with treatment choice among patients with small- to medium-sized tumors was relatively higher for those who underwent observation and stereotactic radiation (96% and 97%, respectively) than microsurgery (85%).[10]

DECISION-MAKING CRITERIA IN VESTIBULAR SCHWANNOMA MANAGEMENT

When counseling to achieve shared decision-making, clinicians present the best available evidence in the context of the patient's personal values and priorities. To do so, the broad range of criteria affecting the risk-benefit profiles of each option are considered.

Major Criteria in Decision-Making

Decision-making criteria in VS management can be categorized into tumor, patient, symptom, and contextual factors (**Fig. 2**). Tumor-related criteria, including size, growth, and location in relation to surrounding structures, are critical in deciding *when* to consider intervention over observation. Generally accepted indications for intervention include tumor size greater than or equal to 15 mm with cerebellopontine angle (CPA) extension, contact with surrounding structures such as brainstem, and significant tumor growth. The probability of less optimal microsurgical outcomes including facial paresis and failure of hearing preservation increase significantly at 14 to 20 mm of CPA extension.[11] Increased morbidity associated with hydrocephalus and cranial neuropathy has been documented for large tumors treated with stereotactic radiation.[12] Tumor growth had been traditionally defined as greater than or equal to

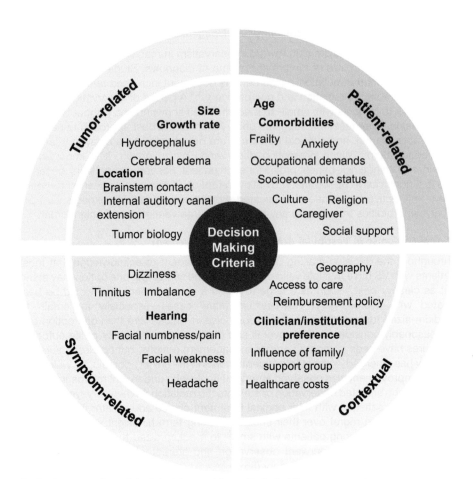

Fig. 2. Conceptual model of decision-making criteria in VS management.

2 mm increase on linear diameter, but recent literature has demonstrated volumetric growth as a more sensitive indicator of tumor growth than linear measurements.[13]

Patient-related major criteria include age and medical comorbidities. When intervention is warranted, advanced age itself does not preclude microsurgery but duration of hospital stay and complication rates are higher among older adults.[14] Risk profiles are most unfavorable for older adults with multiple comorbidities and high baseline frailty.[15] Although stereotactic radiation may be preferred among older adults, the risks of unfavorable events including hydrocephalus and accelerated hearing loss also increase with advanced age and should be incorporated into expectation management.[12]

In the symptom-related context, a major decision-making criterion is residual hearing at presentation. Patients are often surprised to learn that tumor treatment does not restore hearing or resolve tinnitus. It is important to clarify expectations early in the discussion. Although observation is increasingly accepted as an effective strategy for retaining hearing, the goal of hearing preservation *long-term* in the case of a small tumor with serviceable hearing allows for the option of microsurgery. When a patient presents with serviceable hearing, the risk profile involving hearing loss should be discussed for each option including hearing preservation microsurgical approaches.

Surgeon preference and experience factor into decision-making. There is considerable practice variation between skull base centers, and surgeons are likely inherently biased toward their scope of practice, as they are more aware of attainable outcomes from procedures they perform most. It is entirely appropriate to discuss the clinical team's own scope of practice and outcomes based on their experiences. However, it is important to present the entire range of options and place referrals as needed for management options or surgical approaches not used in their practice for patients to be fully informed. Multidisciplinary input is a key tool in reducing referral bias and improving provision of individualized treatment counseling over a single treatment modality. When asked, second opinions should be encouraged, as additional information will reinforce earlier received information and may provide patients with higher confidence and satisfaction in the selected choices.

Setting Priorities and Framing Risks

Modern treatment modalities focus on maximizing patient quality of life and minimizing functional deficits. However, patients and clinicians do not necessarily share the same values or priorities, and motivations vary between patients. Although the outcome measures traditionally considered have been tumor control, facial nerve function, and hearing, recent studies revealed additional parameters including dizziness and headache are more impactful determinants of long-term quality of life.[16] To encourage identification of preferences and priorities, patients may need help understanding what each deficit means and what rehabilitation strategies exist (see **Fig. 1**).

Facial nerve function remains a paramount priority. Rates of facial nerve preservation remain robust, greater than 90%, regardless of treatment option.[6] The rate of anatomic preservation of the facial nerve has been reported to be as high as 93% in microsurgery.[17] Still, dissection of the tumor from the facial nerve is one of the most challenging aspects of VS microsurgery. When framing the risk of facial nerve dysfunction, it is important to consider patient knowledge and prior experiences. A patient who has not encountered facial nerve palsy may need descriptive information to better understand the implications of incomplete eye closure, oral incompetence, or loss of mimetic expression. A prior study assessing disease-specific quality of life and disability demonstrated that the patients with various levels of facial nerve paresis/paralysis (House-Brackmann II–VI) after VS surgery had significantly lower quality-of-life scores than ones with normal facial function. However, the severity of facial nerve paresis/paralysis was not significantly associated with quality-of-life scores.[18]

Dizziness and imbalance have been identified as the strongest predictors of long-term quality of life among patients with VS, more impactful than facial paresis, hearing, or tinnitus.[16] Treatment modality does not influence the prevalence of chronic dizziness.[19] All strategies carry inherent risks to vestibular function. Reviewing the mechanisms of vestibular loss for each option may assist in framing the risks of chronic dizziness. In microsurgery, the vestibular nerve from which the tumor arises is transected by design. With radiation, the vestibular nerve and organs are exposed to long-term radiation effects. Even in observation, vestibular function is expected to deteriorate during the natural course of disease progression. Vestibular rehabilitation can be used at any point regardless of the chosen management option.

Hearing loss influences patient choices in VS management. Hearing preservation via middle fossa or retrosigmoid approach is meaningful only if the hearing preserved is superior to spontaneous hearing preservation during observation. Conversely, there exist risks of hearing deterioration with observation and loss of candidacy for hearing preservation surgery. Hearing preservation rates with microsurgery vary,

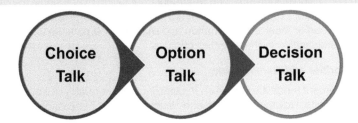

- "What do you expect from treatment of the vestibular schwannoma?"
- "Do you have all the information you think you need to decide?"
- "What do you like about [treatment option]? What concerns do you have about [treatment option]?"

Deliberation

Choice Talk → **Option Talk** → **Decision Talk**

Examples:
"Now that we have talked about vestibular schwannoma and what it does, it's time to think about what to do next."

"You have several reasonable management options available."

Examples:
"What have you heard or read about the treatment of vestibular schwannoma?"

"Some options may have different impact on you compared to other people"

Examples:
"What matters the most to you from your point of view?"

"Are you ready to decide? Would you want more time?"

Fig. 3. Shared decision-making model involving 3 steps. (*Data from* Elwyn G, Frosch D, Thomson R, et al. Shared decision making: a model for clinical practice. *J Gen Intern Med.* 2012;27(10):1361-7.)

approximating 70% for small tumors and less than 5% for large tumors,[20] and based on other factors discussed in later articles. Risks of hearing loss following stereotactic radiation can be framed in a longitudinal context, as it is associated with a potentially accelerated decline in hearing over time. Kaplan-Meier analyses of time from diagnosis to nonserviceable hearing demonstrated that serviceable hearing preservation rates were approximately 80%, 40%, and 20% at 1, 5, and 10 years after stereotactic radiation versus 96%, 62%, and 42% for observation, respectively.[21,22]

COMMUNICATION STRATEGIES IN SHARED DECISION-MAKING

The principles of shared decision-making and its positive impact on health outcomes are well established.[23] Here the authors present several specific communication strategies to successfully accomplish shared decision-making in VS management.

Choice Talk, Option Talk, and Decision Talk

Elwyn and colleagues proposed a model of shared decision-making involving 3 key steps: choice talk, option talk, and decision talk (**Fig. 3**).[1] Choice talk conveys awareness that a choice exists and emphasizes the importance of respecting individual preferences and the role of uncertainty. During option talk, clinicians inform patients about treatment options, first checking patient knowledge followed by listing and describing options. Clinicians should be clear about the pros and cons of different options while framing effects and risks in absolute as well as relative terms. Decision talk allows patients to explore what matters most to them and to move to a decision when ready. Deliberation is supported in all 3 steps. The process may require more than one encounter and time in between to process and consider a range of possible futures.

Best-Case/Worst-Case Scenarios

The Best-Case/Worst-Case framework is an effective strategy for discussing high-stakes management options.[24] Clinicians use stories to describe how patients might experience the range of possible outcomes in the best case, worst case, and most likely scenarios. For example, for a patient considering hearing preservation microsurgery: best case (complete resection, hearing preservation, excellent facial function) and worst case (growing residual tumor, complete hearing loss, facial paralysis); this helps patients evaluate outcomes based on personal goals rather than isolated procedural risks and is especially helpful in preparing patients and families for the possibility of a poor outcome. The framework can be adapted to explore preferences and tolerance by discussing differences in long-term and short-term risk profiles of each VS treatment. For example, risks of complication are highest up-front for microsurgery, whereas radiation complications often present later.

FRAMING THE CONVERSATION FOR SHARED DECISION-MAKING
Starting the Conversation

The success of shared decision-making depends largely on clinician understanding of patient knowledge, readiness to learn, and preferences. Clinicians may open the discussion by reviewing the diagnosis of VS and determining the patient's baseline level of understanding. Some patients are first learning of tumor diagnoses, whereas others are seeking second or third opinions already knowing their preferred treatment option. After assessing *what patients know and want to know*, clinicians fill in knowledge gaps and answering questions. As many patients relate all tumors to cancer, it is important to clarify early on that VS are benign, often grow slowly or display saltatory growth, and cause symptoms by affecting surrounding nerves and the inner ear. When introducing the concept of observation as a medically valid option chosen by many, it helps to review VS natural history. Visualization of radiology images helps patients grasp tumor-related criteria in decision-making, including brainstem contact, internal auditory canal extension, and cranial nerve displacement.

There Are More than Three Options

Although patients may consider observation, stereotactic radiation, and microsurgery as separate entities, numerous combinations of these strategies exist over the long run. To protect neurologic function, incomplete resection may be necessary before administering stereotactic radiation for remaining tumor. Patients with growing tumors after stereotactic radiation may undergo observation or microsurgery. When significant comorbidities preclude resection, a palliative approach may be appropriate. For example, hydrocephalus caused by a VS in a poor surgical candidate can be palliated by placement of a ventriculoperitoneal shunt alone.

Reducing Choice Overload

Patients with VS may experience choice overload, where an increasing number of options lead to decreased motivation to choose or dissatisfaction with the finally chosen option.[25] Thus, the responsibility to inform patients of all available management options without bias needs to be balanced by efforts to present a manageable set of reasonable options within the standard of care. In cases with apparent "best options" (eg, young patients with large tumors), clinicians should feel comfortable presenting reduced sets of choices. Even when patients have multiple reasonable options, clinicians may categorize them into a reduced number of sequential choices to avoid choice overload (see **Fig. 1**).[26]

Decision Support

Decision aids in the form of brochures, worksheets, or videos foster the practice of shared decision-making by improving patient knowledge, enhancing active patient participation, and creating realistic expectations.[27,28] Decision aids have 3 elements: clinical information, values clarification, and preparation for communication with clinicians. Validated tools for VS are lacking, but patient education materials with the core elements are available via government agencies, academic institutions, and support groups.[29,30] Tools incorporating machine-learning based prediction models and mobile applications have been developed to provide supportive information for VS decision-making.[31,32] Pilot implementation reduced decision conflict and improved satisfaction with made decisions.[31]

CULTIVATING INCLUSIVITY IN DECISION-MAKING

The highly interactive process of shared decision-making may be more challenging but no less essential for patients with disabilities or different cultural backgrounds. Supported decision-making is a tool that allows older individuals and patients with disabilities to retain decision-making capacity while choosing supporters to help them make choices[33]; this is different from guardianship or durable powers of attorney that identify substitute decision-makers in case of incapacitation. Although bringing supporters into appointments, supported decision-making preserves patient agency by providing materials using plain language and visual formats, extra discussion time, and role-playing to deepen understanding.

Patients from different racial/ethnic and cultural backgrounds appraise their decision-making process less positively than do white, English-speaking patients in the United States.[34] Further, racial minority patients with VS are less likely to receive surgery and more likely to be managed conservatively despite presenting with large tumors.[4,35] The root causes of racial disparities are complex, involving clinician/institutional/systemic biases, socioeconomics, access to care, patient satisfaction/adherence, and language barriers. When surveyed, only 36% of US surgeons reported awareness of racial/ethnic disparities in health care in general and 11% within their hospital/clinic.[36] Strategies to address disparities in VS decision-making include clinician cultural competency training, improving patient health literacy, incorporation of patient navigators and peer-support networks, and simplifying appointment logistics (eg, multidisciplinary clinics).[37]

SUMMARY

Trends in management of VS have shifted considerably in the past several decades to focus on maximizing functional outcomes and quality of life. Shared decision-making, engaging both clinicians and patients and reaching decisions based on patient values and priorities, has become more important than ever. With the advancement in understanding of the disease and treatment technologies, we have reached an exciting era where clinicians can present various medically reasonable options based on the available evidence and patients can prioritize their values to choose the "best" treatment.

CLINICS CARE POINTS

- Effective shared decision-making in management of vestibular schwannoma requires an investment of time and effort from both the clinician and the patient.

- For clinicians, shared decision making is more than just providing patients with information; it involves building a relationship of trust and learning about the patient's values, preferences, and priorities.

- While various treatment options are available for vestibular schwannoma, all modalities have related risks. It is important to help patients understand what each risk and deficit means and what rehabilitation strategies exist for the symptoms that impact quality of life.

- To avoid choice overload and decision fatigue, clinicians may consider presenting choices in a sequential manner and using a best-case/worst-case framework for discussion of outcomes and risks.

ACKNOWLEDGMENT

JSC is supported by the Lions International Hearing Foundation and American Academy of Otolaryngology - Head and Neck Surgery; ASV is funded by the NIH (NINDS), Burroughs Wellcome Fund, Sontag Foundation, and the V Foundation for Cancer Research; MEA is funded by NIH (NIDCD U24DC020851, NINDS UG3NS107688), Kellogg Charitable Trust, and Lions International Hearing Foundation.

DISCLOSURES

None relevant.

REFERENCES

1. Elwyn G, Frosch D, Thomson R, et al. Shared decision making: a model for clinical practice. J Gen Intern Med 2012;27(10):1361–7.
2. Kemink JL, Langman AW, Niparko JK, et al. Operative management of acoustic neuromas: the priority of neurologic function over complete resection. Otolaryngol Head Neck Surg 1991;104(1):96–9.
3. Carlson ML, Habermann EB, Wagie AE, et al. The Changing Landscape of Vestibular Schwannoma Management in the United States–A Shift Toward Conservatism. Otolaryngol Head Neck Surg 2015;153(3):440–6.
4. Babu R, Sharma R, Bagley JH, et al. Vestibular schwannomas in the modern era: epidemiology, treatment trends, and disparities in management. J Neurosurg 2013;119(1):121–30.
5. Ferri GG, Modugno GC, Pirodda A, et al. Conservative management of vestibular schwannomas: an effective strategy. Laryngoscope 2008;118(6):951–7.
6. Carlson ML, Tveiten OV, Driscoll CL, et al. Long-term quality of life in patients with vestibular schwannoma: an international multicenter cross-sectional study comparing microsurgery, stereotactic radiosurgery, observation, and nontumor controls. J Neurosurg 2015;122(4):833–42.
7. Gauden A, Weir P, Hawthorne G, et al. Systematic review of quality of life in the management of vestibular schwannoma. J Clin Neurosci 2011;18(12):1573–84.

8. Carlson ML, Barnes JH, Nassiri A, et al. Prospective Study of Disease-Specific Quality-of-Life in Sporadic Vestibular Schwannoma Comparing Observation, Radiosurgery, and Microsurgery. Otol Neurotol 2021;42(2):e199–208.

9. Tos T, Caye-Thomasen P, Stangerup SE, et al. Patients' fears, expectations and satisfaction in relation to management of vestibular schwannoma: a comparison of surgery and observation. Acta Otolaryngol 2003;123(5):600–5.

10. Carlson ML, Tveiten OV, Lund-Johansen M, et al. Patient Motivation and Long-Term Satisfaction with Treatment Choice in Vestibular Schwannoma. World Neurosurg 2018;114:e1245–52.

11. Macielak RJ, Wallerius KP, Lawlor SK, et al. Defining clinically significant tumor size in vestibular schwannoma to inform timing of microsurgery during wait-and-scan management: moving beyond minimum detectable growth. J Neurosurg 2021;1–9.

12. Kim JH, Jung HH, Chang JH, et al. Predictive Factors of Unfavorable Events After Gamma Knife Radiosurgery for Vestibular Schwannoma. World Neurosurg 2017; 107:175–84.

13. Lawson McLean AC, McLean AL, Rosahl SK. Evaluating vestibular schwannoma size and volume on magnetic resonance imaging: An inter- and intra-rater agreement study. Clin Neurol Neurosurg 2016;145:68–73.

14. Sylvester MJ, Shastri DN, Patel VM, et al. Outcomes of Vestibular Schwannoma Surgery among the Elderly. Otolaryngol Head Neck Surg Jan 2017;156(1): 166–72. https://doi.org/10.1177/0194599816677522.

15. Dicpinigaitis AJ, Kalakoti P, Schmidt M, et al. Associations of Baseline Frailty Status and Age With Outcomes in Patients Undergoing Vestibular Schwannoma Resection. JAMA Otolaryngol Head Neck Surg 2021;147(7):608–14.

16. Carlson ML, Tveiten OV, Driscoll CL, et al. What drives quality of life in patients with sporadic vestibular schwannoma? Laryngoscope 2015;125(7):1697–702.

17. Samii M, Matthies C. Management of 1000 vestibular schwannomas (acoustic neuromas): the facial nerve-preservation and restitution of function. Neurosurgery 1997;40(4):684–95.

18. Lee J, Fung K, Lownie SP, et al. Assessing impairment and disability of facial paralysis in patients with vestibular schwannoma. Arch Otolaryngol Head Neck Surg 2007;133(1):56–60.

19. Fuentealba-Bassaletti C, Neve OM, van Esch BF, et al. Vestibular Complaints Impact on the Long-Term Quality of Life of Vestibular Schwannoma Patients. Otol Neurotol 2023;44(2):161–7.

20. Ansari SF, Terry C, Cohen-Gadol AA. Surgery for vestibular schwannomas: a systematic review of complications by approach. Neurosurg Focus 2012;33(3):E14.

21. Khandalavala KR, Saba ES, Kocharyan A, et al. Hearing Preservation in Observed Sporadic Vestibular Schwannoma: A Systematic Review. Otol Neurotol 2022;43(6):604–10.

22. Santa Maria PL, Shi Y, Gurgel RK, et al. Long-term hearing outcomes following stereotactic radiosurgery in vestibular schwannoma patients—a retrospective cohort study. Neurosurgery 2019;85(4):550.

23. Shay LA, Lafata JE. Where is the evidence? A systematic review of shared decision making and patient outcomes. Med Decis Making 2015;35(1):114–31.

24. Taylor LJ, Nabozny MJ, Steffens NM, et al. A Framework to Improve Surgeon Communication in High-Stakes Surgical Decisions: Best Case/Worst Case. JAMA Surg 2017;152(6):531–8.

25. Scheibehenne B, Greifeneder R, Todd PM. Can there ever be too many options? A meta-analytic review of choice overload. J. Consume Res. 2010;37(3):409–25.

26. Schwartz MS. Patient Counseling Following Diagnosis of Sporadic Vestibular Schwannoma. In: Carlson ML, Link MJ, Driscoll CLW, et al, editors. *Management of Vestibular Schwannoma*. Thieme; 2019. p. 74–7.
27. Stacey D, Legare F, Lewis K, et al. Decision aids for people facing health treatment or screening decisions. Cochrane Database Syst Rev 2017;4(4):CD001431.
28. Newsome A, Sieber W, Smith M, et al. If you build it, will they come? A qualitative evaluation of the use of video-based decision aids in primary care. Fam Med 2012;44(1):26–31.
29. National Institute on Deafness and Other Communication Disorders. Vestibular Schwannoma (Acoustic Neuroma) and Neurofibromatosis. Available at: https://www.nidcd.nih.gov/sites/default/files/Documents/health/hearing/VestibularSchwannoma-FactSheet.pdf. Accessed Jan 2023.
30. National Health Services. Acoustic Neuroma (Vestibular Schwannoma). 2022. Available at: https://www.nhs.uk/conditions/acoustic-neuroma/. Accessed Jan 2023.
31. La Monte OA, Moshtaghi O, Tang E, et al. Use of a Novel Clinical Decision-Making Tool in Vestibular Schwannoma Treatment. Otol Neurotol 2022;43(10):e1174–9.
32. Gadot R, Anand A, Lovin BD, et al. Predicting surgical decision-making in vestibular schwannoma using tree-based machine learning. Neurosurg Focus 2022;52(4):E8.
33. Shogren KA, Wehmeyer ML, Lassmann H, et al. Supported decision making: A synthesis of the literature across intellectual disability, mental health, and aging. Educ Train Autism Dev Disabil 2017;52(2):144–57.
34. Hawley ST, Morris AM. Cultural challenges to engaging patients in shared decision making. Patient Educ Couns 2017;100(1):18–24.
35. Butterfield JT, Golzarian S, Johnson R, et al. Racial disparities in recommendations for surgical resection of primary brain tumours: a registry-based cohort analysis. Lancet 2022;400(10368):2063–73.
36. Britton BV, Nagarajan N, Zogg CK, et al. US Surgeons' Perceptions of Racial/Ethnic Disparities in Health Care: A Cross-sectional Study. JAMA Surg 2016;151(6):582–4.
37. Natale-Pereira A, Enard KR, Nevarez L, et al. The role of patient navigators in eliminating health disparities. Cancer 2011;117(S15):3541–50.

Intraoperative Cochlear Nerve Monitoring in Vestibular Schwannoma Microsurgery

Kevin Y. Zhan, MD, Cameron C. Wick, MD*

KEYWORDS

- Auditory brainstem response • Cochlear nerve action potential
- Electrocochleography

KEY POINTS

- Auditory brainstem response (ABR) is a far-field recording that requires averaging, thus is not real-time monitoring. Cochlear nerve action potential is a near-field recording with larger amplitudes and is closer to a real-time measurement.
- Alternative nerve monitoring strategies are needed when the hearing is lost or will be lost during the surgical approach.
- Evoked ABR is safe and feasible but is susceptible to electrical interference.

INTRODUCTION

Vestibular schwannoma (VS) is a benign tumor originating from the eighth cranial nerve, with 90% of patients citing hearing loss as their initial symptom.[1] The etiology of the hearing loss remains unknown.[2] Improved screening algorithms for asymmetric sensorineural hearing loss (SNHL) have improved VS detection, but patients still present with various tumor sizes that poorly correlate to functional hearing status.[3,4]

Traditionally, intraoperative eighth nerve monitoring is used during hearing preservation VS microsurgery, affording the surgeon feedback while dissecting near the cochlear nerve.[5] Auditory-evoked auditory brainstem response (eABR) and to a lesser extent direct eighth nerve monitoring/cochlear nerve action potential (CNAP) serve as the core modalities for intraoperative feedback. These tests require intact hearing and an approach that does not violate the otic capsule. There is no consensus for when monitoring should or not be used. It can be considered at the surgeon's discretion when baseline hearing is serviceable and there is potential for preservation. This article

Department of Otolaryngology–Head & Neck Surgery, Washington University, St Louis, MO, USA
* Corresponding author.
E-mail address: cameron.wick@wustl.edu

Otolaryngol Clin N Am 56 (2023) 471–482
https://doi.org/10.1016/j.otc.2023.02.007
0030-6665/23/© 2023 Elsevier Inc. All rights reserved.

reviews the traditional techniques for cochlear nerve monitoring during hearing preservation VS microsurgery and alternative modalities when ABR and CNAP are not feasible.

HEARING PRESERVATION VESTIBULAR SCHWANNOMA MICROSURGERY

A healthy, intact auditory system captures and transduces mechanical sound energy to neural impulses in the cochlea, and then transmits it from the cochlear nerve to the auditory cortex. The electrical potentials generated along the auditory pathway are independent of a patient's state of consciousness; thus, auditory monitoring can be used in conjunction with general anesthesia. Cochlear nerve monitoring serves as an indicator for hearing but is inherently different than the subjective perception of sound. Therefore, on occasion there can be discrepancies between the intraoperative neural measurements and behavioral responses.[6,7]

Auditory Brainstem Response

The usefulness of intraoperative nerve monitoring data relies on the timeframe in which it is received. In this manner, ABR and CNAP are fundamentally different. During ABR, a sound probe in the ipsilateral ear canal produces a loud acoustic click stimulus that gets carried along the auditory pathway. The signal traveling through the brainstem is considered a far-field measurement due to its relative distance from the sound source. These far-field neural transmissions are detected by an active electrode at the scalp vertex, a reference electrode on the contralateral mastoid, and a ground electrode on the forehead (**Fig. 1**). Software then averages the activity of neural generators along the auditory pathway, whereas characteristic and reproducible waveforms are generated.[8] Knowledge of the origin and time latencies of the five ABR waves is paramount for appropriate interpretation (**Table 1**). The five ABR waveforms represent the

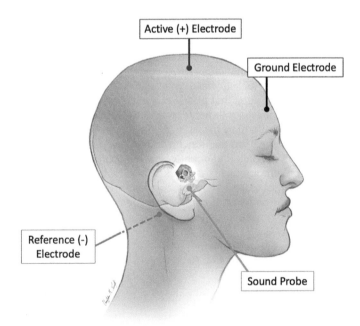

Fig. 1. ABR sound probe and electrode setup.

Table 1		
Auditory brainstem response waveforms		
Waveforms	**Proposed Neural Generator Location**	**Latency (ms)**
I	Cochlear nerve (modiolus/IAC)	1.7 ± 0.15
II	Cochlear nerve (proximal CPA vs cochlear nucleus)	2.8 ± 0.17
III	Cochlear nucleus and superior olive	3.9 ± 0.19
IV	Lateral lemniscus	5.1 ± 0.24
V	Inferior colliculus	5.7 ± 0.25

Abbreviations: CPA, cerebellopontine angle; IAC, internal auditory canal.

vertex of the positive wave deflection. Waves I, III, and V are the most prominent. The small size of the ABR neural response is measured in nanovolts (nV), and the time latency is measured in milliseconds (ms).[9]

Such tiny electrical responses in the ABR must be separated from background brain electrical activity, skeletal muscle activity, and electrical interference in the operating room.[10,11] Intraoperatively, if there is significant 60-Hz electrical interference, one should check for commonly offending sources such as inadequately shielded power strips, mechanical patient beds, or patient warming devices. One thousand to two thousand stimulus response cycles are required to obtain a reliable ABR waveform, requiring greater than 90 seconds or more of averaging time. This is the principal downside to ABR monitoring, as actual feedback is significantly delayed after a potential nerve injury, thus far-field neural data obtained from ABR are not actually real-time monitoring.

There is debate as to what constitutes a significant baseline shift in ABR morphology. When ABR is performed, a baseline measurement is obtained and throughout the procedure additional ABR measurements are recorded to look for changes in wave amplitude or latency (**Fig. 2**). The most widely recognized criteria for concerning waveform changes comes from the American Society for Neurophysiological Monitoring 2007 position statement which states a greater than 50% reduction in amplitude and/or an increase of greater than 1 ms latency from baseline should warn surgeons of potential nerve injury.[12] A latency shift can occur from cochlear nerve stretching via cerebellar retraction. Ischemic injury to the labyrinthine artery can also cause loss of the ABR.[13] Although there are no large, published reports on the predictive values of various ABR response changes, loss of ABR waveforms without recovery is generally considered a poor prognostic factor for residual postoperative hearing.[10,11] In a series of 10 patients, 100% of patients with the loss of ABR had anacusis postoperatively.[14] However, reports of postoperative hearing despite the loss of ABR also exist.[6,7,15] Conversely, the presence of ABR does not guarantee functional hearing. The challenge with universal criteria for ABR measurements stems from significant variability in preoperative hearing status, stimulation/recording paradigms, artifact removal strategies, and end-user interpretation expertise. In general, ABR monitoring is of little risk to the patient and can be useful feedback to the surgeon. Nevertheless, thoughtful consideration of its limitations is germane.

Cochlear Nerve Action Potential

In contrast to ABRs far-field responses, CNAP provides a near-field, essentially real-time measurement obtained from a recording electrode placed directly on the cochlear nerve. This concept was first reported by Silverstein and colleagues[16] in

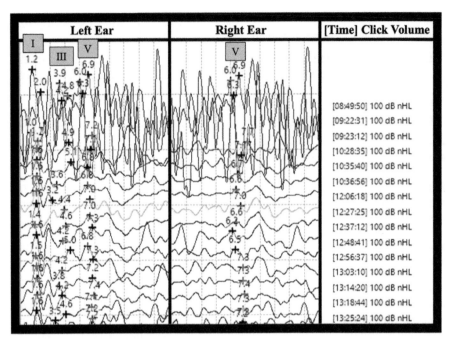

Fig. 2. Maintenance of intraoperative ABR during a left retrosigmoid VS resection.

1985 and the technique has largely remained unchanged. The CNAP stimulus is the same an acoustic ABR. However, in CNAP, the recording electrode is placed directly on the proximal cochlear nerve in the cerebellopontine angle (CPA) or internal auditory canal (IAC). The recorded neural amplitudes are measured in microvolts (μV) and are comparatively much larger than the ABR signal. The larger CNAP signal is secondary to an improved signal-to-noise ratio as the recording electrode makes direct contact with the neural generator (eg, the cochlear nerve). The larger amplitude and cleaner signal mean less averaging (10–300 trials) and essentially a real-time measurement. The more robust signal is also perhaps more predictive, meaning that the CNAP response may be seen even in the absence of conventional ABR waveforms.[9] The CNAP waveforms have four major vertexes: two with a negative deflection (N1, N2) and two with a positive deflection (P1, P2). The N1 negative vertex serves as the primary monitoring wave of interest. Although the CNAP signal is reliable, placement of the electrode can be challenging given the dynamic pulsations of the brain, cerebrospinal fluid, and tumor dissection. Several CNAP electrode designs have been proposed yet no standardized electrode exists.[15,17,18] Manufacturing changes have also limited previously available commercial products.[17] Manipulation of a single-arm subdermal electrode can suffice as the recording electrode (**Fig. 3**). There lacks consensus on what CNAP waveform changes indicate a clinically meaningful difference. Commonly, absolute changes in N1 latencies are used.[5] Several proponents of CNAP have published series showing that CNAP is superior to ABR and results in improved hearing preservation outcomes.[15,19] However, studies that show no difference between ABR and CNAP also exist.[20] CNAP and ABR can be used simultaneously. Regardless of which technique is used, the surgeon and monitoring team should be aware of each system's inherent advantages and disadvantages (**Table 2**).

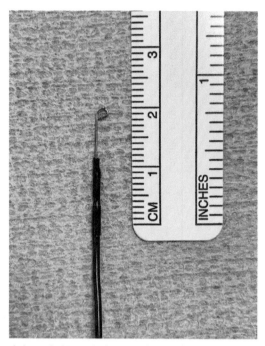

Fig. 3. Single-arm subdermal electrode bent to facilitate CNAP.

Cochlear Implant Advancements

Many patients with a VS eventually develop SNHL. Patients rehabilitated with a contralateral routing of sound hearing aid or osseointegrated implant fail to restore the benefits of binaural hearing. Recent advancement in single-sided deafness Cochlear Implant (CI) indication and magnetic resonance imaging compatible internal receiver magnets have spurred interest in CI placement with VSs. Results from CI rehabilitation after VS resection show wide variability with 80% using their device daily and only 50% achieving open-set speech.[21] If alternative cochlear nerve monitoring strategies could provide feedback on the physiologic status of the nerve during or after tumor resection, it is logical to think that CI outcomes could improve. The remaining portions of this article discuss developments in alternative cochlear nerve monitoring strategies.

ALTERNATIVE MONITORING METHODS DURING MICROSURGERY
Cochlear Function

The etiology of the VS-induced SNHL remains poorly understood. Attempts to distinguish between nerve and cochlear sites of lesion are ongoing. When the cochlea receives sound, the outer hair cells modify the basilar membrane. In doing so, the cochlea creates a noise byproduct that can be measured as an otoacoustic emission (OAE).[22] A VS is thought to have minimal influence on the OAEs if the hearing is intact.[23] Preoperative OAEs have not shown much predictive value for hearing preservation surgery compared with other commonly measured characteristics.[24] Intraoperatively, OAEs show quick response to tumor and cochlear nerve manipulation with some postoperative predictive value if they are lost.[25] When hearing is lost the OAE function is lost, therefore this measurement offers limited value in those who already have SNHL or those undergoing a translabyrinthine approach.

Table 2
Comparison of auditory brainstem response and cochlear nerve action potential

Parameter	ABR	CNAP
Active electrode location	Scalp vertex; ground on forehead	Cochlear nerve in the IAC or CPA
Stimulus	Acoustic stimulus (click or pure tone; >70 dB HL) delivered via ipsilateral ear canal	
Relative distance from the stimulus	Far-field	Near-field
Wave of interest	I, III, and V	N1
Amplitude measurement	Nanovolts	Microvolts
Latency	Variable	Variable
Runs to average the signal	1000–2000	10–300
Time delay	Minutes	Seconds

Abbreviations: ABR, auditory brainstem response; CNAP, cochlear nerve action potential; CPA, cerebellopontine angle; IAC, internal auditory canal.

Electrocochleography (ECochG) is another marker of cochlear function and more sensitive than pure-tone audiometry. The measurement is a complex interplay of outer hair cell function measured by the cochlear microphonic, inner hair cell function measured by the summating potential, and proximal cochlear nerve function measured by the action potential.[26] ECochG has recently found clinical utility in predicting CI outcomes and hearing preservation.[27,28] The other benefit of ECochG is its ability to differentiate between neural versus hair cell etiologies of SNHL. Applying ECochG for VS and lateral skull base microsurgery has been limited thus far, but initial studies are underway. One report of round window ECochG during translabyrinthine VS microsurgery showed variability in the total response measurements ranging from 0.1 to 100 μV. The recordings also identified different sites of hearing loss with some cases showing a reduced SP suggesting an intracochlear deficit, whereas other cases showed more neural detriments. Despite a moderate correlation ($r = 0.67$) of ECochG to preoperative word recognition score (WRS), two patients with 0% WRS showed good cochlear function on ECochG suggesting their SNHL was a neural etiology.[29] This important study highlights the complexity of SNHL associated with VSs. It also suggests that predictive modeling with ECochG might provide insight into the site of lesion whether the cochlear nerve is healthy enough to carry the CI signal.

Electrically Evoked Monitoring

Although not economically sustainable, CIs have been used for cochlear nerve stimulation and electrically evoked monitoring. Neurofibromatosis type-2 (NF2) is characterized by bilateral VSs; therefore, preservation of a cochlear nerve during tumor resection can have profound rehabilitative benefit. One such case series demonstrated feasibility of electrically eABR in three patients with NF2.[30] Intraoperative eABR was measured in two patients but limited in the third patient secondary to facial nerve stimulation. eABR helped during tumor dissection, and all three patients had sound awareness on initial CI activation. Performance declined in one user, likely from residual tumor growth. Like acoustic ABR, eABR requires thousands of cycles to compute a reliable waveform. The electrical artifact also degrades waves I and III, making wave V the only reliable waveform in eABR.

Adding cochlear measurements to CI-eABR has also been described. CIs have proprietary telemetry function that can record spiral ganglion neural activity. In a case of a unilateral, sporadic VS resection, neural response imaging was added to eABR to provide real-time, near-field measurements.[31] Another measure of cochlear nerve integrity is the stapedial reflex. The feasibility of electrical stimulation of the stapedial reflex has been described as an adjunct to eABR and telemetry.[32] Further studies are necessary to see to assess the full benefit of these techniques.

To make intraoperative eABR more cost-effective, MED-EL has developed a stimulating platform with a disposable electrode array. The Auditory Nerve Test System (ANTS) comprises three parts: Auditory Nerve Test Electrode (ANTE), connector cable, and stimulator box (**Fig. 4**). The device is commercially available in Europe but not yet approved by the Food & Drug Administration (FDA). The initial report using ANTS during VS microsurgery came in 2019 by Kasbekar and colleagues.[33] They used ANTS during a translabyrinthine approach for a 2 cm NF2-associated VS and stopped dissecting when the eABR was lost. The patient did not get sound with a CI but eABR recordings were feasible.

The first published series using ANTS during translabyrinthine VS microsurgery with simultaneous CI reported on five patients, all with severe-to-profound SNHL and poor WRS.[34] Preoperative eABR was measurable in all patients but required a wide range of

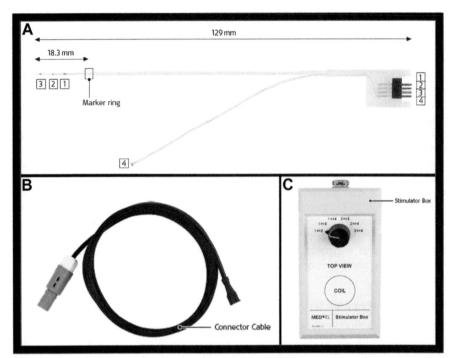

Fig. 4. Auditory Nerve Test System (ANTS) (*A*) Auditory Nerve Test Electrode (ANTE) measuring 18 mm with three intracochlear contacts and one extracochlear ground. (*B*) Connector cable. (*C*) Stimulator box. Photos used with permission from MED-EL.

stimulating levels. Intraoperatively, wave V was absent in one patient and weak in another, notably both patients had previously undergone retrosigmoid surgery and had a growing residual tumor. Intraoperative electrical artifact also added to interpretation difficulties in one patient. All five patients received a CI as the surgeons felt the cochlear nerves were intact. The authors found that the eABR data, when available, correlated with CI performance. The three patients with intact eABR after tumor dissection all obtained open-set speech, whereas those with absent or weak eABR had no sound perception. Another series of 14 patients also showed promising predictive value to intraoperative eABR.[35] Of the nine patients with an eABR, all received auditory perception with their CI. Only one of the five patients without an eABR heard sound with the CI, leading the authors to conclude a 93% diagnostic accuracy in this small series.

In the United States, ANTS has only been available via an investigator-initiated device exemption (Clinicaltrail.gov Identifier: NCT04241679). The clinical trial is designed for ANTE insertion for baseline eABR before IAC and CPA opening (**Fig. 5**). eABR is measured throughout tumor dissection (**Figs. 6** and **7**). After tumor removal, a final eABR is recorded and cochlear implantation is performed if the cochlear nerve is deemed intact. The ANTS has not been associated with any perioperative complications. On-going studies are needed to determine the predictive value of intraoperative eABR and the impact of SSD rehabilitation on quality of life. CI outcomes following VS microsurgery should also account for baseline hearing characteristics measured by audiograms or ECochG. Of note, studies with better baseline auditory function have shown superior CI outcomes.[36] Further studies are needed before the use of CI in patients with unilateral VS can be widely advocated.

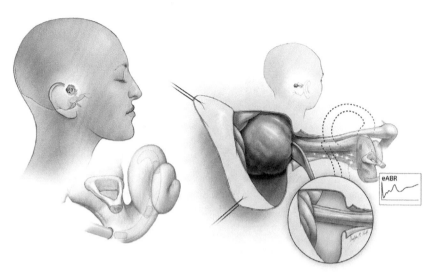

Fig. 5. Illustration of the ANTS system for eABR recordings. The test electrode is placed in the cochlea to facilitate cochlear nerve stimulation and eABR recording during tumor dissection.

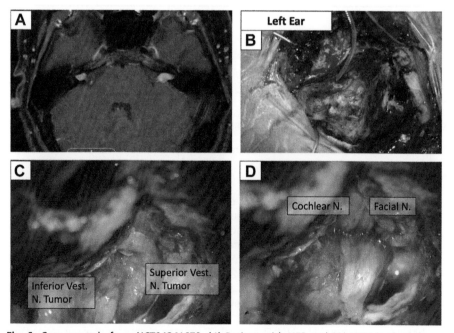

Fig. 6. Case example from NCT04241679. (*A*) Patient with NF2 and 0% WRS in the left ear. (*B*) Intraoperative placement of the ANTE. (*C*) Tumors in the IA. (*C*, *D*) Tumors are resected while keeping the cochlear nerve and facial nerve intact. *Red arrow* points to the tumor of interest, shown in *B*, *C*, and *D*.

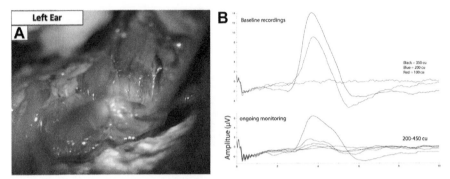

Fig. 7. Case example from NCT04241679. (*A*) Tumor dissection in the IAC. (*B*) Wave V measurements at and during tumor dissection (CU, current unit and is equivalent to current level).

CLINICS CARE POINTS

- Auditory brainstem response (ABR) measures waves I, III, and V.
- Evoked ABR measures one wave V.
- Cochlear nerve action potential measures N1.
- The best estimate for a significant change in ABR waveforms is a greater than 50% reduction in amplitude and/or an increase in 1 ms latency from baseline.

CONTRIBUTIONS

K.Y. Zhan—Article preparation, editing, analysis; C.C. Wick—Study design, article preparation, editing, analysis.

DISCLOSURES

K.Y. Zhan—None; C.C. Wick—Consultant for Stryker and Cochlear Ltd.

REFERENCES

1. Matthies C, Samii M. Management of 1000 vestibular schwannomas (acoustic neuromas): clinical presentation. Neurosurgery 1993;40(1):1–10.
2. Ren Y, Chari DA, Vasilijic S, et al. New developments in neurofibromatosis type 2 and vestibular schwannoma. Neurooncol Adv 2021;3(1):vdaa153.
3. Durakovic N, Valente M, Goebel JA, et al. What defines asymmetric sensorineural hearing loss? Laryngoscope 2019;129(5):1023–4.
4. Brown A, Early S, Vasilijic S, et al. Sporadic vestibular schwannoma size and location do not correlate with the severity of hearing loss at initial presentation. Front Oncol 2022;12:836504.
5. Vivas E.X., Carlson M.L., Neff B.A., et al., Congress of neurological surgeons systematic review and evidence-based guidelines on intraoperative cranial nerve monitoring in vestibular schwannoma surgery, *Neurosurgery*, 82 (2), 2018, E44-E46.

6. Mustain WD, al-Mefty P, Anand VK. Inconsistencies in the correlation between loss of brain stem auditory evoked response waves and postoperative deafness. J Clin Monit 1992;8(3):231–5.
7. James ML, Husain AM. Brainstem auditory evoked potential monitoring: when is change in wave V significant? Neurology 2005;65(10):1551–5.
8. Mastronardi L, Campione A, Zomorodi A, et al. Hearing preservation. In: Mastronardi L, Fukushima T, Campione A, editors. Advances in vestibular schwannoma microneurosurgery: improving results with new technologies. Cham: Springer International Publishing; 2019. p. 95–103.
9. Cueva RA. Preoperative, intraoperative, and postoperative auditory evaluation of patients with acoustic neuroma. Otolaryngol Clin North Am 2012;45(2):285–90.
10. Legatt AD. Mechanisms of intraoperative brainstem auditory evoked potential changes. J Clin Neurophysiol 2002;19(5):396–408.
11. Colletti V, Fiorino FG. Vulnerability of hearing function during acoustic neuroma surgery. Acta Otolaryngol 1994;114(3):264–70.
12. Martin WH, Stecker MM. ASNM position statement: intraoperative monitoring of auditory evoked potentials. J Clin Monit Comput 2008;22(1):75–85.
13. Levine RA, Ojemann RG, Montgomery WW, et al. Monitoring auditory evoked potentials during acoustic neuroma surgery. Insights into the mechanism of the hearing loss. Ann Otol Rhinol Laryngol 1984;93(2 Pt 1):116–23.
14. Neu M, Strauss C, Romstöck J, et al. The prognostic value of intraoperative BAEP patterns in acoustic neurinoma surgery. Clin Neurophysiol 1999;110(11):1935–41.
15. Yamakami I, Yoshinori H, Saeki N, et al. Hearing preservation and intraoperative auditory brainstem response and cochlear nerve compound action potential monitoring in the removal of small acoustic neurinoma via the retrosigmoid approach. J Neurol Neurosurg Psychiatr 2009;80(2):218–27.
16. Silverstein H, McDaniel AB, Norrell H. Hearing preservation after acoustic neuroma surgery using intraoperative direct eighth cranial nerve monitoring. Am J Otol 1985;Suppl:99–106.
17. Cueva RA, Morris GF, Prioleau GR. Direct cochlear nerve monitoring: first report on a new atraumatic, self-retaining electrode. Am J Otol 1998;19(2):202–7.
18. Antezana LA, Carlson ML, Hoffman EM, et al. Electrode alternative for eighth nerve monitoring during vestibular schwannoma resection. Laryngoscope 2021;131(3):E759–63.
19. Danner C, Mastrodimos B, Cueva RA. A comparison of direct eighth nerve monitoring and auditory brainstem response in hearing preservation surgery for vestibular schwannoma. Otol Neurotol 2004;25(5):826–32.
20. Piccirillo E, Hiraumi H, Hamada M, et al. Intraoperative cochlear nerve monitoring in vestibular schwannoma surgery–does it really affect hearing outcome? Audiol Neuro Otol 2008;13(1):58–64.
21. Wick CC, Butler MJ, Yeager LH, et al. Cochlear implant outcomes following vestibular schwannoma resection: systematic review. Otol Neurotol 2020;41(9):1190–7.
22. Abdala C, Visser-Dumont L. Distortion product otoacoustic emissions: a tool for hearing assessment and scientific study. Volta Rev 2001;103(4):281–302.
23. Ferri GG, Modugno GC, Calbucci F, et al. Hearing loss in vestibular schwannomas: analysis of cochlear function by means of distortion-product otoacoustic emissions. Auris Nasus Larynx 2009;36(6):644–8.
24. Brackmann DE, Owens RM, Friedman RA, et al. Prognostic factors for hearing preservation in vestibular schwannoma surgery. Am J Otol 2000;21(3):417–24.

25. Morawski K, Namyslowski G, Lisowska G, et al. Intraoperative monitoring of cochlear function using distortion product otoacoustic emissions (DPOAEs) in patients with cerebellopontine angle tumors. Otol Neurotol 2004;25(5):818–25.

26. Eggermont JJ. Cochlea and auditory nerve. Handb Clin Neurol 2019;160:437–49.

27. Walia A, Shew MA, Kallogjeri D, et al. Electrocochleography and cognition are important predictors of speech perception outcomes in noise for cochlear implant recipients. Sci Rep 2022;12(1):3083.

28. Giardina CK, Brown KD, Adunka OF, et al. Intracochlear electrocochleography: response patterns during cochlear implantation and hearing preservation. Ear Hear 2019;40(4):833–48.

29. Riggs WJ, Fitzpatrick DC, Mattingly JK, et al. Electrocochleography During Translabyrinthine Approach for Vestibular Schwannoma Removal. Otol Neurotol 2020;41(3):e369–77.

30. Butler MJ, Wick CC, Shew MA, et al. Intraoperative cochlear nerve monitoring for vestibular schwannoma resection and simultaneous cochlear implantation in neurofibromatosis type 2: A case series. Oper Neurosurg 2021;21(5):324–31.

31. Patel NS, Saoji AA, Olund AP, et al. Monitoring cochlear nerve integrity during vestibular schwannoma microsurgery in real-time using cochlear implant evoked auditory brainstem response and streaming neural response imaging. Otol Neurotol 2020;41(2):e201–7.

32. Kocharyan A, Daher GS, Nassiri AM, et al. Intraoperative use of electrical stapedius reflex testing for cochlear nerve monitoring during simultaneous translabyrinthine resection of vestibular schwannoma and cochlear implantation. Otol Neurotol 2022;43(4):506–11.

33. Kasbekar AV, Tam YC, Carlyon RP, et al. Intraoperative monitoring of the cochlear nerve during Neurofibromatosis Type-2 vestibular schwannoma surgery and description of a "test intracochlear electrode". J Neurol Surg Rep 2019;80(1):e1–9.

34. Dahm V, Auinger A, Honeder C, et al. Simultaneous vestibular schwannoma resection and cochlear implantation using electrically evoked auditory brainstem response audiometry for decision-making. Otol Neurotol 2020;41(9):1266–73.

35. Medina MM, Polo R, Amilibia E, et al. Diagnostic accuracy of intracochlear test electrode for acoustic nerve monitoring in vestibular schwannoma surgery. Ear Hear 2020;41(6):1648–59.

36. Conway RM, Tu NC, Sioshansi PC, et al. Early outcomes of simultaneous translabyrinthine resection and cochlear implantation. Laryngoscope 2021;131(7):E2312–7.

Translabyrinthine Approach for Sporadic Vestibular Schwannoma

Patient Selection, Technical Pearls, and Patient Outcomes

Zachary G. Schwam, MD*, Maura K. Cosetti, MD,
George B. Wanna, MD

KEYWORDS

• Translabyrinthine approach • Vestibular schwannoma • Acoustic neuroma
• Cerebellopontine angle tumor • Asymmetric hearing loss

KEY POINTS

- The translabyrinthine approach for vestibular schwannoma resection is a versatile surgical corridor and can be used for tumors of any size.
- We recommend the translabyrinthine approach for patients with nonserviceable hearing or in those with low probability of hearing preservation based on a variety of factors and the experience of the surgical team.
- Careful review of the preoperative CT scan is necessary to ensure feasibility and ease of approach.

INTRODUCTION
Historical Perspective

Although the translabyrinthine approach to resection of vestibular schwannomas is a popular approach utilized by lateral skull base surgeons, it has only been performed with some regularity since the 1960s when William House published his initial series of 41 cases.[1–4] Although the exact dates are up for some debate,[5,6] vestibular schwannomas have been resected only since the mid-1890s, and a transtemporal approach was first proposed in 1904 by Panse.[2,3] Due to high initial mortality rates and advances in antibiotics, equipment, and anesthesia that did not manifest until the mid-twentieth century, the translabyrinthine approach was largely abandoned for decades.[1–8]

Department of Otolaryngology-Head and Neck Surgery, Icahn School of Medicine at Mount Sinai, 1 Gustave L. Levy Place, Box 1189, New York, NY 10029, USA
* Corresponding author.
E-mail address: Zachary.schwam@mountsinai.org

Otolaryngol Clin N Am 56 (2023) 483–493
https://doi.org/10.1016/j.otc.2023.02.008
0030-6665/23/© 2023 Elsevier Inc. All rights reserved.

A Brief Overview of the Translabyrinthine Approach

The translabyrinthine approach consists of a wide postauricular incision, raising of an anteriorly based periosteal flap, drilling a large mastoidectomy, removing all bone over the middle fossa and posterior fossa dura, decompressing the sigmoid sinus, exenterating the labyrinth, exposing the internal auditory canal (IAC), drilling superior and inferior troughs around it, opening the posterior fossa and IAC dura, identifying the facial nerve, and dissecting the lesion off of critical neurovascular structures (**Figs. 1–4**). Abdominal fat is harvested and used to pack the IAC and mastoidectomy defect as reapproximation of the dura is not usually practical.[2,9]

The translabyrinthine approach sacrifices hearing in exchange for wide facial nerve exposure from brainstem to stylomastoid foramen, extradural drilling, lack of cerebellar retraction, and routine opening of the IAC along its length from porus to fundus.[1,10] Although a routine approach for a neurotologist, many neurosurgeons are more comfortable with alternate approach corridors. Closure of the bony defect with grafts such as abdominal fat also exposes one to additional potential morbidity.[10]

DISCUSSION
Patient Selection

The translabyrinthine approach is primarily used for the removal of cerebellopontine angle (CPA) tumors that have rendered patients without serviceable hearing or in those lesions in which maintenance of serviceable hearing is unlikely after surgical resection[1] because the approach causes unilateral profound hearing loss. Unilateral profound hearing loss impairs sound localization and limits speech understanding in noise.[11] Although the definition of "serviceable" has evolved over time, it is now commonly accepted to be defined as a pure-tone average (PTA) of 50 dB or lesser hearing level

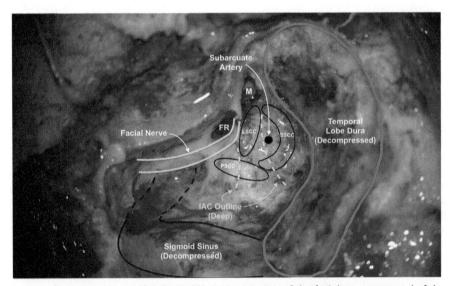

Fig. 1. Left temporal bone after mastoidectomy, opening of the facial recess, removal of the incus, and decompression of the sigmoid sinus and middle fossa dura complete. Next steps include labyrinthectomy, opening of the IAC and posterior fossa, and dissection of the tumor from the critical neurovascular structures. Dashed lines indicate deeper structures not yet uncovered. FR, Facial recess; IAC, Internal auditory canal; LSCC, Lateral semicircular canal; M, Malleus; PSCC, Posterior semicircular canal; SSCC, Superior semicircular canal.

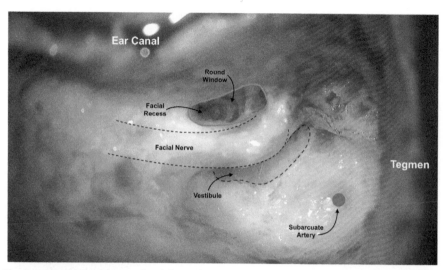

Fig. 2. Left temporal bone after labyrinthectomy and opening of the facial recess for later eustachian tube obliteration. The vestibule is open; the ampulla of the superior semicircular canal is a good anatomic landmark for the superior aspect of the IAC.

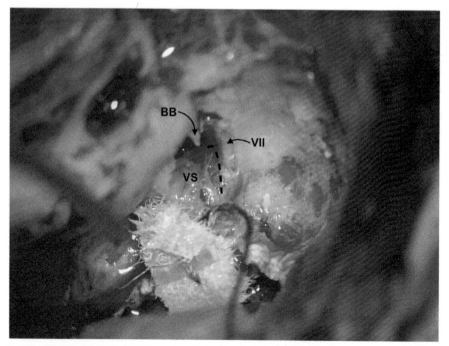

Fig. 3. The dura over the IAC is open and a plane is developed between the tumor and facial nerve (dashed *line*). Bill's bar is a vertical bony landmark that is usually just posterior to the facial nerve. BB, Bill's bar, VII, facial nerve, VS, vestibular schwannoma.

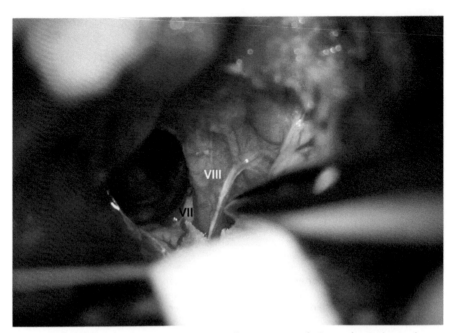

Fig. 4. At the brainstem, the facial nerve typically emanates inferior and anterior to the vestibulocochlear nerve.

and a word recognition score (WRS) 50% or greater.[11] With greater sensitivity in imaging, earlier detection has identified progressively smaller tumors in patients with increasingly better preoperative hearing. According to a national cohort study from Denmark, mean overall tumor size decreased from 26 mm to 7 mm between 1976 and 2015, with a large increase in the numbers of intracanalicular tumors at diagnosis.[11,12] A corresponding increase in "good" hearing (speech discrimination $\geq$70%) from 20% to 60% was found during the same time frame using the same national cohort.[12] Surgical hearing outcomes must always be weighed against alternate modalities, with retention of serviceable hearing in only 55% of patients with observed tumors[13,14] and in 23% after radiotherapy at 10-year follow-up.[13,15]

One of the primary predictors of hearing preservation microsurgery is limited extension into the CPA. In Wallerius' series of 244 patients, hearing preservation was achieved in 64% of IAC tumors without CPA extension, 28% in those with less than 15 mm CPA extension, and 9% in those with 15 mm or lesser CPA extension.[11] Yates and colleagues had similar findings analyzing 64 patients undergoing retrosigmoid approach to vestibular schwannomas and good preoperative hearing; only 6.3% retained their hearing postoperatively, and this occurred in none with a CPA component of 25 mm or greater.[16] In Post's series of 46 patients, if the extracanalicular component was less than 2 cm, there was a 52% chance of hearing preservation, whereas it was significantly higher at 83% if the extracanalicular component was 1 cm or lesser.[17] Other predictors of adverse hearing outcomes include deep impaction of the tumor in the fundus or cochlea, lack of fundal fluid cap, and origin from the inferior vestibular nerve.[10,11,18]

Although many authors prefer not to attempt hearing preservation microsurgery above a certain size threshold,[1,11,13,16] it is important for the skull base team to analyze their own results and to counsel patients using their own data. The fact that there are multiple divergent opinions on the matter suggests that results are very center-dependent and surgeon-dependent; these factors should be weighed against the literature, with all of its attendant biases and variations in measurements that may render studies uncomparable.[10,11]

Comparing Skull Base Approaches

According to guidelines published by the Congress of Neurological Surgeons, there is not enough evidence to recommend one surgical approach over another when considering the factors of complete resection or facial nerve function in the setting of nonserviceable hearing.[19] There are many ingrained opinions among various centers and experts, and we encourage teams to use the approach with the greatest success in their hands along with patient buy-in.[10,11] Recent research has shown that complication rates as well as quality of life measures are not significantly different among the various surgical approaches.[20,21]

The classic teaching dictates that patients undergoing retrosigmoid craniotomy have a higher risk of significant headache secondary to irritation from bone dust during drilling or adhesions between the dura and suboccipital muscles.[7,22,23] In a survey administered by Carlson and colleagues, their group found that there were no differences in long-term severe headache incidence among the various surgical approaches but was more likely codependent with anxiety, depression, and younger age.[21] In spite of this finding, they found that patients with a positive headache history had more difficulty with respect to headache in the first 3 to 6 months postoperatively after retrosigmoid approach.[21] Similarly, Ruckenstein found significantly worse headache outcomes in the first 6 months for retrosigmoid as compared with translabyrinthine approaches, with no significant differences at 1 year.[24]

In terms of facial function, there is no clear consensus as to the best approach.[10] Ansari found that tumors with greater than 15 mm of extracanalicular extension had better facial function using a retrosigmoid approach[7]; Isaacson, Wiet, and Ren found no differences in facial function when comparing translabyrinthine to retrosigmoid or middle fossa approaches[25–27]; and Jacob found lower rates of good facial function in their translabyrinthine versus retrosigmoid patients (88% vs 96%).[28] In Ansari's systematic review examining 35 studies and 5064 patients, there were no significant differences in facial function between retrosigmoid, middle fossa, and translabyrinthine approaches (4%, 16.7%, 0%, respectively). However, when performing a subgroup analysis, they found that the retrosigmoid approach had significantly lower rates of facial dysfunction than middle fossa or translabyrinthine approaches for tumors 1.5 to 3.0 cm (6.1%, 11.5%, 7.2%) and better rates than the translabyrinthine approach for tumors greater than 3.0 cm (30.2% vs 42.5%).[7] In Brackmann's large series of 580 translabyrinthine approaches, excellent facial nerve function was strongly tied to tumor size; if the tumor was less than 3.5 cm, 84% had House-Brackmann grade I/II facial function at 1-year follow-up compared with only 53% for patients with tumors greater than 3.5 cm.[29] Another important factor potentially confounding facial nerve reporting outcomes is the degree of tumor resection; Gurgel's systematic review of 30 studies including 1390 patients with tumors 2.5 cm or greater showed comparable rates of good facial function between the translabyrinthine and retrosigmoid approaches but when stratified by the degree of resection, subtotal resection had far better rates than near-total or gross-total resection (92.5% vs 74.6% vs 47.3%, respectively).[30] It is therefore important to interpret facial function results with an eye toward extent of resection, realizing that definitions of extent of resection may be inconsistent and vary across centers.[31]

Cerebrospinal fluid (CSF) leak after vestibular schwannoma resection may manifest as either otorhinorrhea or as a pseudomeningocele depending on the approach and site of leak. The retrosigmoid approach potentially exposes air cells off the craniotomy and the IAC, which must be meticulously waxed and closed (in some cases with abdominal fat), as compared with the translabyrinthine approach where the open communication between the mastoid and CPA is nearly always closed with abdominal fat. In Ansari's aforementioned systematic review, they found a significantly higher rate of CSF leak after retrosigmoid craniotomy (10.3%) compared with 5.3% middle fossa and 7.1% translabyrinthine approach.[7] In contrast, Selesnick's meta-analysis of nearly 6000 vestibular schwannoma resections found no differences among the 3 major approaches (all between 9.5% and 10.6%),[32] and Sughrue and Copeland found higher rates of CSF leak in patients undergoing translabyrinthine approaches.[33,34]

Some authors prefer the translabyrinthine approach in patients who were previously radiated or in those already operated on using an alternate approach due to the relatively wide exposure and early potential access to the facial nerve at the labyrinthine segment.[2] Other factors, including amount of residual tumor, tumor recurrence, mortality rates, and prevalence of other complications were not found to vary widely between the approaches.[7]

Technical Aspects and Special Circumstances

Although a brief, general overview of the approach was mentioned earlier, there are several technical pearls and tips with regard to patient selection worth mentioning. The translabyrinthine approach is challenging in patients with small, sclerotic mastoids or in those with very anterior sigmoid sinuses because it crowds the field and minimizes access to the IAC and CPA (**Fig. 5**). The translabyrinthine approach should also be avoided in those with active chronic ear disease due to risk of infection seeding the intracranial space. In the event of a very high, obstructive jugular bulb, it can be compressed as long as one is careful to avoid the lower cranial nerves on the medial aspect. Some authors prefer a retrosigmoid approach if the tumor is ipsilateral to the significantly asymmetric, dominant sigmoid to avoid intracranial venous hypertension.[2,10]

Our group avoids the use of pins and advocates for aggressive strapping to the bed as need for significant rotation is common. We make a semilunar skin incision approximately 3 to 4 cm from the postauricular sulcus superiorly and posteriorly, and the incision is brought closer as one goes toward the mastoid tip. The periosteal flap is

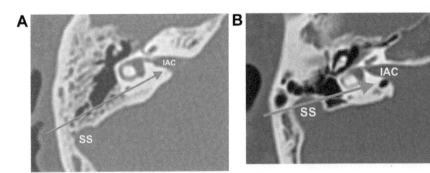

Fig. 5. (*A*) Computed tomography scan showing an ideal temporal bone for a translabyrinthine approach. The sigmoid sinus is posterior and the drilling corridor (*arrow*) is direct to the IAC. Contrast this to (*B*), which has a large and anteriorly placed sigmoid sinus, obstructing the drilling corridor. IAC, internal auditory canal; SS, sigmoid sinus.

elevated carefully and with minimal cautery to prevent shrinkage; this layer can be used to achieve a multilayer closure. Additionally, the periosteal incisions are designed not to lie directly under the skin incision; in the event of pseudomeningocele, this ensures an indirect, rather than a direct path of fluid egress. In older patients with more adherent dura, we may leave very small, thin islands of bone on the middle fossa and posterior fossa dura/sigmoid to avoid significant bleeding. We visualize the second genu and descending portion of the facial nerve well so that a safe and efficient labyrinthectomy can be performed; the ampulla of the posterior semicircular canal comes quite close to the vertical segment of the facial nerve. An advantage of the translabyrinthine approach includes the possibility of early access to the labyrinthine portion of the facial nerve even before identifying the IAC fundus; identification of the nerve in the lateral aspect of the IAC may facilitate tumor dissection especially in cases where there is a large burden of disease. Although gross total resection and perfect facial nerve function are ideal, this is often not possible for various reasons. In those cases, we favor subtotal or near-total resection to avoid unnecessary morbidity in these benign tumors, particularly in the way of facial nerve paralysis.[2,35,36]

In an attempt to prevent CSF rhinorrhea, we prophylactically drill a facial recess, remove the incus, and pack the eustachian tube with fat, surgicel, temporalis fascia, and muscle. Although this step is effective in our hands and used frequently by high volume skull base surgeons,[9] Jacob and colleagues reported no difference in CSF leak rates between those patients whose eustachian tubes were packed and those whose were not.[28] Other authors advocate for not opening the antrum, packing temporalis around the incus, and putting fascia to block off the antrum.[9,28,37] Cases of CSF leak even in the setting of eustachian tube packing are possible in the setting of peritubal air cells that drain distal to the site of packing.[28,38] We check the tympanic membrane with a speculum at the end of the case to ensure there are no perforations. When packing the mastoid and IAC defect with fat, we encourage multiple smaller pieces to achieve more effective obliteration of dead space.[37,39] If feasible, we reapproximate the dural flaps in the posterior fossa with a stitch to facilitate tight packing of fat. To ensure adequate compression of the abdominal fat in the mastoid cavity and to aid in preventing cosmetically untoward asymmetry, we often place a mesh cranioplasty plate over the bony defect and attempt a tight, multilayer closure that includes the periosteum. Hunter and colleagues reported a significant decrease in their CSF leaks using this method (1.9% vs 11.6% in nearly 1500 cases).[40]

Postoperatively, we encourage early ambulation and aggressive control of nausea. Postoperative antibiotics and steroids are frequently given, and a compressive headwrap is often left on until the day of discharge.[9]

Concomitant Cochlear Implantation

Although an in-depth discussion as to the efficacy of simultaneous cochlear implantation at the time of vestibular schwannoma resection is beyond the scope of this article, the translabyrinthine approach is the most well suited to this technique for appropriately selected patients with intact cochlear nerves. Ongoing studies demonstrate novel monitoring techniques using intracochlear electrodes to guide whether stimulation may be successful. Additionally, simultaneous placement of the implant at the time of tumor resection limits the impact of possible delayed cochlear ossification that would preclude future electrode placement. A second procedure is avoided, and there is theoretically less spiral ganglion degeneration the sooner the implant is placed and the neural elements stimulated. It should be noted that even in MRI-compatible implants, significant artifact is expected and can preclude effective imaging-based tumor surveillance particularly in cases of subtotal resection.[40–48]

SUMMARY

The translabyrinthine approach to vestibular schwannoma resection is effective in patients without serviceable hearing and in those in which hearing preservation is unlikely. Anatomic and tumor-related factors in addition to team experience and patient preferences must be considered when choosing this approach.

CLINICS CARE POINTS

- The translabyrinthine approach is best for patients without serviceable hearing or in patients in whom hearing preservation is unlikely to be successful. Extracanalicular extent of the tumor is one of a few important prognostic variables for hearing preservation.
- Anatomic factors such as a sclerotic mastoid and very anterior or dominant sigmoid sinus may make the translabyrinthine craniotomy an inconvenient approach.
- Skeletonizing the second genu and mastoid segments of the facial nerve is key to a safe and efficient labyrinthectomy.
- To prevent CSF leak, we recommend tight (but not compressive) packing of small strips of fat into the cavity, routine obliteration of the eustachian tube, and placement of a cranioplasty plate as a rigid buttress.
- The translabyrinthine approach is ideal for simultaneous cochlear implantation in well-selected patients.

DECLARATION OF INTERESTS

George Wanna has no disclosures. Maura Cosetti has received travel grants from MED-EL, Austria, Cochlear, Australia, Stryker, United States, educational research grants from Advanced Bionics, and has done clinical research with Advanced Bionics, Cochlear, and Otonomy. She is on the surgical advisory board of Cochlear.

REFERENCES

1. Arriaga MA, Lin J. Translabyrinthine approach: indications, techniques, and results. Otolaryngol Clin North Am 2012;45:399–415.
2. Chen BS, Brackmann DE. Translabyrinthine Approach for Vestibular Schwannoma Resection. In: Carlson ML, Link MJ, Driscoll CL, et al, editors. Comprehensive management of vestibular schwannoma. New York: Thieme; 2019. p. 225–34.
3. Panse R. Klinische und pathologische Mitteilungen. Eu Arch Otorhinolaryngol 1904;61:251–5.
4. House WF. Transtemporal bone microsurgical removal of acoustic neuromas. Evolution of transtemporal bone removal of acoustic tumors. Arch Otolaryngol 1964;80:731–42.
5. Nguyen-Huynh AT, Jackler RK, Pfister M, et al. The aborted early history of the translabyrinthine approach: a victim of suppression or technical prematurity? Otol Neurotol 2007;28:269–79.
6. Gibson G. Remarks on the results of surgical measures in a series of cerebral cases. Edinb Med J 1896;41:689–92.
7. Ansari SF, Terry C, Cohen-Gadol AA. Surgery for vestibular schwannomas: a systematic review of complications by approach. Neurosurg Focus 2012;33:E14.

8. Cushing H. Tumors of the nervus acusticus and the syndrome of the cerebello-pontine angle. Philadelphia: WB Saunders; 1917.
9. Van Gompel JJ, Carlson ML, Wiet RM, et al. A Cross-sectional Survey of the North American Skull Base Society on Vestibular Schwannoma, Part 2: Perioperative Practice Patterns of Vestibular Schwannoma in North America. J Neurol Surg B Skull Base 2018;79:297–301.
10. Sweeney A, Carlson ML, Driscoll CL. Surgical Approach Selection for Vestibular Schwannoma Microsurgery. In: Carlson ML, Link MJ, Driscoll CL, et al, editors. Comprehensive management of vestibular schwannoma. New York: Thieme; 2019. p. 208–18.
11. Wallerius KP, Macielak RJ, Lawlor SK, et al. Hearing Preservation Microsurgery in Vestibular Schwannomas: Worth Attempting in "Larger" Tumors? Laryngoscope 2022;132:1657–64.
12. Reznitsky M, Petersen M, West N, et al. Epidemiology of vestibular schwanno-mas—prospective 40-year data from an unselected national cohort. Clin Epide-miol 2019;11:981–6.
13. Saliba J, Friedman RA, Cueva RA. Hearing preservation in vestibular schwan-noma surgery. J Neurol Surg B Skull Base 2019;80:149–55.
14. Stangerup SE, Thomsen J, Tos M, et al. Long-term hearing preservation in vestib-ular schwannoma. Otol Neurotol 2010;31:271–5.
15. Coughlin AR, Willman TJ, Gubbels SP. Systematic review of hearing preservation after radiotherapy for vestibular schwannoma. Otol Neurotol 2018;39:273–83.
16. Yates PD, Jackler RK, Satar B, et al. Is it worthwhile to attempt hearing preserva-tion in larger acoustic neuromas? Otol Neurotol 2003;24:460–4.
17. Post KD, Eisenberg MB, Catalano PJ. Hearing preservation in vestibular schwan-noma surgery: what factors influence outcome? J Neurosurg 1995;83:191–6.
18. Cohen NL, Lewis WS, Ransohoff J. Hearing preservation in cerebellopontine angle tumor surgery: the NYU experience 1974–1991. Am J Otol 1993;14:423–33.
19. Hadjipanayis CG, Carlson ML, Link MJ, et al. Congress of Neurological Surgeons systematic review and evidence-based guidelines on surgical resection for the treatment of patients with vestibular schwannomas. Neurosurgery 2018;82:E40–3.
20. Carlson ML, Barnes JH, Nassiri A, et al. Prospective study of disease-specific quality-of-life in sporadic vestibular schwannoma comparing observation, radio-surgery, and microsurgery. Otol Neurotol 2021;42:e199–208.
21. Carlson ML, Tveiten OV, Driscoll CL, et al. Long-term quality of life in patients with vestibular schwannoma: an international multicenter cross-sectional study comparing microsurgery, stereotactic radiosurgery, observation, and nontumor controls. J Neurosurg 2015;122:833–42.
22. Cerullo LJ, Grutsch JF, Heiferman K, et al. The preservation of hearing and facial nerve function in a consecutive series of unilateral vestibular nerve schwannoma surgical patients (acoustic neuroma). Surg Neurol 1993;39:485–93.
23. Schessel DA, Nedzelski JM, Rowed D, et al. Pain after surgery for acoustic neu-roma. Otolaryngol Head Neck Surg 1992;107:424–9.
24. Ruckenstein MJ, Harris JP, Cueva RA, et al. Pain subsequent to resection of acoustic neuromas via suboccipital and translabyrinthine approaches. Am J Otol 1996;17:620–4.
25. Isaacson B, Telian S, El-Kashlan H. Facial nerve outcomes in middle cranial fossa vs. translabyrinthine approaches. J Otol Head Neck Surg 2005;133:906–10.

26. Wiet RJ, Mamikoglu B, Odom L, et al. Long-term results of the first 500 cases of acoustic neuroma surgery. Otolaryngol Head Neck Surg 2001;124:645–51.
27. Ren Y, MacDonald BV, Tawfik KO, et al. Clinical predictors of facial nerve outcomes after surgical resection of vestibular schwannoma. Otolaryngol Head Neck Surg 2021;164:1085–93.
28. Jacob A, Bortman JS, Robinson LL Jr, et al. Does packing the eustachian tube impact cerebrospinal fluid rhinorrhea rates in translabyrinthine vestibular schwannoma resections? Otol Neurotol 2007;28:934–8.
29. Brackmann DE, Cullen RD, Fisher LM. Facial nerve function after translabyrinthine vestibular schwannoma surgery. Otolaryngol Head Neck Surg 2007;136:773–7.
30. Gurgel RK, Dogru S, Amdur RL, et al. Facial nerve outcomes after surgery for large vestibular schwannomas: do surgical approach and extent of resection matter? Neurosurg Focus 2012;33:E16.
31. Carlson ML, Link MJ, Wanna GB, et al. Management of sporadic vestibular schwannoma. Otolaryngol Clin North Am 2015;48:407–22.
32. Selesnick SH, Liu JC, Jen A, et al. The incidence of cerebrospinal fluid leak after vestibular schwannoma surgery. Otol Neurotol 2004;25:387–93.
33. Sughrue ME, Yang I, Aranda D, et al. Beyond audiofacial morbidity after vestibular schwannoma surgery. J Neurosurg 2011;114:367–74.
34. Copeland WR, Mallory GW, Neff BA, et al. Are there modifiable risk factors to prevent a cerebrospinal fluid leak following vestibular schwannoma surgery? J Neurosurg 2015;122:312–6.
35. Schwartz MS, Kari E, Strickland BM, et al. Evaluation of the increased use of partial resection of large vestibular schwannomas: facial nerve outcomes and recurrence/regrowth rate. Otol Neurotol 2013;34:1456–64.
36. Perkins EL, Manzoor NF, Totten DJ, et al. The influence of extent of resection and tumor morphology on facial nerve outcomes following vestibular schwannoma surgery. Otol Neurotol 2021;42:e1346–52.
37. Goddard JC, Oliver ER, Lambert PR. Prevention of cerebrospinal fluid leak after translabyrinthine resection of vestibular schwannoma. Otol Neurotol 2010;31:473–7.
38. Grant IL, Welling DB, Oehler MC, et al. Transcochlear repair of persistent cerebrospinal fluid leaks. Laryngoscope 1999;109:1392–6.
39. House JL, Hitselberger WE, House WF. Wound closure and cerebrospinal fluid leak after translabyrinthine surgery. Am J Otol 1982;4:126–8.
40. Hunter JB, Sweeney AD, Carlson ML, et al. Prevention of Postoperative Cerebrospinal Fluid Leaks After Translabyrinthine Tumor Resection With Resorbable Mesh Cranioplasty. Otol Neurotol 2015;36:1537–42.
41. Conway RM, Tu NC, Sioshansi PC, et al. Early outcomes of simultaneous translabyrinthine resection and cochlear implantation. Laryngoscope 2021;131:E2312–7.
42. Wick CC, Butler MJ, Yeager LH, et al. Cochlear implant outcomes following vestibular schwannoma resection: systematic review. Otol Neurotol 2020;41:1190–7.
43. Feng Y, Lane JI, Lohse CM, et al. Pattern of cochlear obliteration after vestibular schwannoma resection according to surgical approach. Laryngoscope 2020;130:474–81.
44. Sanna M, Piccirillo E, Kihlgren C, et al. Simultaneous cochlear implantation after translabyrinthine vestibular schwannoma resection: a report of 41 cases. Otol Neurotol 2021;42:1414–21.

45. Carswell V, Crowther JA, Locke R, et al. Cochlear patency following translabyrinthine vestibular schwannoma resection: implications for hearing rehabilitation. J Laryngol Otol 2019;133:560–5.
46. Delgado-Vargas B, Medina M, Polo R, et al. Cochlear obliteration following a translabyrinthine approach and its implications in cochlear implantation. Acta Otorhinolaryngol Ital 2018;38:56–60.
47. Klenzner T, Glaas M, Volpert S, et al. Cochlear implantation in patients with single-sided deafness after the translabyrinthine resection of the vestibular schwannoma-Presented at the Annual Meeting of ADANO 2016 in Berlin. Otol Neurotol 2019;40:e461–6.
48. Kuo SC, Gibson WP. The role of the promontory stimulation test in cochlear. Cochlear Implants Int 2002;3:19–28.

Middle Cranial Fossa Approach for Sporadic Vestibular Schwannoma

Patient Selection, Technical Pearls, and Hearing Results

Rustin G. Kashani, MD, Armine Kocharyan, MD, Alexander D. Claussen, MD, Bruce J. Gantz, MD, Marlan R. Hansen, MD*

KEYWORDS

- Vestibular schwannoma • Middle fossa approach • Hearing preservation
- Resection • Surgical outcomes

KEY POINTS

- Microsurgical resection of vestibular schwannoma through the middle fossa approach offers the opportunity for total tumor resection in patients who have serviceable hearing and tumors that do not significantly contact the brainstem.
- Optimal surgical exposure requires robust knowledge of middle fossa anatomy.
- Middle fossa resection can provide excellent hearing outcomes with long-term durability.

INTRODUCTION

The middle cranial fossa (MCF) technique is one of the primary surgical approaches for removing lesions involving the internal auditory canal (IAC). Much of the pioneering work in developing this procedure was tediously performed by William F. House, who described the complicated anatomy of the middle fossa and corridor to accessing the IAC in 1961.[1] At that time, the MCF approach was largely used for vestibular nerve section in patients suffering from intractable vertigo, although House hypothesized the procedure could be used to remove small vestibular schwannomas (VS) confined to the IAC. Testing this conjecture, House and colleagues[2] subsequently published initial outcomes from the MCF approach in 1968. Among 5 patients with tumors confined to the IAC, all underwent gross total resection and 4 patients had

Department of Otolaryngology–Head and Neck Surgery, University of Iowa Hospitals and Clinics, University of Iowa, Iowa City, IA 52242, USA
* Corresponding author.
E-mail address: marlan-hansen@uiowa.edu

Otolaryngol Clin N Am 56 (2023) 495–507
https://doi.org/10.1016/j.otc.2023.02.009
0030-6665/23/© 2023 Elsevier Inc. All rights reserved.

preserved or improved hearing. Outcomes were not as favorable for tumors extending into the cerebellopontine angle (CPA), where hearing was preserved in 3 of 14 patients. This led the authors to conclude that "the middle fossa approach has its most ideal application in the management of those tumors that are confined to the internal auditory canal."[2] More than 5 decades later, the MCF approach has been extensively studied and elaborated on, leading to a more nuanced understanding of its utility and optimal execution. Although this article focuses on MCF excision of VS, the MCF exposure is useful for a variety of other skull base neoplasms and pathologic conditions, highlighting the importance of mastering the technique.[3,4]

PATIENT SELECTION

The MCF approach is appropriate for patients who still have serviceable hearing, often defined as pure tone average (PTA) of 50 decibels or less and word recognition score (WRS) of at least 50%.[5] It should be considered in the context of contemporary hearing preservation therapies for VS: observation, stereotactic radiosurgery (SRS), and microsurgery. Observation with serial imaging is typically pursued in patients who have tumors with little to no symptoms, advanced age, or poor health. If observed tumors grow, patients may opt for SRS, which will typically arrest growth in smaller tumors.[6] However, many patients will ultimately choose microsurgery with the retrosigmoid or MCF approaches; the majority of observed patients eventually lose hearing and, following SRS, serviceable hearing rates drop from 80% at 1-year post-therapy to 48% at 5 years and 23% at 10 years.[7,8] With increased availability of magnetic resonance imaging (MRI), intracanalicular tumors are more frequently diagnosed, often in patients with WRS exceeding 70%.[9–12] Thus, a reasonable argument can be made to pursue hearing preservation microsurgery in these circumstances. In addition to PTA and WRS, preoperative auditory brainstem response (ABR) testing can be performed, which can prognosticate hearing outcomes.[5] We perform preoperative ABR as a baseline comparison to intraoperative ABR. As such, preoperative absent or diminished waveform does not influence our decision to recommend MCF excision.

Size and location are additional factors in selecting the MCF approach, which offers excellent exposure of the lateral IAC and labyrinthine segment of the facial nerve. At numerous centers, the technique has become the preferred hearing preservation approach for intracanalicular tumors.[4,5,12–15] It is typically used for VS involving the IAC without significant brainstem involvement, similar to the lesion depicted in **Fig. 1**. Tumors with significant CPA involvement (<1 cm) may be better addressed by the retrosigmoid approach.[16–19] Additionally, high-resolution heavily weighted T2 sequences can aid in identifying the relationship between the lesion and the seventh and eighth cranial nerves. Some studies have found that a preoperative fundal cerebrospinal fluid (CSF) cap on T2 sequence may portend preserved hearing but the strength of this association has been inconsistent.[3,20,21] A preserved cochlear fluid T2 signal has been correlated with hearing preservation, despite no relationship between the presence of the fluid signal and preoperative hearing status.[22]

A special consideration with the MCF approach is that tumor removal requires temporal lobe retraction and dural elevation, which can predispose patients to temporary aphasia, seizures, long-term processing difficulties, and rarely hemorrhage or hematoma formation.[23] Hence, many advocate against using the approach in patients above age 65 due to decreased resiliency of the temporal lobe and a tendency for the dura to be thinner and more adherent.[23] These complications have been rare in our experience at the University of Iowa.

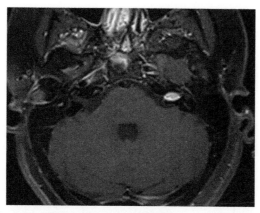

Fig. 1. MRI, axial view, T1-weighted sequence following intravenous gadolinium, displaying an enhancing lesion occupying the left IAC measuring 1 cm in a 40-year-old woman. The patient underwent gross total MCF resection with preservation of hearing and facial nerve function.

In summary, the MCF approach can generally be recommended for patients with the following.

1. Intracanalicular tumors without significant cerebellopontine extension (>1 cm) or brainstem contact
2. Serviceable hearing, ideally with greater than 70% WRS
3. Age younger than 65 years

Based on our institutional experience, we counsel patients with tumors 1 cm or smaller and greater than 70% WRS that we have about a 75% chance of preserving at least 75% WRS; patients with greater than 70% WRS and no brainstem contact have a 50% chance of maintaining at least 70% WRS.[12]

SURGICAL TECHNIQUE AND PEARLS

The MCF approach is performed under general anesthesia. An arterial line is placed and the bed is rotated 180°. The patient is laid supine; arms are tucked and the patient is strapped to allow for full bed rotation. The head is placed on a gel headrest and turned. Pinning is not necessary. Facial nerve monitoring is used thus long-acting paralytics are avoided. Intraoperative audiologic monitoring can be performed by placing an insert earphone in the external auditory canal (EAC) to enable cochlear nerve action potential (CNAP) recordings and scalp/mastoid electrodes for far field ABR recording, a technique that has been previously described.[3] Intravenous steroids and antibiotics are given before incision. To ease temporal lobe retraction, mannitol is administered at time of incision and the patient is hyperventilated.

A posteriorly based skin flap measuring 6 × 8cm is designed in the temporal hairline, beginning in the postauricular crease and extending anteriorly as shown in **Fig. 2**. To avoid injury to the frontal branch of the facial nerve, the incision should not extend beyond the temporal hairline. The skin flap is elevated off the temporalis fascia and a 4 × 4cm segment of fascia is harvested. The temporalis muscle flap is anteriorly/inferiorly based and staggered from the skin incisions. A cuff of fascia is left on each side of the muscle flap incisions to ensure watertight muscle flap closure at the end of the case. The muscle is elevated off the squamous temporal bone inferiorly and the EAC and zygomatic root are identified.

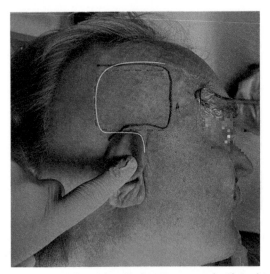

Fig. 2. Marked ink skin incision for right-sided MCF approach. The white line denotes an alternate anteriorly based skin incision. The dashed blue line represents the design for the temporalis muscle flap, which is anteriorly based and staggered inferiorly with respect to the skin flap.

The craniotomy, depicted in **Fig. 3**, measures 4 × 6cm and is positioned one-third posterior and two-thirds anterior to the EAC. The width of the craniotomy must be limited to ensure that the self-retaining middle fossa retractor can be secured. The vertical bone cuts of the craniotomy must also be parallel to give the retractor stable

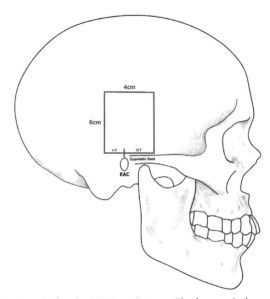

Fig. 3. Anatomic landmarks for the MCF craniotomy. The bone window measures 4 × 6 cm; its inferior border lies at the zygomatic root, and it is positioned one-third anterior to and two-thirds posterior to the EAC.

purchase on bone. A 4-mm cutting burr is initially used followed by a 4-mm diamond burr as the dura is approached. The anteroinferior corner of the craniotomy can be angled if mobilizing the temporalis proves difficult. The bone flap is separated from dura with a curved periosteal elevator then set aside. Elevation of the dura at the margins of the craniotomy for 1 to 2 cm reduces the pressure on the temporal lobe under the retractor blade. Next, the inferior border of the craniotomy is brought down to the level of the middle fossa floor using a rongeur or drill.

Dural elevation is performed in a posterior to anterior and lateral to medial fashion. This prevents injury to the greater superficial petrosal nerve (GSPN) and geniculate ganglion, which can be dehiscent in up to 15% of patients.[24] Anatomic landmarks are illustrated in **Fig. 4**. Anteriorly, the limit of dissection is foramen spinosum, from which the middle meningeal artery emerges. The artery can be sacrificed by cauterizing it on the dural side and cutting it free, then packing the foramen. Foramen ovale and the mandibular division of the trigeminal nerve will be found just anterior to foramen spinosum. The true petrous ridge must be identified posteromedially, which may require mobilization of the petrosal sinus out of a lateral false ridge. The arcuate eminence and GSPN are identified. It should be noted that an arcuate eminence might

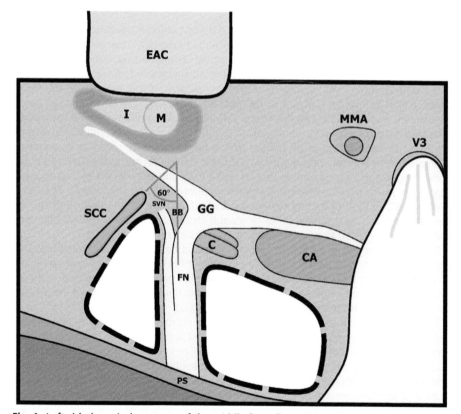

Fig. 4. Left-sided surgical anatomy of the middle fossa floor. The white regions with dashed borders represent the areas of drilling for trough creation. The IAC is typically found at a 60° angle to the SSC. BB, Bill Bar; C, cochlea; CA, carotid artery; EAC, external auditory canal; FN, facial nerve; GG, geniculate ganglion; I, incus; M, malleus; MMA, middle meningeal artery; PS, petrosal sinus; SCC, superior semicircular canal; SVN, superior vestibular nerve; V3, mandibular division of trigeminal nerve.

not be evident or the prominence might not provide a true landmark for the superior semicircular canal (SCC). As elevation proceeds anteromedially along the petrous ridge, a lip of bone is often encountered that corresponds to the approximate location of porus acousticus, which is in line with the EAC. The IAC lies in a plane that bisects the GSPN and SCC. The blade tip of the House-Urban retractor is placed at the medial margin of the ridge in line with IAC. It can be helpful to gently cauterize the dura as elevation proceeds because this causes the dura to retract.

There are 2 different strategies to identify the IAC. Fisch described identifying the SCC by slowly removing bone over the canal until a blue or gray line is seen.[25] The SCC is always perpendicular to the petrous ridge. If the arcuate eminence is poorly defined, whitish membranous bone can be removed until a more-dense yellow otic capsule bone is recognized. Once the position of the SSC is established, the IAC is found in a plane 60° anterior and medial. Identifying the position of the SSC enables one to remove the bone between the IAC posterior margin and the SSC. In another method used by our institution, the IAC can be identified medially by drilling in the plane that bisects the GSPN and SCC. The SCC is blue-lined using a broad diamond burr. This enables the surgeon to expose the entire IAC and provide a large posterior corridor to remove the tumor. The surgeon must exercise caution in this maneuver to avoid iatrogenic SCC dehiscence.

The IAC is then completely exposed. Anterior and posterior troughs afford 270° access around the IAC. The posterior trough extends to the SCC; the ampullated end of the SCC is blue-lined as well. The anterior trough is created by drilling through the petrous apex. The anterior edge of the IAC should be closely followed to avoid entry into the basal turn of the cochlea and identify the labyrinthine segment of the facial nerve, which lies within 0.5 mm of the cochlea. Following the anterior edge helps ensure that dissection follows the lateral IAC into the labyrinthine facial nerve rather than inadvertently following the superior vestibular nerve into the ampullated end of the SCC. Careful drilling is performed at the fundus laterally until the labyrinthine segment, vertical crest, and superior vestibular nerve can be appreciated through bone. A right-angle probe can be placed under the bony ledge of the IAC to approximate how much bone is present along the anterior edge and the fundus. The bone over the IAC is then delicately removed using a flap knife or fine right-angle hook. The entrance to the fallopian canal or meatal foramen contains a fibrous ligament that should be incised to prevent swelling and injury to the facial nerve.

The dura of the IAC is opened longitudinally with a beaver blade and reflected. The facial, cochlear, and vestibular nerves are identified; the identity of the facial nerve can be confirmed with a nerve stimulator. Both vestibular nerves are transected. A modified electromyography needle electrode is placed in the anterior trough of the IAC for continuous CNAP monitoring during tumor dissection.

Tumor is meticulously peeled away from the surrounding nerves in atraumatic fashion with fine microinstruments and fenestrated suction. Medial to lateral dissection prevents disruption of fragile auditory nerve fibers entering the cribrosa. Continuous irrigation helps to identify the plane of dissection between tumor and nerve. Additionally, dissecting in a subcapsular plane can further minimize trauma to the facial and auditory nerves. Before tumor extirpation, the course of the facial nerve is fully identified. A right-angle 2.5-mm hook is an ideal instrument to separate the facial nerve from the tumor capsule. Slowly debulking the tumor posteriorly will enable separation of the tumor from the anteriorly compressed facial nerve. Upon tumor removal, the operative field is copiously irrigated and hemostasis is confirmed.

The IAC defect is plugged with temporalis muscle or abdominal fat based on surgeon preference. Any opened apical or mastoid air cells are occluded with muscle or bone wax. Temporalis fascia is draped over the dural defect and middle fossa floor. The posterior aspect of the fascia can be tucked in between the petrous ridge and temporal lobe, then unfurled laterally. Next, the dura is tacked laterally to soft tissue with 4-0 Nurolon suture to obliterate the epidural space. The craniotomy flap is secured with plates. The temporalis and subcutaneous tissue layers are each closed with buried interrupted 3-0 Vicryl suture. The skin layer is approximated with 3-0 Nylon suture. All layers are closed in watertight fashion. A tight mastoid pressure dressing is applied.

COMPLICATIONS AND RISKS

CSF leak is the most common complication following MCF resection, with rates ranging from 3% to 10%.[26,27] Leaks can be managed with the placement of a lumbar drain. Sequela of temporal lobe retraction includes aphasia, seizures, and processing difficulties; these are rare complications affecting less than 1% of patients.[12,13] Epidural hematoma, cerebral edema, and pneumoencephalus pose significant morbidity but are also very uncommon, as are wound infection, meningitis, deep venous thrombosis, pulmonary embolism, and death.

Facial nerve function is preserved in the vast majority of MCF cases, with studies reporting House-Brackmann I-II scores in 90% to 100% of patients, as seen in **Table 1**.[20,28–33] Comparisons of facial nerve outcome between tumor approaches suggest that MCF resection may have a higher risk of immediate short-term facial nerve injury, because a superiorly effaced facial nerve can be subject to more manipulation during tumor, and equivalent rates of delayed short-term paresis.[34–36] However, long-term studies have found that outcomes can become equivalent between approaches with time.[34]

HEARING OUTCOMES

Rates of hearing preservation following the MCF approach range from 48% to 96%.[12,13,37–45] Data from contemporary studies are summarized in **Table 1**.[20,28–33] Most authors define serviceable hearing as 50 dB PTA or less and at least 50% WRS, which falls within class A and B of the American Academy of Otolaryngology-Head and Neck Surgery system.[46–50] Of these measures, we rely most heavily on WRS as the most important indicator of functional hearing. Preserved WRS can be aided with amplification even with an elevated PTA. The wide range in reported hearing preservation outcomes may stem from variation in definitions of hearing level, reported follow-up period, characteristics of patients and tumors between series, and degree of institutional experience with the MCF approach.[51] Smaller tumor size, anteroposterior tumor position, slower rate of growth, presence of preoperative ABR, and better preoperative WRS and PTA have all been associated with an increased likelihood of hearing preservation.[20,33,52–59] Despite the numerous risk factors identified, it is difficult to predict the chance of hearing preservation for a given patient, possibly due to a complex and nonlinear interaction between factors. It has been suggested that the degree of adhesion between the cochlear nerve and tumor may be the most significant prognostic factor with respect to hearing preservation.[16] A recent study used a machine learning algorithm to predict hearing preservation after MCF resection in 144 patients; the authors reported a 60% rate of hearing preservation with predictive model accuracy of 0.68.[33] It is also important to consider the durability of hearing preservation outcomes over time. Long-term data have demonstrated 49% to 84% rate of serviceable hearing several years after resection, suggesting sustained results.[4,39,43,60,61] We have previously reported hearing preservation rates of 81% in

Table 1
Summary of contemporary studies using the middle fossa approach for sporadic vestibular schwannoma resection

Study	Number of Patients	Mean Follow-Up (mo)	Mean Patient Age (y)	Mean Tumor Size (mm)	Preoperative Serviceable Hearing[a]	Hearing Preservation Rate	Postoperative AAO-HNS		Functional Facial Nerve Preservation[b]	Complications (N)		
							A	B		Infection	CSF Leak	Other
Ahmed et al,[29] 2018	159	-	49	9.3	145 (93.5%)	101 (70%)	50 (32%)	51 (32.9%)	132 (93%)	-	-	-
Arts et al,[13] 2006	73	-	-	8.9	62 (85%)	45 (72%)	21 (33%)	24 (39%)	69 (96%)	1	-	4 aseptic meningitis; 1 transient aphasia; 1 DVT 1 transient ulnar neuropathy
Dixon et al,[33] 2022	144	-	47	9.6	133 (93.4%)	86 (60%)	-	-	-	-	-	-
Kosty et al,[19] 2018	63	21	50	10	47 (76%)	22 (54%)	9 (22%)	13 (32%)	62 (98%)	3	2	1 CVA; 1 epidural hematoma; 3 DVT
Kohlberg et al,[31] 2021	67	18.2	50.2	10.1	51 (76%)	32 (47.7%)	-	-	60 (89.5%)	3	3	1 CVA; 2 DVT
La Monte et al,[20] 2022	63	-	47.4	11.5	63 (100%)	37 (58.7%)	29 (46%)	8 (12.7%)	-	-	-	-
Meyer et al,[12] 2006	162	-	49	<10[c]	124 (77%)	75 (60%)	46 (37%)	29 (23%)	157 (96%)	-	9	2 aseptic meningitis; 2 aphasia; 2 seizures
Raheja et al,[28] 2016	78	15.1	49	7.5	61 (78%)	38 (63%)	14 (23%)	24 (40%)	59 (90%)	3	0	0

Study														
Ren et al,[32] 2021	60	-	46.4	9.2	59 (98.3%)	31 (51.7%)	19 (31.7%)	12 (20.0%)	-	-	-	-	-	-
Roche et al,[45] 2017	13	169.2	67.1	8.7	13 (100%)	10 (77%)[d]	1 (7.6%)	2 (15.3%)	-	-	-	-	-	-
Vincent et al,[62] 2012	77	102	49	9	73 (95%)	46 (60%)	25 (32%)	21 (27%)	74 (96%)	-	-	-	-	-
Woodson et al,[37] 2010	49	70.5	48	<10[e]	46 (94%)	38 (83%)	16 (35%)[f]	22 (48%)[f]	49 (100%)	-	-	-	-	-

Abbreviations: AAO-HNS, American Academy of Otolaryngology-Head and Neck Surgery; CSF, cerebrospinal fluid leak; CVA, cerebrovascular accident; DVT, deep vein thrombosis.

[a] Serviceable hearing defined as WRS ≥50% and PTA ≤ 50 dB HL.

[b] Functional facial nerve preservation defined as House-Brackmann grade I or II.

[c] The authors reported tumor sizes in ranges, the majority (57%) were <10 mm in size, 21% were 11–14 mm, and 22% were 15 mm or larger.

[d] This rate of hearing preservation is based on WRS.

[e] All tumors in this series were less than 10 mm in size; mean size was not reported.

[f] PTA in the operated ear was adjusted for the change in PTA due to bilateral progressive sensorineural hearing loss seen in the nonoperated ear.

tumors less than 1 cm in size, with intact serviceable hearing at an average 14 years of follow-up.[4,12] For patients with a preserved auditory nerve following tumor removal that fail to maintain adequate hearing levels, a cochlear implant may provide auditory rehabilitation in appropriate cases.

SUMMARY

The MCF approach is an excellent technique for removing primarily intracanalicular VS in patients with serviceable hearing. Knowledge of the intricate middle fossa anatomy is essential to performing the procedure safely. With proper execution, the technique offers the ability for total tumor removal and preservation of hearing, with durable long-term results.

CLINICS CARE POINTS

- Ideal surgical candidates are patients with intracanalicular tumors, serviceable hearing with WRS >70%, and age <65 years.
- Identification of the superior semicircular canal is a key operative step, as this landmark keeps the surgeon oriented to the complex anatomy of the middle fossa.
- Craniotomy and temporal lobe retraction are generally well tolerated with rare sequelae.

DISCLOSURE

The authors disclose no conflicts of interest.

REFERENCES

1. House WF. Surgical exposure of the internal auditory canal and its contents through the middle, cranial fossa. Laryngoscope 1961;71:1363–85.
2. House WF, Gardner G, Hughes RL. Middle cranial fossa approach to acoustic tumor surgery. Arch Otolaryngol 1968;6:631–41.
3. Sun DQ, Sullivan CB, Kung RW, et al. How well does intraoperative audiologic monitoring predict hearing outcome during middle fossa vestibular schwannoma resection? Otol Neurotol 2018;39(7):908–15.
4. Roche JP, Woodson EA, Hansen MR, et al. Ultra long-term audiometric outcomes in the treatment of vestibular schwannoma with the middle cranial fossa approach. Otol Neurotol 2018;39:e151–7.
5. Brackmann DE, Owens RM, Friedman RA, et al. Prognostic factors for hearing preservation in vestibular schwannoma surgery. Am J Otol 2000;21:417–24.
6. Fouad A, Tran ED, Feng AY, et al. Stereotactic radiosurgery for vestibular schwannoma outcomes in patients with perfect word recognition-a retrospective cohort study. Otol Neurotol 2021;42:755–64.
7. Stangerup SE, Tos M, Thomsen J, et al. Hearing outcomes of vestibular schwannoma patients managed with 'wait and scan': predictive value of hearing level at diagnosis. J Laryngol Otol 2010;124:490–4.
8. Carlson ML, Jacob JT, Pollock BE, et al. Long-term hearing outcomes following stereotactic radiosurgery for vestibular schwannoma: patterns of hearing loss and variables influencing audiometric decline. J Neurosurg 2013;118:579–87.

9. Cohen NL, Lewis WS, Ransohoff J. Hearing preservation in cerebellopontine angle tumor surgery: the NYU experience 1974–1991. Am J Otol 1993;14: 423–33.

10. Nadol JB Jr, Levine R, Ojemann RG, et al. Preservation of hearing in surgical removal of acoustic neuromas of the internal auditory canal and cerebellar pontine angle. Laryngoscope 1987;97:1287–94.

11. Stangerup SE, Caye-Thomasen P, Tos M, et al. Change in hearing during 'wait and scan' management of patients with vestibular schwannoma. J Laryngol Otol 2008;122:673–81.

12. Meyer TA, Canty PA, Wilkinson EP, et al. Small acoustic neuromas: surgical outcomes versus observation or radiation. Otol Neurotol 2006;27:380–92.

13. Arts HA, Telian SA, El-Kashlan H, et al. Hearing preservation and facial nerve outcomes in vestibular schwannoma surgery: results using the middle cranial fossa approach. Otol Neurotol 2006;27:234–41.

14. Jacob A, Robinson LL Jr, Bortman JS, et al. Nerve of origin, tumor size, hearing preservation, and facial nerve outcomes in 359 vestibular schwannoma resections at a tertiary care academic center. Laryngoscope 2007;117:2087–92.

15. Shelton C, Brackmann DE, House WF, et al. Acoustic tumor surgery. Prognostic factors in hearing preservation. Arch Otolaryngol Head Neck Surg 1989;115: 1213–6.

16. Sameshima T, Fukushima T, McElveen JT Jr, et al. Critical assessment of operative approaches for hearing preservation in small acoustic neuroma surgery: retrosigmoid vs middle fossa approach. Neurosurgery 2010 Sep;67(3):640–4 [discussion: 644-5].

17. Misra BK, Purandare HR, Ved RS, et al. Current treatment strategy in the management of vestibular schwannoma. Neurol India 2009;57:257–63.

18. Peng KA, Wilkinson EP. Optimal outcomes for hearing preservation in the management of small vestibular schwannomas. J Laryngol Otol 2016;130:606–10.

19. Irving RM, Jackler RK, Pitts LH. Hearing preservation in patients undergoing vestibular schwannoma surgery: comparison of middle fossa and retrosigmoid approaches. J Neurosurg 1998;88(5):840–5.

20. La Monte OA, Tawfik KO, Khan U, et al. Analysis of hearing preservation in middle cranial fossa resection of vestibular schwannoma. Otol Neurotol 2022;43:395–9.

21. Goddard JC, Schwartz MS, Friedman RA. Fundal fluid as a predictor of hearing preservation in the middle cranial fossa approach for vestibular schwannoma. Otol Neurotol 2010;31:1128–34.

22. Prabhu V, Kondziolka D, Hill TC, et al. Preserved cochlear CISS signal is a predictor for hearing preservation in patients treated for vestibular schwannoma with stereotactic radiosurgery. Otol Neurotol 2018;39(5):628–31.

23. Patil CG, Veeravagu A, Lad SP, et al. Craniotomy for resection of meningioma in the elderly: a multicentre, prospective analysis from the National Surgical Quality Improvement Program. J Neurol Neurosurg Psychiatr 2010;81:502–5.

24. Rhoton AL Jr, Pulec JL, Hall GM, et al. Absence of bone over the geniculate ganglion. J Neurosurg 1968;28(1):48–53.

25. Fisch U. Transtemporal surgery of the internal auditory canal: report of 92 cases, technique indications, and results. Adv Oto-Rhino-Laryngol 1970;17:203–40.

26. Scheich M, Ginzkey C, Ehrmann-Müller D, et al. Management of CSF leakage after microsurgery for vestibular schwannoma via the middle cranial fossa approach. Eur Arch Oto-Rhino-Laryngol 2016;273(10):2975–81.

27. Lipschitz N, Kohlberg GD, Tawfik KO, et al. Cerebrospinal fluid leak rate after vestibular schwannoma surgery via middle cranial fossa approach. J Neurol Surg B Skull Base 2019;80(4):437–40.
28. Raheja A, Bowers CA, MacDonald JD, et al. Middle fossa approach for vestibular schwannoma: good hearing and facial nerve outcomes with low morbidity. World Neurosurg 2016;92:37–46.
29. Ahmed S, Arts HA, El-Kashlan H, et al. Immediate and long-term hearing outcomes with the middle cranial fossa approach for vestibular schwannoma resection. Otol Neurotol 2018;39:92–8.
30. Kosty JA, Stevens SM, Gozal YM, et al. Middle fossa approach for resection of vestibular schwannomas: a decade of experience. Oper Neurosurg (Hagerstown). 2019;16:147–58.
31. Kohlberg GD, Lipschitz N, Raghavan AM, et al. Middle cranial fossa approach to vestibular schwannoma resection in the older patient population. Otol Neurotol 2021;42:e75–81.
32. Ren Y, Merna CM, Tawfik KO, et al. Auditory brain stem response predictors of hearing outcomes after middle fossa resection of vestibular schwannomas. J Neurol Surg B Skull Base 2021;83:496–504.
33. Dixon PR, Wojdyla L, Lee J, et al. Machine learning to predict hearing preservation after middle cranial fossa approach for sporadic vestibular schwannomas. Otol Neurotol 2022;43:1072–7.
34. Sweeney AD, Carlson ML, Driscoll CLW. Surgical approach selection for vestibular schwannoma microsurgery. In: Carlson ML, Driscoll CLW, Link MJ, editors, editors. Comprehensive management of vestibular schwannoma. New York, 208–218, Stuttgart; Delhi; Rio de Janeiro: Thieme; 2019.
35. Seo JH, Jun BC, Jeon EJ, et al. Predictive factors influencing facial nerve outcomes in surgery for small-sized vestibular schwannoma. Acta Otolaryngol 2013;133(7):722–7.
36. Arriaga MA, Chen DA. Facial function in hearing preservation acoustic neuroma surgery. Arch Otolaryngol Head Neck Surg 2001;127(5):543–6.
37. Woodson EA, Dempewolf RD, Gubbels SP, et al. Long-term hearing preservation after microsurgical excision of vestibular schwannoma. Otol Neurotol 2010;31:1144–52.
38. Staecker H, Nadol JB Jr, Ojeman R, et al. Hearing preservation in acoustic neuroma surgery: middle fossa versus retrosigmoid approach. Am J Otol 2000;21:399–404.
39. Hilton CW, Haines SJ, Agrawal A, et al. Late failure rate of hearing preservation after middle fossa approach for resection of vestibular schwannoma. Otol Neurotol 2011;32:132–5.
40. Kutz JW Jr, Scoresby T, Isaacson B, et al. Hearing preservation using the middle fossa approach for the treatment of vestibular schwannoma. Neurosurgery 2012;70:334–40 [discussion: 40–1].
41. Chee GH, Nedzelski JM, Rowed D. Acoustic neuroma surgery: the results of long-term hearing preservation. Otol Neurotol 2003;24:672–6.
42. Holsinger FC, Coker NJ, Jenkins HA. Hearing preservation in conservation surgery for vestibular schwannoma. Am J Otol 2000;21:695–700.
43. Wang AC, Chinn SB, Than KD, et al. Durability of hearing preservation after microsurgical treatment of vestibular schwannoma using the middle cranial fossa approach. J Neurosurg 2013;119:131–8.
44. Shelton C, Hitselberger WE, House WF, et al. Hearing preservation after acoustic tumor removal: long-term results. Laryngoscope 1990;100:115–9.

45. Roche JP, Goates AJ, Hasan DM, et al. Treatment of Lateral Skull Base and Posterior Cranial Fossa Lesions Utilizing the Extended Middle Cranial Fossa Approach. Otol Neurotol 2017;38:742–50.
46. Angeli S. Middle fossa approach: indications, technique, and results. Otolaryngol Clin North Am 2012;45:417–38.
47. House JW. Translabyrinthine approach. In: Brackman DE, Shelton C, Arriaga MA, editors. Otologic Surgery. Philadelphia: W.B. Saunders; 1994. p. 606–16.
48. Filipo R, Delfini R, Fabiani M, et al. Role of transient-evoked otoacoustic emissions for hearing preservation in acoustic neuroma surgery. Am J Otol 1997;18: 746–9.
49. Hecht CS, Honrubia VF, Wiet RJ, et al. Hearing preservation after acoustic neuroma resection with tumor size used as a clinical prognosticator. Laryngoscope 1997;107:1122–6.
50. Monsell EM, Balkany TA, Gates GA, et al. Committee on Hearing and Equilibrium guidelines for the evaluation of hearing preservation in acoustic neuroma (vestibular schwannoma). American Academy of Otolaryngology Head and Neck Surgery Foundation, INC. Otolaryngol Head Neck Surg 1995;113:179–80.
51. Sughrue ME, Yang I, Aranda D, et al. Hearing preservation rates after microsurgical resection of vestibular schwannoma. J Clin Neurosci 2010;17:1126–9.
52. Stidham KR, Roberson JB. Implementation of a clinical pathway in management of the postoperative vestibular schwannoma patient. Laryngoscope 2001;111: 1938–43.
53. Cueva RA, Chole RA. Maximizing exposure of the internal auditory canal via the retrosigmoid approach: an anatomical, radiological, and surgical study. Otol Neurotol 2018;39:916–21.
54. Gjuric M, Rudic M. What is the best tumor size to achieve optimal functional results in vestibular schwannoma surgery? Skull Base 2008;18:317–25.
55. Hadjipanayis CG, Carlson ML, Link MJ, et al. Congress of neurological surgeons systematic review and evidence-based guidelines on surgical resection for the treatment of patients with vestibular schwannomas. Neurosurgery 2018;82: E40–3.
56. Nguyen QT, Wu AP, Mastrodimos BJ, et al. Impact of fundal extension on hearing after surgery for vestibular schwannomas. Otol Neurotol 2012;33:455–8.
57. Preet K, Ong V, Sheppard JP, et al. Postoperative hearing preservation in patients undergoing retrosigmoid craniotomy for resection of vestibular schwannomas: a systematic review of 2034 patients. Neurosurgery 2020;86:332–42.
58. Robinette MS, Bauch CD, Olsen WO, et al. Nonsurgical factors predictive of postoperative hearing for patients with vestibular schwannoma. Am J Otol 1997;18: 738–45.
59. Colletti V, Fiorino FG, Carner M, et al. Mechanisms of auditory impairment during acoustic neuroma surgery. Otolaryngol Head Neck Surg 1997;117:596–605.
60. Friedman RA, Kesser B, Brackmann DE, et al. Long-term hearing preservation after middle fossa removal of vestibular schwannoma. Otolaryngol Head Neck Surg 2003;129:660–5.
61. Quist TS, Givens DJ, Gurgel RK, et al. Hearing preservation after middle fossa vestibular schwannoma removal: are the results durable? Otolaryngol Head Neck Surg 2015;152:706–11.
62. Vincent C, Bonne NX, Guérin C, et al. Middle fossa approach for resection of vestibular schwannoma: impact of cochlear fossa extension and auditory monitoring on hearing preservation. Otol Neurotol 2012;33(5):849–52.

Retrosigmoid Approach for Sporadic Vestibular Schwannoma

Patient Selection, Technical Pearls, and Hearing Results

Jacob C. Lucas, MD[a], Caleb J. Fan, MD[a], Jeffrey T. Jacob, MD[b],
Seilesh C. Babu, MD[a],*

KEYWORDS

- Vestibular schwannoma • Acoustic neuroma • Retrosigmoid • Neurotology

KEY POINTS

- The retrosigmoid corridor provides the most broadly applied approach for resection of sporadic vestibular schwannoma.
- It may be utilized for any size tumor and for patients with intact hearing with the intention of hearing preservation.
- For larger tumors, the skull base surgeon must weigh the benefits the retrosigmoid approach against those of the translabyrinthine route. For smaller tumors where hearing preservation is a goal, the retrosigmoid approach is contrasted to the middle fossa route.
- Hearing preservation is most likely for patients with small and medially located intracanalicular tumors with minimal extension into the cerebellopontine angle, and excellent preoperative hearing.

INTRODUCTION, HISTORICAL CONTEXT, AND BACKGROUND

Microsurgical management of vestibular schwannoma (VS) has evolved over the past century and includes 3 primary neurotologic surgical approaches. The retrosigmoid (RS) corridor to the cerebellopontine angle (CPA) allows for generous anatomic exposure and the theoretical possibility of hearing preservation following complete extirpation of tumor. The first described route to the CPA was a variation of the RS approach, which used a unilateral suboccipital craniectomy associated with exceedingly high mortality, owing to the disruption of the principal blood supply to the brainstem, the

[a] Michigan Ear Institute, 30055 Northwestern Highway, Suite 101, Farmington Hills, MI 48334, USA; [b] Michigan Head and Spine Institute, 29275 Northwestern Highway, #100, Southfield, MI 48034, USA
* Corresponding author.
E-mail address: sbabu@michiganear.com

Otolaryngol Clin N Am 56 (2023) 509–520
https://doi.org/10.1016/j.otc.2023.02.010
0030-6665/23/© 2023 Elsevier Inc. All rights reserved.

need for cerebellar resection, and poor sterile technique[1]. Harvey Cushing popularized a bilateral suboccipital approach along with enucleation and subtotal resection of tumor to decrease mortality from greater than 84% down to around 4%. The wide decompression allowed for improved exposure along with decreased cerebral pressure, and subtotal resection was used to debulk tumor and limit damage to surrounding structures.[2] Walter Dandy further improved on this approach and began advocating for total resection resulting in similar mortalities but decreased recurrence.[3] Despite these advances in surgical technique, facial paralysis was the accepted norm, and a small price to pay for the removal of large compressive tumors. As stated by Dandy in his monograph, *Results of Removal of Acoustic Tumors by the Unilateral Approach* (1941):

> *Paralysis of the facial nerve must usually be accepted as a necessary sequel of the operation... Preservation of this nerve would be a most welcome addition to the operation, but its greatly attenuated size and its long course around the posterior wall of the tumor make this exceedingly difficult, for the present at least.*

William House[4] popularized the translabyrinthine (TL) and middle fossa (MF) approaches within the nascent field of neurotology, whereas the suboccipital approach remained the preferred technique within the neurosurgical community. As mortalities have declined and facial nerve outcomes have improved, a new focus on hearing preservation has emerged as a captivating outcome measure to the neurotologic community. The use of the RS approach has continued to hold favor among skull base surgeons as a hearing preservation approach, in contrast to its earlier role for radical resection of larger tumors. Its versatility for both large and small tumors makes this an attractive option when considering microsurgical removal of a vestibular schwannoma.

DISCUSSION
Surgical Indications

Any treatment discussion centered on vestibular schwannoma should revolve around 3 primary management options:

- Observation
- Microsurgical resection
- Gamma knife radiosurgery

The patient is counseled on the risks, benefits, and alternatives to proceeding with treatment (compared with observation with serial imaging).

- Observation remains a valid option for nearly all patients who are asymptomatic or minimally symptomatic, excepting patients with large tumors causing brainstem compression or hydrocephalus.
- In the authors' experience, gamma knife radiosurgery is reserved for patients with small to medium tumors demonstrating growth and without compression on the brainstem, who wish to avoid surgery or who are too frail to undergo surgical removal. However, some centers advocate for radiosurgical treatment as first-line management.[5]
- The decision to proceed with surgery is patient-centered, and the choice of approach is based on tumor size, location within the CPA, and internal auditory canal (IAC), hearing status, and surgeon preference.

The Surgical Approach: General Considerations

- For most tumors larger than 15 mm, there will be significant extension into the CPA necessitating either the RS or the TL approach.

- The primary advantage of the RS approach over the TL approach is preservation of the labyrinth and theoretical preservation of hearing. The RS approach allows for early entry into the CPA and identification of critical neurovascular elements. Cerebellar retraction and intradural drilling are necessary. Up to 3 mm of the lateral IAC will be obscured owing to the labyrinth and transverse crest.[6,7]
- As a hearing preservation approach, smaller tumors in the medial IAC with limited extension to the CPA are amenable to removal,[8] although most series cite an overall preservation rate less than 50%.
- Staged removal of very large or "giant" tumors (>4 cm) may be performed with a combination of RS and TL routes, with initial debulking followed by definitive removal of the IAC component. Facial outcomes may be more favorable when a planned staged approach is used.[9]

Preoperative Assessment

- A hearing evaluation, including pure tone audiometry and speech discrimination score, should always be obtained, especially in cases whereby hearing preservation is a goal.
- Preoperative imaging should include a gadolinium contrast MRI scan of the brain and IAC wherever possible. The route of the sigmoid and transverse sinuses and height of the jugular bulb are noted.
- The anticipated risks to proceeding with surgery are discussed and documented at length. The principal risks to hearing and the facial nerve are discussed. Additional risks include persistent postoperative headache, vestibular loss necessitating rehabilitation, cerebrospinal fluid (CSF) leak, stroke, and death.
- The pros and cons of the 3 principal approaches to the CPA are weighed with the patient. The ideal patient for a hearing preservation attempt with RS approach has a small tumor with limited extension toward the fundus, an anteriorly based sigmoid, a hypo-pneumatized mastoid and petrous bone, and excellent preoperative hearing. Hearing preservation is most likely if the tumor is limited to the IAC, or with minimal extension to the CPA.[10] **Fig. 1** demonstrates the MRI appearance and preoperative hearing status of a candidate patient for a hearing preservation attempt.

Patient Positioning

- The patient is positioned as per surgeon preference. The most common positioning is in the supine position. The head is flexed and turned with the shoulder extended to facilitate exposure of the suboccipital area. The Mayfield (Integra LifeSciences, Princeton, NJ) holder is used to pin the patient in position. Care is taken to avoid vascular compression, which can exacerbate cerebellar swelling.
- A "park bench" lateral decubitus position may be used with the head rotated contralaterally, flexed toward the chest, and flexed laterally toward the contralateral shoulder (**Fig. 2**A, B). This is the authors' preferred positioning. The patient is turned onto the contralateral side with slight flexion at the hips and knees. Blankets or padding can be placed in front of the patient with the ipsilateral arm draped over them. The contralateral arm is placed onto an arm board with ample padding. An axillary roll is helpful for arm positioning. All pressure points are padded.
- The "beach chair" semi-sitting position is an additional positioning consideration that is less frequently used owing to the extensive preparation time and increased risk of venous air embolism (VAE). However, there are some distinct advantages for the interested surgeon.[11,12] Additional intraoperative monitoring

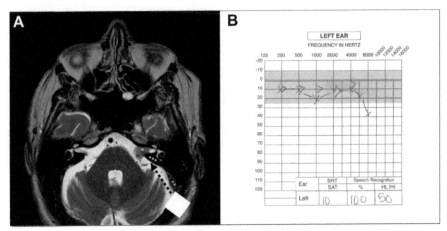

Fig. 1. A candidate patient for hearing preservation surgery via RS approach. (*A*) T2-weighted MRI sequence shows a mass consistent with vestibular schwannoma centered on the IAC with minimal extension into the CPA. Note the fundal fluid signal lateral to the tumor as well as the relationship of the vestibule and posterior semicircular canal to the IAC. (*asterisk*) Vestibular schwannoma; (*2 asterisks*) sigmoid sinus; (*3 asterisks*) IAC bone removed during intradural drilling. (*white box*) Craniotomy site; (*dashed arrow*) approach path from craniotomy site to tumor through the CPA. (*B*) The patient demonstrated excellent preoperative hearing with PTA of 10 dB and WRS (*inset*) of 100%. HL, hearing loss; SAT, speech attention threshold; SRT, speech reception threshold; WRS, word recognition score.

with transesophageal ultrasound allows for monitoring of air in the venous circulation so that VAE can be prevented.

Perioperative and Anesthetic Considerations

- Facial nerve electromyogram (EMG), auditory brainstem responses (ABR), and somatosensory potentials are monitored intraoperatively by a neuromonitoring team. Lower cranial nerves (eg, vagus nerve) may be monitored for large tumors through the use of an EMG-equipped endotracheal tube.
- Perioperative maneuvers to decrease swelling and intracranial pressure are used. Six to 10 mg of Dexamethasone and appropriate weight-based antibiotics are given preoperatively. Intracranial pressure is reduced with Mannitol 0.5 to 1 g/kg and hyperventilation to reach an end-tidal CO_2 between 25 and 30 mm Hg.
- Long-term paralytics are avoided owing to the need for continuous cranial nerve and somatosensory monitoring.

Preparation

- Hair posterior to the postauricular sulcus is liberally shaved toward the occiput. A C-shaped incision is marked posterior to the estimated location of the sigmoid sinus, approximately 4 to 5 cm back from the sulcus (see **Fig. 2A**).
- Local anesthetic with epinephrine is infiltrated.

Operative steps

- Incision is carried down through the skin and subcutaneous tissue exposing the deeper muscle and periosteal layer. A thick anteriorly based skin flap will help to facilitate water-tight closure at the conclusion of the case.

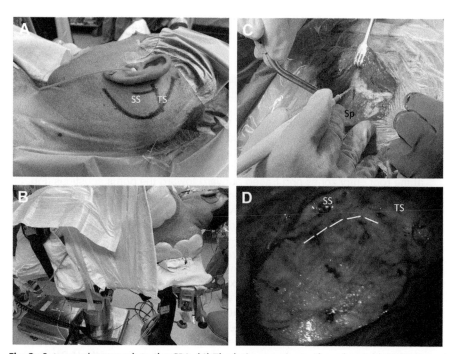

Fig. 2. Setup and approach to the CPA. (*A*) The hair posterior to the sulcus is liberally shaved 4 to 5 cm. A C-shaped incision is marked. The location of the transverse and sigmoid sinuses is estimated. (*B*) The patient is positioned in the lateral decubitus "park bench" position with adequate padding, and the Mayfield holder is secured. (*C*) The soft tissue exposure is performed by raising an anteriorly based skin flap. The splenius muscle is identified and reflected as an inferiorly based flap. (*D*) An approximately 3 × 3 cm craniotomy is designed. The junction of the transverse and sigmoid sinuses is identified to define the anteriosuperior limit of dissection. (*dotted line*) Durotomy incision just posterior to sigmoid sinus. Sp, splenius muscle; SS, sigmoid sinus; TS, transverse sinus.

- The bony cortex is further exposed by reflecting the splenius as an inferiorly based muscle flap (**Fig. 2**C). Care is taken to limit blind electrocautery dissection into the deeper inferior muscle attachments, as the vertebral artery is at risk of injury.
- A mastoid emissary vein is commonly encountered and can be controlled with electrocautery or bone wax.
- The craniotomy is bounded by the sigmoid sinus anteriorly and its confluence with the transverse sinus superiorly. The window size is based on surgeon preference but is generally around 3 × 3 cm (**Fig. 2**D).
- The craniotomy is drilled first with a large cutting bur and copious irrigation. As it is deepened, a diamond drill is used to eggshell the bone overlying the dura. Finally, the dura is elevated gently to avoid tearing. The junction of the transverse and sigmoid sinuses is most easily identified early during bony dissection and allows inferior tracing down along the sigmoid anteriorly. Neurotologists tend to have an affinity for skeletonization of the sigmoid during transtemporal approaches. To prevent excessive air cell exposure, however, the sigmoid is approached posteriorly, only exposing what is necessary for defining the bounds of the craniotomy. Alternatively, a bone flap craniectomy is developed with the

drill and craniotome footplate for later replacement. Burr holes can be placed and connected using rongeur forceps, with bone fragments saved for later use.

- The dura is opened, and tacking sutures are placed to secure the edges for later closure.
- The arachnoid is sharply lysed to begin drainage of the cisternal CSF fluid. Allowing adequate egress of CSF will facilitate relaxation of the cerebellar hemisphere and exposure of the CPA.
- At this point the CPA component of the tumor is identified, and dissection can begin. Use of a stimulating probe can help to identify the facial nerve, which may be draped on the surface of the tumor. The tumor is centrally debulked with an ultrasonic aspirator. The seventh and eighth nerves can then be identified at the root entry zones and traced outward toward the porus acusticus (**Fig. 3**). The cochlear nerve should be preserved as long as possible during the course of dissection even if hearing preservation is not a goal; this prevents the full weight of the tumor from causing traction on the facial nerve, especially through the cisternal segment.
- With the root entry zones dissected free and the tumor at least partially debulked within the cistern, the IAC component may be addressed. H-flaps are designed along the posterior petrous face to expose the bony IAC. As in all approaches to the IAC, wide exposure is achieved with careful drilling of superior and inferior troughs to provide 270° or more of IAC dura. The featureless petrous face forces careful and steady drilling to blue-line the IAC and identify the superior and inferior troughs. Laterally, the posterior semicircular canal and vestibule are at risk of violation and may be blue-lined with the drill as well. The dura of the IAC is sharply opened; tumor dissection continues within the intracanalicular segment, and the vestibular nerves are identified and sharply transected. At this point, there is frequently some blind dissection performed, as the most lateral aspect of the tumor may not be visible through direct line of sight. As the IAC component is rolled

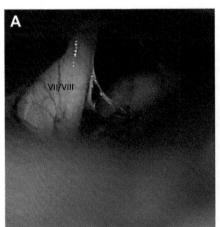 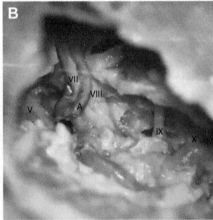

Fig. 3. CPA as viewed through RS craniotomy. (*A*) Intraoperative photograph of the cistern as the IAC is approached. The 7/8 nerve complex is seen bridging from the root entry zone to the porus acusticus. (*B*) Cadaveric depiction of the CPA through an RS view; porus drilled to highlight the relationship of the facial and vestibulocochlear nerve. A, AICA loop; IX, glossopharyngeal nerve; V, trigeminal nerve; VII, facial nerve; VIII, vestibulocochlear nerve; X, vagus nerve.

medially, the lateral surface of the tumor is seen to confirm adequate removal. If the smooth edge of the tumor is not visualized, there may be a transected component of the tumor left behind.

- With the CPA and IAC components mobilized, the last of the tumor is dissected from the cisternal facial nerve and cochlear nerve if preserved.
- The CPA is irrigated copiously to clear any remaining blood, bone dust, and debris.
- Open air cells within the IAC should be sealed off with bone wax to achieve as tight a closure as possible and prevent CSF fistula.
- A water-tight dural closure is performed with Nurolon (Ethicon, Somerville, NJ) suture. Collagen-based dural grafting material can be used to augment this closure along with a synthetic dural glue.
- The authors again emphasize the importance of sealing off any exposed mastoid air cells with bone wax. A highly pneumatized mastoid compartment may extend as far posteriorly as the RS craniotomy site. Waxing these cells is critical to prevent CSF fistula.
- A cranioplasty is finally performed, with either titanium plate, replacement of bone flap, or hydroxyapatite sealant. The authors frequently use hydroxyapatite cement to perform a water-tight cranioplasty with excellent results.
- The periosteal and muscle layers are closed tightly overlying the craniotomy with buried absorbable Vicryl (Ethicon, Somerville, NJ) sutures. Resuspension of the splenius muscle can provide an additional deep layer of closure. The dermis of the skin flap is closed tightly in a similar fashion. The skin is closed with nonabsorbable Prolene (Ethicon, Somerville, NJ) suture in a running locking fashion.

Complications

- The RS approach is associated with an increased incidence of headache (17%) and CSF leak (10%) as compared with the other approaches in one systematic review.[13]
- Vascular complications are fortunately rare but include postoperative hemorrhage or hematoma formation in the CPA, Anterior Inferior Cerebellar Artery (AICA) infarction causing disruption of the cerebellar peduncle and pons, and intrapontine hemorrhage or infarction.
- Facial nerve outcomes are similar to the TL approach and may be superior to the MF approach, with greater than 90% of patients achieving House-Brackmann I or II at 1-year follow-up.[14]

SELECTED HEARING PRESERVATION RESULTS

As tumor size increases, the likelihood of hearing preservation decreases in a predictable fashion.[15,16] Patient factors, such as a fundal fluid "cap," lateral tumor extension, and preoperative hearing status, all may play variable roles in the success of hearing preservation attempts in both microsurgical and radiosurgical management. [17–19] However, tumor size seems to be the predominant factor in hearing preservation likelihood.[10,20] The removal of very small tumors, especially in asymptomatic patients, is an area of intense controversy and debate within the neurotologic community; the treatment paradigm for these tumors is constantly changing, and in recent years, there has been a distinct shift in thinking toward observation rather than microsurgical removal, with similar long-term hearing preservation rates to microsurgery.[21]

The bulk of hearing preservation data comes from single-institution case series. A recent systematic review by Preet and colleagues[10] seems to be among the most

Table 1
Recently reported hearing preservation rates for retrosigmoid approach

Study	Design	No. of Patients	Hearing Preservation Rate	Author Conclusions
Zhu et al,[22] 2018	Retrospective case series	110 patients with small vs undergoing retrosigmoid (RS) approach vs 160 patients undergoing serial observation	Surgery: Serviceable hearing, 59.3% Observation: Serviceable hearing, 48.7% at 7 y follow-up	Tumor removal should be first-line treatment for young patients with small tumors and good preoperative hearing
Mazzoni et al,[23] 2018	Retrospective case series	100 patients underwent RS approach for VS	52% maintained serviceable hearing in the overall cohort; 91% of patients with word recognition score of >70, PTA <30, and tumor size <10 mm maintained serviceable hearing	Hearing preservation was dependent on tumor size and preoperative hearing status
Breun et al,[24] 2019	Retrospective case series	367 patients with small, medium, or large tumors had preoperative serviceable hearing	31.6% maintained serviceable hearing	Functional hearing preservation is possible but dependent on size and preoperative hearing status
Huo et al,[25] 2019	Retrospective case series	138 patients with small or medium tumors and serviceable preoperative hearing (MF and RS approaches were pooled)	58% maintained serviceable hearing in the RS group, 56% in the MF group. There was no statistically significant difference between MF and RS approaches	Better preoperative hearing, shorter hearing loss period, tumors from superior vestibular nerve, and normal wave I on ABR were associated with serviceable postoperative hearing
Tawfik et al,[26] 2020	Retrospective case series	153 patients with word recognition score of at least 50%	41.8% overall maintained serviceable hearing, 57.6% with intracanalicular tumors maintained serviceable hearing	Smaller tumors and class A preoperative hearing were positive predictors of hearing preservation

Zanoletti et al,[27] 2020	Retrospective case series	100 patients with serviceable preoperative hearing (93 with AAO class A or B)	47% of patients with preoperative class A or B hearing maintained serviceable postoperative hearing	Preoperative hearing status and tumor size were correlated with postoperative hearing outcome
Wallerius et al,[28] 2022	Retrospective case series	243 patients with serviceable hearing (RS or MF approach)	Tumor confined to IAC: 64% Tumor with <15 mm CPA extension: 28% Tumor with >15 mm CPA extension: 9%	The strongest predictor of hearing preservation after microsurgery is tumor size
Yancey et al,[29] 2022	Retrospective case series	130 patients underwent treatment with gamma knife or surgery	40% preservation with gamma knife 69% preservation with MF 31% preservation with RS	Surgery provided more durable hearing preservation than gamma knife at long-term follow-up
Bozhkov et al,[30] 2022	Retrospective case series	138 patients underwent RS approach	83% preservation for tumors <12 mm 30% preservation for tumors between 12 and 25 mm 5% preservation for tumors >25 mm	Surgery on small tumors can achieve excellent hearing preservation. Size is more important than anatomic relationship
Preet et al,[10] 2019	Systematic review and meta-analysis	2034 pooled patients across 26 studies with preoperative serviceable hearing underwent RS approach for VS	57% preservation for intracanalicular tumors; 37% for small tumors; 12% for large tumors	Hearing preservation rates ranged from 0% to 100%. Using a random effects model, the aggregate hearing preservation rate for RS was 35%

comprehensive examinations of the RS approach for hearing preservation, having examined 2034 patients with preoperative serviceable hearing from a total of 26 studies over a span of 20 years. Overall hearing preservation of the pooled cohort was 35% in a random effects model. Based on tumor size, preservation of hearing occurred in 57%, 37%, and 12% for intracanalicular, small, and large tumors, respectively. The reported hearing preservation rates from this and a selection of recent (within the past 5 years) larger series are included in **Table 1**.[10,22–30] Overall rates of serviceable hearing are modest when contrasted to the best case series for the MF approach.

Patients with small, ideally intracanalicular tumors and excellent, ideally American Academy of Otolaryngology - Head and Neck Surgery (AAO-HNS) class A hearing (>70% word recognition and <30 dB pure tone average)[31] are the best candidates for a hearing preservation approach. A conservative *general* estimate for any given patient in this group is a 50/50 chance of serviceable hearing following surgical removal. The most widely accepted definition of "serviceable hearing" is a word discrimination score of 50% and a pure tone average of less than 50,[32] corresponding to 1995 AAO-HNS class A and B hearing. Of note, the 1995 A to D classification system continues to be used in outcomes reporting, although the updated 2012 system[33] now encourages outcome reporting in a raw scattergram so that the data granularity may be better preserved and standardized across studies. Despite this, the imperfect "50/50" rule has endured.

In the outcomes reporting, a patient with excellent preoperative hearing may have a postoperative hearing outcome of 50% speech discrimination and a pure tone average of 50 dB—this would be considered a success! Clearly, outcomes are imperfectly reported; nonetheless, for an appropriately selected patient, the promise of preserved hearing after surgery remains enticing to both patients and surgeons alike.

In the discussion of hearing outcomes following acoustic tumor surgery, the authors disclose one additional caveat. Hearing rehabilitation with cochlear implantation is emerging as an effective and durable option in any patient with an intact cochlear nerve following surgery.[34] Cochlear implantation can be performed concurrent with tumor removal, for example, during a TL approach, or as a staged rehabilitative procedure following any approach to the IAC as long as the cochlear nerve is preserved. Although native hearing is not preserved, the possibility of hearing rehabilitation is an emerging option further complicating discussion.

CLINICS CARE POINTS

- The retrosigmoid approach is versatile and widely applied to any sporadic vestibular schwannoma. It can be used for small tumors for hearing preservation, large tumors, or as part of a staged resection for very large tumors.
- Hearing preservation rates following microsurgery are similar to that of the middle fossa approach.
- Tumor size and preoperative hearing status are the most important predictors of success with a hearing preservation attempt.

DISCLOSURE

The authors have no disclosures or financial interests related to the present article.

REFERENCES

1. Krause F. Zur Freilegung der hinteren Felsenbeinflache und des Kleinhirns. Beitr Klin Chir 1903;37:728–64.
2. Cushing H.,Tumors of the Nervus Acusticus and the Syndrome of the cerebello-pontile angle, Saunders Company, Philedelphia and London.
3. Dandy WE. Results of Removal of Acoustic Tumors by the Unilateral Approach. Arch Surg 1941;42(6):1026.
4. House WF. Transtemporal Bone Microsurgical Removal of Acoustic Neuromas. Arch Otolaryngol 1964;80:731–42.
5. Johnson S, Kano H, Faramand A, et al. Long term results of primary radiosurgery for vestibular schwannomas. J Neuro Oncol 2019;145(2):247–55.
6. Haberkamp TJ, Meyer GA, Fox M. Surgical exposure of the fundus of the internal auditory canal: anatomic limits of the middle fossa versus the retrosigmoid trans-canal approach. Laryngoscope 1998;108(8 Pt 1):1190–4.
7. Kartush JM, Telian SA, Graham MD, et al. Anatomic basis for labyrinthine preservation during posterior fossa acoustic tumor surgery. Laryngoscope 1986;96(9 Pt 1):1024–8.
8. Yamakami I, Yoshinori H, Saeki N, et al. Hearing preservation and intraoperative auditory brainstem response and cochlear nerve compound action potential monitoring in the removal of small acoustic neurinoma via the retrosigmoid approach. J Neurol Neurosurg Psychiatry 2009;80(2):218–27.
9. Porter RG, LaRouere MJ, Kartush JM, et al. Improved facial nerve outcomes using an evolving treatment method for large acoustic neuromas. Otol Neurotol 2013;34(2):304–10.
10. Preet K, Ong V, Sheppard JP, et al. Postoperative Hearing Preservation in Patients Undergoing Retrosigmoid Craniotomy for Resection of Vestibular Schwannomas: A Systematic Review of 2034 Patients. Neurosurgery 2020;86(3):332–42.
11. Scheller C, Rampp S, Tatagiba M, et al. A critical comparison between the semi-sitting and the supine positioning in vestibular schwannoma surgery: subgroup analysis of a randomized, multicenter trial. J Neurosurg 2019;3:1–8.
12. Arambula AM, Wichova H, Lucas JC, et al. Analysis of Imaging Results for Semi-sitting Compared with Supine Positioning in the Retrosigmoid Approach for Resection of Cerebellopontine Angle Vestibular Schwannomas. Otol Neurotol 2023;21. https://doi.org/10.1097/MAO.0000000000003814.
13. Ansari SF, Terry C, Cohen-Gadol AA. Surgery for vestibular schwannomas: a systematic review of complications by approach. Neurosurg Focus 2012;33(3):E14.
14. Lalwani AK, Butt FY, Jackler RK, et al. Facial nerve outcome after acoustic neuroma surgery: a study from the era of cranial nerve monitoring. Otolaryngol Head Neck Surg 1994;111(5):561–70.
15. Yates PD, Jackler RK, Satar B, et al. Is it worthwhile to attempt hearing preservation in larger acoustic neuromas? Otol Neurotol 2003;24(3):460–4.
16. Gjuric M, Rudic M. What is the best tumor size to achieve optimal functional results in vestibular schwannoma surgery? Skull Base 2008;18(5):317–25.
17. Goddard JC, Schwartz MS, Friedman RA. Fundal fluid as a predictor of hearing preservation in the middle cranial fossa approach for vestibular schwannoma. Otol Neurotol 2010;31(7):1128–34.
18. Bojrab DI, Fritz CG, Lin KF, et al. A Protective Cap: Fundal Fluid Cap Facilitates a Reduction in Inner Ear Radiation Dose in the Radiosurgical Treatment of Vestibular Schwannoma. Otol Neurotol 2021;42(2):294–9.

19. La Monte OA, Tawfik KO, Khan U, et al. Analysis of Hearing Preservation in Middle Cranial Fossa Resection of Vestibular Schwannoma. Otol Neurotol 2022; 43(3):395–9.
20. Mohr G, Sade B, Dufour JJ, et al. Preservation of hearing in patients undergoing microsurgery for vestibular schwannoma: degree of meatal filling. J Neurosurg 2005;102(1):1–5.
21. Khandalavala KR, Saba ES, Kocharyan A, et al. Hearing Preservation in Observed Sporadic Vestibular Schwannoma: A Systematic Review. Otol Neurotol 2022;43(6):604–10.
22. Zhu W, Chen H, Jia H, et al. Long-Term Hearing Preservation Outcomes for Small Vestibular Schwannomas: Retrosigmoid Removal Versus Observation. Otol Neurotol 2018;39(2):e158–65.
23. Mazzoni A, Zanoletti E, Denaro L, et al. Retrolabyrinthine meatotomy as part of retrosigmoid approach to expose the whole internal auditory canal: rationale, technique, and outcome in hearing preservation surgery for vestibular schwannoma. Oper Neurosurg Hagerstown Md 2018;14(1):36–44.
24. Breun M, Nickl R, Perez J, et al. Vestibular Schwannoma Resection in a Consecutive Series of 502 Cases via the Retrosigmoid Approach: Technical Aspects, Complications, and Functional Outcome. World Neurosurg 2019;129:e114–27.
25. Huo Z, Chen J, Wang Z, et al. Prognostic Factors of Long-Term Hearing Preservation in Small and Medium-Sized Vestibular Schwannomas After Microsurgery. Otol Neurotol 2019;40(7):957–64.
26. Tawfik KO, Alexander TH, Saliba J, et al. The Effect of Tumor Size on Likelihood of Hearing Preservation After Retrosigmoid Vestibular Schwannoma Resection. Otol Neurotol 2020;41(10):e1333–9.
27. Zanoletti E, Mazzoni A, Frigo AC, et al. Hearing Preservation Outcomes and Prognostic Factors in Acoustic Neuroma Surgery: Predicting Cutoffs. Otol Neurotol 2020;41(5):686–93.
28. Wallerius KP, Macielak RJ, Lawlor SK, et al. Hearing Preservation Microsurgery in Vestibular Schwannomas: Worth Attempting in "Larger" Tumors? Laryngoscope 2022;132(8):1657–64.
29. Yancey KL, Barnett SL, Kutz W, et al. Hearing Preservation After Intervention in Vestibular Schwannoma. Otol Neurotol 2022;43(8):e846–55.
30. Bozhkov Y, Shawarba J, Feulner J, et al. Prediction of Hearing Preservation in Vestibular Schwannoma Surgery According to Tumor Size and Anatomic Extension. Otolaryngol Head Neck Surg 2022;166(3):530–6.
31. Committee on Hearing and Equilibrium guidelines for the evaluation of hearing preservation in acoustic neuroma (vestibular schwannoma). J Am Acad Otolaryngol-Head Neck Surg 1995;113(3):179–80.
32. Wade PJ, House W. Hearing preservation in patients with acoustic neuromas via the middle fossa approach. Otolaryngol Head Neck Surg 1984;92(2):184–93.
33. Gurgel RK, Jackler RK, Dobie RA, et al. A new standardized format for reporting hearing outcome in clinical trials. Otolaryngol Head Neck Surg 2012;147(5):803–7.
34. Conway RM, Tu NC, Sioshansi PC, et al. Early Outcomes of Simultaneous Translabyrinthine Resection and Cochlear Implantation. Laryngoscope 2021;131(7):E2312–7.

Radiation for Sporadic Vestibular Schwannoma

An Update on Modalities, Emphasizing Hearing Loss, Side Effects, and Tumor Control

Erika Woodson, MD, FACS

KEYWORDS

- Vestibular schwannoma • Stereotactic radiosurgery • Gamma knife
- Acoustic neuroma • Hearing preservation • LINAC • Cyberknife

KEY POINTS

- Stereotactic radiosurgery is a well-established modality to control vestibular schwannoma growth. Most patients receive durable tumor control. Tumor control is relatively consistent among modalities.
- Stereotactic radiosurgery does not improve survival of serviceable hearing above natural history.
- Potential sequalae of stereotactic radiosurgery include hearing loss, facial nerve dysfunction (paresis or spasm), trigeminal neuralgia, hydrocephalus, and rarely, brain edema or necrosis.
- Differentiating between true treatment failure and pseudoprogression requires serial imaging for several years after initial treatment.
- Stereotactic radiosurgery has an emerging role in the adjuvant treatment of vestibular schwannoma after subtotal and near-total resection.

INTRODUCTION

Vestibular schwannomas (VS) are benign tumors of the vestibulocochlear nerve that frequently present with hearing loss. Historically, VS were typically diagnosed when large and surgical removal was the only available method of treatment.

Stereotactic radiosurgery (SRS) emerged in the late 1970s as a treatment modality for VS. Claims data in the United States have demonstrated that the use of SRS has increased, whereas the number of tumors receiving microsurgery or being observed has been relatively static. Bashjawish and colleagues[1] determined that treatment

The author has no financial relationships to disclose.
Kaiser Permanente—Southern California, San Diego, 5893 Copley Drive, San Diego, CA 92111, USA
E-mail address: Erika.x.woodson@kp.org

Otolaryngol Clin N Am 56 (2023) 521–531
https://doi.org/10.1016/j.otc.2023.02.011
0030-6665/23/© 2023 Elsevier Inc. All rights reserved.

trends were based on tumor size, with 1- to 2-cm tumors more likely to be treated with SRS than observation or microsurgery.

When counseled of their treatment options, patients with a new diagnosis of a small- or medium-sized VS are typically given 3 options: observation, microsurgery, and SRS. Stratifying which of those options may be best for the individual patient is the duty of the entire skull base team in conjunction with the patient through a process of shared decision making. This stratification is based on several factors, including patient age, comorbidities, tumor size and growth rate (if known), symptoms of or imaging findings of mass effect, hearing status, and patient preference.

DEFINITIONS

Several definitions are important to understand before embarking on a discussion of SRS with respect to VS treatment.

- *Stereotactic radiosurgery:* As defined by the National Cancer Institute, "A type of external radiation therapy that uses special equipment to position the patient and precisely give a... single fraction of radiation to a tumor."[2] Traditionally, the term SRS referred to single-fraction treatment. However, now SRS may also refer to 3 to 5 fractions delivered via stereotaxis.
- *Hypofractionation:* Radiation prescriptions call for delivery of a certain number of Gray delivered over a certain number of treatment days. Frequently, SRS is delivered as a single fraction, compared with conventional external beam radiation, which is divided into 25 or 30 fractions (treatment dates). Hypofractionation refers to treatments delivered over 3 to 5 days (fractions), and it is frequently used with linear accelerator modalities.
- *Cochlear dose:* The cochlear dose is the dose of radiation delivered to the cochlea during SRS treatment. It is calculated in the planning software and can be expressed in several ways: point dose to the modiolus, average dose, and maximal dose are the most common. The accuracy of calculating cochlear dose will be dependent on accurate delineation of the cochlea and modiolus in the planning software (**Fig. 1**).

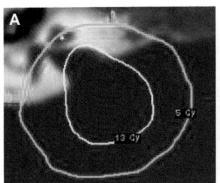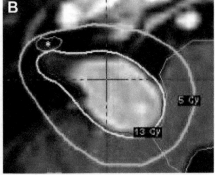

Fig. 1. Cochlear dose shown in treatment planning software (Gamma Knife). (*A*) The author prefers to use the bone window on the computed tomographic scan for coregistration to most accurately map out the cochlea (*) and modiolus. Despite the medial location of the tumor, the majority of this modiolus received 5 Gy. (*B*) One can appreciate that there is poor definition of the cochlea (*) on the MRI sequence. This basal turn of cochlea (*) also received 5 Gy.

- *Serviceable hearing:* Serviceable hearing is defined by the patient's ability to successfully listen and understand with the tumor ear. Hearing at serviceable levels predicts that a patient would generally benefit from hearing amplification. Serviceable hearing is most commonly defined by 2 classification schemes: the Gardner-Robertson Scale and the American Academy of Otolaryngology Head and Neck Surgery reporting standard for VS.[3,4] Although there are differences between scales in assessing grades of hearing based on pure tone average (PTA), and speech discrimination score (SDS), both systems typically designate hearing better than 50-dB PTA and 50% SDS as serviceable.

TECHNIQUES
Modalities and Biological Differences

Several modalities of SRS are used today. The most common modality is Gamma Knife (GK) radiosurgery, followed by linear accelerator (LINAC), and proton beam strategies. Rarely, intensity-modulated radiation therapy is used.

Gamma knife

Gamma Knife (Elekta, Stockholm, Sweden) is a treatment modality that uses gamma decay of Cobalt 60 sources arranged spherically within the unit. The SRS is delivered by precise louvres that open and shut, exposing the sources in varying degrees and times, delivering up to 192 beams of gamma radiation to converge in a precise target with a single-shot margin of error of less than 0.1 mm.[5] Classically, GK is delivered as a single fraction, using a headframe and pins to secure the patient position for the treatment. Treatment times for GK vary according to the age of the cobalt sources, size, and shape of the tumor. The dose is typically 12 to 13 Gy to the 50% isodose line.

Gamma Knife's chief advantage is its precision. It has a very sharp dose fall-off, which minimizes radiation to the surrounding tissue. A relative disadvantage of the GK is head frame fixation. Although it allows for secure patient positioning, frame placement demands local anesthetic and anxiolysis, such as intravenous midazolam. Patients with significant kyphosis or prior craniectomies may be challenging frame placements. These systems are also limited in their ability to access a tumor extending into the neck, for example, a cervical schwannoma or jugular paraganglioma.

The newest iteration of GK, the Leksell Gamma Knife Icon, has an integrated cone-beam computed tomography that allows treatment to be delivered via mask fixation. Treatment can then be hypofractionated or delivered in a single fraction. Because the radiation sources are fixed in position, the tolerance for patient movement is very low. The cone beam detects patient movement such that if patient movement falls out of the parameters for precise delivery (1 mm), the machine will stop treatment. With such low tolerance for movements, not all patients may be able to lay still enough for mask-based GK treatment.

Linear accelerator

LINAC is commonly used to deliver single-fraction or hypofractionated treatment. Common examples of LINAC include Novalis (Varian Medical Systems, Palo Alto, CA, USA, and BrainLAB, Feldkirchen, Germany) and Cyberknife (Accuray, Sunnyvale, CA, USA; using a robotic arm-mount multileaf collimator). Photons are delivered by a gantry that moves around the patient. Mask fixation is used rather than frame. Cyberknife touts submillimeter precision for its treatment delivery system; however, a 1-mm margin of error is more reasonable to expect.[6]

LINAC is typically delivered in a hypofractionated scheme of 3 to 5 treatments for VS, with total doses of 18 to 24 and 20 to 25 Gy, respectively. The prescription delivers a higher total dose of radiation to the tumor than a single-fraction GK scheme, because the hypofractionation allows for some normal tissue recovery between treatment doses.

Proton beam

Proton beam therapy (PBT) is a modality of stereotactic radiation that may be delivered in a single fraction or fractionated scheme. Protons are generated in a particle accelerator and delivered by a gantry that moves around the patient and also requires mask fixation. There are major biological differences between protons and photons (LINAC) worth noting. One major difference between protons and gamma rays or photons is how the particle behaves after it enters the body. Protons penetrate a certain distance into the tissue and then release energy (Bragg peak).[7] If a plan is designed well, the Bragg peak will cause maximal energy delivery to the tumor with negligible "exit dose" to normal tissue. In contrast, gamma rays and photon (LINAC) rays travel completely through the body and therefore expose normal tissue along the entire beam route to the radiation (constant albeit small amounts).

In the skull base, the Bragg peak has a potential disadvantage: the proton beam penetration is more erratic and less consistent than in supratentorial intra-axial lesions. The highly variable density of tissues in the beam's path (eg, mastoid and otic capsule) cause lateral scattering of the protons and unavoidable range uncertainties.[8] If the energy peak occurs at the perimeter of or outside the tumor, then toxicity to normal tissue will occur. These density factors affect scatter and target delivery for gamma and photon beams as well, but they have less potential for harm, as these beams do not release a burst of energy along their paths.

HEARING RESULTS

Initial enthusiasm for SRS stemmed from its promise as a potentially less-invasive modality that permitted hearing preservation (HP). Although reports indicated good short-term HP rates, evidence indicated that rates of serviceable hearing at 5 and 10 years or beyond are less encouraging. Coughlin and colleagues[9] determined that the overall 10-year survival of serviceable hearing after SRS was 29% in a systematic review.

Multiple series of pooled outcomes have identified predictive factors for maintaining hearing after SRS. These risk factors include marginal tumor dose ≤12 Gy, cochlear dose less than 4 Gy, and the related size of the lateral cerebrospinal fluid fundal cap, pretreatment hearing thresholds, tumor size, and pretreatment growth rate.[10–12] Perhaps the most important predictor of serviceable HP after SRS is pretreatment hearing thresholds: people with more residual hearing at baseline have more hearing that can be lost before acquiring nonserviceable hearing. In addition, much scrutiny has been placed on treatment dose, modality, and fractionation scheme as possible factors without consistent conclusions. The most recent systematic review and meta-analysis concluded that HP at mean follow-up of 6.7 years was 59% overall, with no statistically significant difference between LINAC and GK modalities.[10] High heterogenicity between studies has been noted throughout the literature, in addition to bias, which hinders strong conclusions from the multiple systematic reviews and meta-analyses on the topic.

Some radiosurgeons promote an upfront approach to treating VS immediately at the time of diagnosis, arguing that patients treated at time of diagnosis rather than after a period of observation had better hearing results.[13] However, this premise ignores the fact that patients undergoing SRS after observation are doing so for a reason, typically growth. If one radiates both growing and quiescent tumors indiscriminately, hearing results should be better than if only growing tumors were selected for treatment. Data however suggest that observed patients experiencing growth trend toward better long-term HP after SRS compared with continued observation.[14]

Importantly, the same factors that render a tumor favorable with regards to HP for one modality also render it favorable for others. If one extrapolates the natural history of hearing in an observed intracanalicular tumor, which presents with class A/GR 1 hearing, that individual is likely to retain class A hearing over time without treatment: 81% at a mean of 8.9 years.[15] Similarly, 88% of patients with normal pretreatment hearing retained GR 1 levels after GK.[16] Furthermore, HP for these ideal patients after microsurgery via middle cranial fossa also do very well. Thus far, evidence-based guidelines suggest that SRS, natural history, and microsurgery each have a moderately high probability of preserving hearing at 5 years in this best-case-scenario patient.[12]

In other words, if cared for by an experienced center, patient- and tumor-related factors predict long-term HP best, compared with which management strategy is used. This brings up the very important consideration of selection bias seen from single-center experiences. Centers that favor one modality, such as SRS or microsurgery for HP, will tend to select optimal patients for this treatment and report good outcomes, whereas potentially similar outcomes may be observed with other modalities in that same population. Importantly, no randomized controlled trials have been completed comparing all 3 management strategies for small VS, and it is unlikely that this study will ever take place given patients' and providers' reluctance to allocate treatment pathway to chance.

Symptoms and Side Effects of Stereotactic Radiosurgery

An informed discussion with the patient about their treatment options must include symptoms and side effects of each modality, and a careful comparison to other treatment options for a tumor of similar size, in a patient with similar hearing and symptoms.

Dizziness/imbalance

Most patients do not present with bothersome dizziness or vertigo when their tumor diagnosis is made; however, if present, dizziness or vertigo is a prominent predictor for reduced long-term overall quality of life (QOL).[17] Observed patients will notice balance changes over time, although typically there is no acute or abrupt change in function or QOL score. Patients treated with SRS will likewise report dizziness and balance changes affecting their QOL over time, like patients being observed.[18] In contrast, microsurgery tends to cause acute vertigo and imbalance owing to the ablation of any residual vestibular function. This postoperative change can have a lasting effect on dizziness handicap inventory as well as Penn Acoustic Neuroma Quality-of-Life scores.[19] SRS rarely has such an effect on vestibular function, meaning that there is no abrupt drop in QOL. The long-term differences in QOL for dizziness and imbalance are statistically worse (but clinically equivocal) for microsurgery versus observation and SRS.[20] Therefore, avoidance of the expected vestibular symptoms after microsurgery may steer the recommendation toward SRS, especially for those individuals who may not compensate well, such as those with poor vision, peripheral neuropathy, or other central confounders, such as Parkinsonism or poor baseline functional status.

Facial nerve dysfunction

Facial paralysis or paresis is a risk to any patient with VS undergoing treatment, especially microsurgery. As tumor size increases, the likelihood of postoperative facial paresis increases. Overall, primary SRS has significantly lower odds of causing facial nerve dysfunction after treatment, which meta-analyses have demonstrated even with intracanalicular tumors at long-term follow-up (1% vs 11).[21]

Marginal dose appears to be a factor in facial nerve dysfunction. Risk of facial neuropathy after SRS is higher after LINAC versus GK and highest in fractionated stereotactic radiotherapy (proton or photon) (**Table 1**).[10,22,23] A high rate of facial paresis was noted after fractionated PBT (28%, in a single-institution study); however, patients receiving PBT in this study had significantly larger tumors—another risk factor for posttreatment dysfunction.[8] Although facial nerve paresis is relatively uncommon after SRS, temporary facial spasm occurs in approximately 5% of people, most typically between 4 and 12 months after treatment. This typically resolves with time and potential medical therapy.

Trigeminal neuralgia

Trigeminal neuropathy typically refers to hemifacial hypoesthesia, whereas trigeminal neuralgia (TN) indicates sharp, electric shock–like pain. Like hemifacial spasm, TN may also be a complication/side effect of SRS. Patients with preexisting mass effect on the root entry zone of the trigeminal nerve are at particular risk for developing new TN posttreatment. Like facial nerve dysfunction, the risk of TN posttreatment is higher in fractionated treatments with higher total doses (**Table 2**).[10,22,23]

Trigeminal symptoms pretreatment should trigger the skull base surgeon to recommend microsurgery over SRS for relief, as SRS is unlikely to resolve these symptoms. A meta-analysis looking specifically at VS-related TN yielded only a 50% rate of resolution after SRS and noted that tumor shrinkage posttreatment did not improve clinical outcome.[24]

Communicating hydrocephalus

Communicating hydrocephalus (CH) is a unique risk of SRS. Risk of both obstructive hydrocephalus increases with tumor size, but CH can occur with medium-sized tumors with minimal mass effect. Recent meta-analysis indicated the incidence similar between treatment modalities (2%–3%), with an intervention rate (shunting) of 68% to 88% in such situations.[25]

Treatment failure

Pseudoprogression is noted in the first few years posttreatment during which the tumor exhibits enlargement on serial imaging. Deciding whether enlargement is

Table 1
Facial nerve dysfunction after radiation therapy

	Study Type	Gamma Knife	Linear Accelerator	Fractionated Proton Therapy	Fractionated Radiotherapy
		N (%)	N (%)	N (%)	N (%)
Balossier et al,[10] 2023	Meta-analysis/ systematic review	2093 (0.9)[a]	374 (8.8)[a]		
Persson et al,[22] 2017	Systematic review	74 (3.6)			40 (11.2)
Gawish et al,[23] 2021	Meta-analysis/ systematic review	2002 OR 0.71	247 OR 1.13		

Abbreviations: %, FND incidence posttreatment; N, number of patients in that arm of the study; OR, odds ratio.
[a] Statistically significant.

Table 2
Trigeminal neuropathy after radiation therapy

	Study Type	Gamma Knife	Linear Accelerator	Fractionated Proton Therapy	Fractionated Radiotherapy
		N (%)	N (%)	N (%)	N (%)
Balossier et al,[10] 2023	Meta-analysis/ systematic review	1864 (2.0)[a]	424 (8.4)[a]		
Persson et al,[22] 2017	Systematic review	125 (6.0)			30 (8.4)
Gawish et al,[23] 2021	Meta-analysis/ systematic review	1706 OR 0.55[a]	392 OR 1.45		

[a] Statistically significant.

treatment failure or pseudoprogression is an imprecise art. At 6 months posttreatment, MRI typically reveals enlargement, loss of central enhancement, and increased mass effect (**Fig. 2**). Almost half of tumors will continue to measure larger over the first 1 to 3 years posttreatment.[26] Three years posttreatment is a commonly used timeframe in which to accept enlargement; however, some centers have adapted an even larger window. Breshears and colleagues[26] showed that patience paid off: 77% of tumors with pseudoprogression still at 3.5 years had demonstrated regression 6 years posttreatment.

ROLE IN TREATING LARGE TUMORS
Stereotactic Radiosurgery as Adjuvant Therapy

Although gross total resection (GTR) represents the gold standard for VS microsurgery, subtotal (STR) or near total resection (NTR) has become more commonly performed to optimize facial nerve outcomes with tumor control. Recent meta-analysis concluded what most surgeons suspected—risk of tumor regrowth is proportional to the residual tumor volume, whereas age and preoperative tumor volume were not.[27] The likelihood of tumor regrowth is as high as 50% post-STR.[28–30]

The best timing of adjuvant SRS to tumor remnant is still unknown, but it may not matter. Data suggest that immediate postsurgical SRS has no advantage or disadvantage over waiting 1 year.[31] One advantage of delaying adjuvant SRS is to get an accurate picture of residual tumor on MRI. In a third of cases following STR or NTR, residual tumor may not be visible on the immediate postoperative MRI.[32] This same study demonstrated that tumor remnants shrink an average of 46% at 1 year postoperative. Akinduro and colleagues[33] additionally suggested that tumor remnants may continue to regress over the first 2 years postoperative and thus concluded SRS can be delayed until 2 years post-STR.

Ultimately, SRS as an adjuvant after STR gives good tumor control. A meta-analysis in 2018 pooled 9 studies to conclude that tumor control equaled after GTR (93% at mean 46 months' follow-up).[34] Patients with large volumes of residual tumor, however, did not fare as well. Lee and colleagues[35] suggested that residual tumor volume greater than 6.4 cm^3 predicted a 5-year control rate of 69%.

Adjuvant SRS after STR also favors better facial nerve outcomes than GTR for larger tumors, with a House-Brackmann I or II in 96% of patients in this same pooled study. A

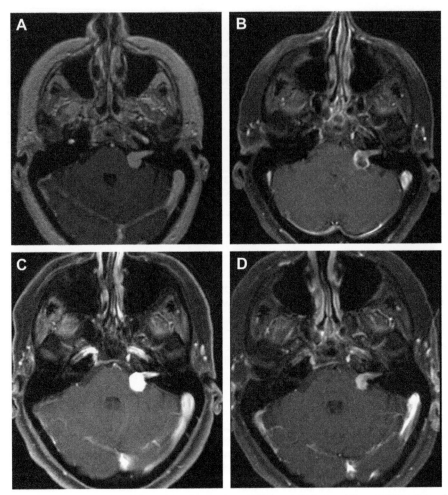

Fig. 2. Serial MRI scanning demonstrating early pseudoprogression and then stabilization of a VS after GK. (*A*) Treatment planning scan. (*B*) Six months postoperative: note the increase in volume and loss of central enhancement. (*C*) One year posttreatment with stabilization of tumor to pretreatment levels. (*D*) Two years posttreatment with visible regression of tumor.

more recent meta-analysis concluded that facial nerve outcomes are not statistically different after adjuvant SRS than prior.[36]

Stereotactic Radiosurgery for Large Tumors

The upper limit of tumor size for SRS is evolving beyond the popular wisdom of a 2.5-cm cerebellopontine angle component.[37] Multiple studies have recently reported on outcomes of patients with Koos IV grade VS undergoing SRS. A multicenter retrospective series reported tumor control in 94% at a median of 38 months of follow-up.[38] Notably, 11% of patients experienced early growth, which was a risk factor for facial paralysis and ultimate treatment failure, and 5% of patients required shunting for hydrocephalus. These same investigators subsequently evaluated the elderly and young subsets of their case series. Elderly patients (>65 years) were more likely to develop hydrocephalus than patients less than 40 years (8% vs 4%), although overall tumor control rates were similar (86% at 10 years).[39,40]

SUMMARY

Multiple modalities for SRS are capable of delivering safe and effective treatment to VS and should be an option discussed with patients pursuing treatment of their tumor. Tumor control is generally good, but poorer than after GTR microsurgery. HP appears to be more dependent on tumor- and patient-related factors rather than modality. Although facial nerve paresis can occur, it is less frequent than after microsurgery. Hybrid approaches with tailored STR and adjuvant SRS appear to offer the patient the advantage of low facial nerve paresis with tumor control similar to GTR. Conventional wisdom placed an upper limit on tumor size for SRS, but data are emerging that SRS for tumors larger than 2.5 cm in CPA diameter has an acceptable-enough risk profile to be discussed as an alternative to microsurgery for selected patients.

CLINICS CARE POINTS

- Stereotactic radiosurgery is a safe and effective management option for most patients pursuing treatment of small- and medium-sized vestibular schwannoma.
- Hearing preservation after stereotactic radiosurgery is best in small, intracanalicular vestibular schwannomas with good baseline hearing.
- Facial paresis is less common after stereotactic radiosurgery than after microsurgery for vestibular schwannoma. The risk is higher in larger tumors and with higher total doses of radiation, such as hypofractionated proton and photon schemes versus single-fraction stereotactic radiosurgery.

Trigeminal neuralgia/neuropathy is more common after stereotactic radiosurgery than microsurgery, and risk is higher in larger tumors and with higher total doses of radiation, such as used in hypofractionated plans versus single-fraction stereotactic radiosurgery.

REFERENCES

1. Bashjawish B, Kılıç S, Baredes S, et al. Changing trends in management of vestibular schwannoma: a National Cancer Database study. Laryngoscope 2019;129(5):1197–205.
2. Available at: https://www.cancer.gov/publications/dictionaries/cancer-terms/def/stereotactic-radiosurgery, Accessed Februrary 9, 2023.
3. Gardner G, Robertson JH. Hearing preservation in unilateral acoustic neuroma surgery. Ann Otol Rhinol Laryngol 1988;97:55–66.
4. American Academy of Otolaryngology Head and Neck Surgery Foundation, Inc. Committee on Hearing and Equilibrium guidelines for the evaluation of hearing preservation in acoustic neuroma (vestibular schwannoma). Otolaryngol Head Neck Surg 1995;113(3):179–80.
5. Available at: https://www.elekta.com/patients/gamma-knife-treatment/, Accessed February 9, 2023.
6. Available at: https://cyberknife.com/brain-tumors/brain-cancer-side-effects/, Accessed Februrary 9, 2023.
7. Desouky O, Zhou G. Biophysical and radiobiological aspects of heavy charged particles. J Taibah Univ Sci 2016;10(2):187–94.

8. Küchler M, El Shafie RA, Adeberg S, et al. Outcome after radiotherapy for vestibular schwannomas (VS)-differences in tumor control, symptoms and quality of life after radiotherapy with photon versus proton therapy. Cancers 2022;14(8):1916.

9. Coughlin AR, Willman TJ, Gubbels SP. Systematic review of hearing preservation after radiotherapy for vestibular schwannoma. Otol Neurotol 2018;39(3):273–83.

10. Balossier A., Tuleasca C., Delsanti C., et al., Long-term hearing outcome after radiosurgery for vestibular schwannoma: a systematic review and meta-analysis, Neurosurgery, 2023. Online published ahead of print.

11. Berger A, Alzate JD, Bernstein K, et al. Modern hearing preservation outcomes after vestibular schwannoma stereotactic radiosurgery. Neurosurgery 2022; 91(4):648–57.

12. Carlson ML, Vivas EX, McCracken DJ, et al. Congress of Neurological Surgeons systematic review and evidence-based guidelines on hearing preservation outcomes in patients with sporadic vestibular schwannomas. Neurosurgery 2018; 82(2):E35–9.

13. Akpinar B, Mousavi SH, McDowell MM, et al. Early radiosurgery improves hearing preservation in vestibular schwannoma patients with normal hearing at the time of diagnosis. Int J Radiat Oncol Biol Phys 2016;95(2):729–34.

14. Milner TD, Locke RR, Kontorinis G, et al. Audiological outcomes in growing vestibular schwannomas managed either conservatively, or with stereotactic radiosurgery. Otol Neurotol 2018;39(2):e143–50.

15. Reznitsky M, Cayé-Thomasen P. Systematic review of hearing preservation in observed vestibular schwannoma. J Neurol Surg B Skull Base 2019;80(2):165–8.

16. Kirchmann M, Karnov K, Hansen S, et al. Ten-year follow-up on tumor growth and hearing in patients observed with an intracanalicular vestibular schwannoma. Neurosurgery 2017;80(1):49–56.

17. Deberge S, Meyer A, Le Pabic E, et al. Quality of life in the management of small vestibular schwannomas: Observation, radiotherapy and microsurgery. Clin Otolaryngol 2018;43(6):1478–86.

18. Barnes JH, Patel NS, Lohse CM, et al. Impact of treatment on vestibular schwannoma-associated symptoms: a prospective study comparing treatment modalities. Otolaryngol Head Neck Surg 2021;165(3):458–64.

19. Fuentealba-Bassaletti C, Neve OM, van Esch BF, et al. Vestibular complaints impact on the long-term quality of life of vestibular schwannoma patients. Otol Neurotol 2023;44(2):161–7.

20. Chweya CM, Tombers NM, Lohse CM, et al. Disease-specific quality of life in vestibular schwannoma: a national cross-sectional study comparing microsurgery, radiosurgery, and observation. Otolaryngol Head Neck Surg 2021;164(3):639–44.

21. Neves Cavada M, Fook-Ho Lee M, Jufas NE, et al. Intracanalicular vestibular schwannoma: a systematic review and meta-analysis of therapeutics outcomes. Otol Neurotol 2021;42(3):351–62.

22. Persson O, Bartek J Jr, Shalom NB, et al. Stereotactic radiosurgery vs. fractionated radiotherapy for tumor control in vestibular schwannoma patients: a systematic review. Acta Neurochir 2017;159(6):1013–21.

23. Gawish A, Walke M, Röllich B, et al. Vestibular schwannoma hypofractionated stereotactic radiation therapy in five fractions. Clin Oncol 2023;35(1):e40–7.

24. Peciu-Florianu I, Régis J, Levivier M, et al. Trigeminal neuralgia secondary to meningiomas and vestibular schwannoma is improved after stereotactic radiosurgery: a systematic review and meta-analysis. Stereotact Funct Neurosurg 2021; 99(1):6–16.

25. De Sanctis P, Green S, Germano I. Communicating hydrocephalus after radiosurgery for vestibular schwannomas: does technique matter? A systematic review and meta-analysis. J Neuro Oncol 2019;145(2):365–73.
26. Breshears JD, Chang J, Molinaro AM, et al. Temporal dynamics of pseudoprogression after gamma knife radiosurgery for vestibular schwannomas-a retrospective volumetric study. Neurosurgery 2019;84(1):123–31.
27. Egiz A, Nautiyal H, Alalade AF, et al. Evaluating growth trends of residual sporadic vestibular schwannomas: a systematic review and meta-analysis. J Neuro Oncol 2022;159(1):135–50.
28. Luryi AL, Kveton JF, Babu S, et al. Evolving role of non-total resection in management of acoustic neuroma in the gamma knife era. Otol Neurotol 2020;41(10): e1354–9.
29. Kasbekar AV, Adan GH, Beacall A, et al. Growth patterns of residual tumor in preoperatively growing vestibular schwannomas. J Neurol Surg B Skull Base 2018; 79(4):319–24.
30. Manzoor NF, Nassiri AM, Sherry AD, et al. Predictors of recurrence after sub-total or near-total resection of vestibular schwannoma: importance of tumor volume and ventral extension. Otol Neurotol 2022;43(5):594–602.
31. Dhayalan D, Perry A, Graffeo CS, et al. Salvage radiosurgery following subtotal resection of vestibular schwannomas: does timing influence tumor control? J Neurosurg 2022;138(2):420–9.
32. Heller RS, Joud H, Flores-Milan G, et al. Changing enhancement pattern and tumor volume of vestibular schwannomas after subtotal resection. World Neurosurg 2021;151:e466–71.
33. Akinduro OO, Lundy LB, Quinones-Hinojosa A, et al. Outcomes of large vestibular schwannomas following subtotal resection: early post-operative volume regression and facial nerve function. J Neuro Oncol 2019;143(2):281–8.
34. Starnoni D, Daniel RT, Tuleasca C, et al. Systematic review and meta-analysis of the technique of subtotal resection and stereotactic radiosurgery for large vestibular schwannomas: a "nerve-centered" approach. Neurosurg Focus 2018; 44(3):E4.
35. Lee WJ, Lee JI, Choi JW, et al. Optimal volume of the residual tumor to predict long-term tumor control using stereotactic radiosurgery after facial nerve-preserving surgery for vestibular schwannomas. J Korean Med Sci 2021; 36(16):e102.
36. Tosi U, Lavieri MET, An A, et al. Outcomes of stereotactic radiosurgery for large vestibular schwannomas: a systematic review and meta-analysis. Neurooncol Pract 2021;8(4):405–16.
37. Carlson ML, Van Gompel JJ, Wiet RM, et al. A cross-sectional survey of the North American Skull Base Society: current practice patterns of vestibular schwannoma evaluation and management in North America. J Neurol Surg B Skull Base 2018; 79:289–96.
38. Pikis S, Mantziaris G, Kormath Anand R, et al. Stereotactic radiosurgery for Koos grade IV vestibular schwannoma: a multi-institutional study. J Neurosurg 2022; 138(2):405–12.
39. Dumot C, Pikis S, Mantziaris G, et al. Stereotactic radiosurgery for Koos grade IV vestibular schwannoma in patients ≥ 65 years old: a multi-institutional retrospective study. Acta Neurochir 2023;165(1):211–20.
40. Dumot C, Pikis S, Mantziaris G, et al. Stereotactic radiosurgery for Koos grade IV vestibular schwannoma in young patients: a multi-institutional study. J Neuro Oncol 2022;160(1):201–8.

Management of Neurofibromatosis Type 2-Associated Vestibular Schwannomas

Pawina Jiramongkolchai, MD, MSCI[a], Marc S. Schwartz, MD[b],
Rick A. Friedman, MD, PhD[a,b],*

KEYWORDS

- Neurofibromatosis type 2 • Vestibular schwannomas
- Hearing preservation strategies • Hearing outcomes

KEY POINTS

- Bilateral vestibular schwannomas (VSs) are the hallmark of neurofibromatosis type 2 (NF2) and present unique challenges in management.
- Management of NF2-associated VSs is highly individualized and must take into consideration patient's age, comorbidities, hearing status, and expectations.
- Proactive early hearing preservation surgery for small VSs especially in pediatric NF2 patients should be considered to maintain and even prolong hearing function and quality of life.

INTRODUCTION

Neurofibromatosis type 2 (NF2) is caused by mutations of the *NF2* gene on chromosome 22 and is characterized by benign tumors of the peripheral and central nervous system. The incidence of NF2 is approximately one in 25,000 to 60,000 with no gender, ethnic, or racial predilections.[1] Although the disease is inherited in an autosomal dominant fashion, approximately half of NF2 patients have de novo mutations. Bilateral vestibular schwannomas (VSs) are the hallmark of NF2. Unlike sporadic VSs, bilateral NF2-associated VSs present unique management dilemmas because of their multifocal nature, presence of other tumors, mass effect on critical neurovascular structures, and risk of total deafness.

[a] Division of Otolaryngology–Head and Neck Surgery, University of California San Diego School of Medicine, 200 West Arbor Drive, MC 8895, San Diego, CA 92103, USA; [b] Department of Neurosurgery, University of California San Diego School of Medicine, 9300 Campus Point Drive, Mail Code 7893, La Jolla, CA 92037, USA
* Corresponding author. Campus Point Drive, #7220, La Jolla, CA 92037.
E-mail address: rafriedman@ucsd.edu

Otolaryngol Clin N Am 56 (2023) 533–541
https://doi.org/10.1016/j.otc.2023.02.012
0030-6665/23/© 2023 Elsevier Inc. All rights reserved.

oto.theclinics.com

Current management options include observation, surgery, and stereotactic radio-surgery (SRS). Although there are no Food and Drug Administration (FDA)-approved pharmacotherapies, clinical trials are underway for the use of medical therapies. Because the goal in managing NF-2 associated VSs is to preserve current function and minimize morbidity, treatment options are highly individualized. This review aims to present current management strategies for NF2-associated VSs with a focus on surgical considerations.

EVALUATION

Although there are several proposed diagnostic criteria for NF2, the Manchester criteria (**Box 1**) is the most widely used.[2] Approximately 90% to 95% of NF2 patients will develop bilateral VSs, the majority by the age of 30 years. Although benign, NF-2-associated VSs are generally more aggressive than sporadic VSs and often invade or may develop from the cochlear nerve.[3] As a result, hearing loss is the most common presenting symptom, with NF2 patients at risk for progressive bilateral hearing deterioration and eventual profound hearing loss. The growth of NF2-associated VSs is highly variable ranging from 0.4 to 8.9 mm/year[4,5] and tend to decrease with increasing age. However, paralleling sporadic VSs, there is an absence in correlation between tumor size and hearing function.[4,6–8]

A complete neurologic examination should be conducted for NF2 patients with particular attention paid to the lower cranial nerves. Lower cranial nerve schwannomas carry a poor prognosis, and lower cranial nerve dysfunction is the most common cause of mortality in NF2 patients.[9] In addition, a neuro-ophthalmologic evaluation should be performed as NF2 patients present with common ocular findings of cataracts, epiretinal membranes, and optic nerve sheath meningiomas.[10] Last, all NF2 patients should receive MRIs of the entire brain and spine with and without gadolinium. Tumors of the spine are almost as common as VSs with the prevalence of spinal tumors as high as 90% at the time of initial diagnosis.[11]

MANAGEMENT
Observation

Patients with small or stable tumors with either good hearing or an only hearing ear are candidates for observation alone. If a "watch and wait" approach is elected, an MRI 6 months after the initial diagnosis followed by annual MRIs and serial audiograms is recommended. Surgery is indicated when there is rapid growth in the tumor causing associated compressive symptoms or significant decline in hearing.

Box 1
Manchester criteria

Bilateral vestibular schwannoma

First-degree relative with NF2 *and* unilateral vestibular schwannoma

First-degree relative with NF2 *and* any of the two NF2-associated lesions: meningioma, schwannoma, ependymoma, and juvenile cataracts

Unilateral vestibular schwannoma *and* any of the two NF2-associated lesions: meningioma, schwannoma, ependymoma, and juvenile cataracts

Multiple meningiomas *or* unilateral vestibular schwannoma *or* any of the two NF2-associated lesions: schwannoma, ependymoma, and juvenile cataracts

Surgery

Unlike sporadic VSs, NF2-associated VSs are more vascular and are frequently in collision with other nearby tumors, such as meningiomas and schwannomas of the fifth and seventh cranial nerves and jugular foramen,[12] factors which the surgeon must take into consideration when counseling patients and selecting surgical approach. Current surgical management includes (1) internal auditory canal decompression via middle fossa craniotomy; (2) tumor removal with attempted hearing preservation surgeries; and (3) tumor removal with non-hearing preservation surgeries with concurrent or subsequent auditory rehabilitation.

Hearing Preservation Surgeries

Like small sporadic VSs, the management of small NF-2 associated VSs is under debate. In NF2 patients with good hearing and bilateral small NF2-associated VSs with favorable radiographic findings, such as a cerebrospinal fluid (CSF) fundal cap, hearing preservation should be a priority. With the high risk of profound bilateral hearing loss over time and associated poor quality of life, hearing preservation surgeries play a larger role especially in younger NF2 patients than those with sporadic VSs. Furthermore, because any level of preserved hearing is important for NF2 patients, the audiologic threshold to attempt hearing preservation is lower compared with patients with sporadic VSs. This approach is further supported by the potential viability of a cochlear implant if the cochlear nerve is preserved, if hearing is lost immediately following surgery or later.

Middle fossa decompression

Although not curative, decompression of the internal auditory canal via a middle cranial fossa approach is a viable surgical option to prolong useful hearing in NF2 patients. In this approach, a middle fossa craniotomy is performed, and the internal auditory canal is widely decompressed. In doing so, pressure exerted by the tumor on the seventh and eighth cranial nerves is relieved. In order to minimize risk to the facial and cochlear nerves, however, the tumor is generally not removed. Several studies have shown that in select NF2 patients, hearing can be preserved and even prolonged with excellent facial nerve outcomes.[13–15] In the largest retrospective cohort study to date of 45 NF2 patients undergoing middle fossa decompression, Slattery and colleagues[15] reported a mean duration of 2.1 years for hearing preservation with some patients having even up to 10 years of meaningful hearing following surgery. Forty-one of the 45 patients (91%) had only one hearing ear and the average tumor size was 19 mm (range 3–41 mm) at the time of surgery.[15]

Middle fossa craniotomy

The middle fossa approach was first described in 1904 for vestibular nerve section in a patient with Meniere's disease.[16] It would not be until nearly 60 years later through the sentinel work of Dr William House that this approach would be used for tumors of the internal auditory canal and cerebellopontine angle. In 1968, Dr Hitselberger described the use of this approach to remove VSs in a series of 12 NF2 patients.[17] Since then, technical refinements in this approach has led to improved postoperative hearing and facial nerve outcomes in this patient population. Although the retrosigmoid approach can be used for hearing preservation, the middle fossa craniotomy is the senior author's preferred approach for attempted hearing preservation for small intracanalicular VSs with minimal extension into the cerebellopontine angle (<2 cm).

In a retrospective series of 28 NF2 patients who underwent middle cranial fossa craniotomies, Brackmann and colleagues[18] found that proactive surgical intervention resulted in high rates of hearing preservation and facial nerve function. The average tumor size was 1.1 cm (range 0.5–3.2 cm) with the majority of tumors smaller than 1.5 cm. Gross total resection was achieved in all cases. With a mean audiologic follow-up time of 12.8 months (range 3–16 months), hearing was preserved within 15 dB pure-tone average (PTA) and 15% speech discrimination score (SDS) in 42.5% of cases, and 70% of cases had some degree of measurable hearing. Of the 11 NF2 patients who underwent bilateral surgery, 8 achieved bilateral hearing preservation. Furthermore, 92% of patients maintained normal facial function postoperatively.[18] In a subsequent study with 55 NF2 patients with a mean tumor size of 1.0 cm (range 0.3–2.1 cm) and average postoperative follow-up of 32.5 months, Friedman and colleagues[19] found that nearly two-thirds of patients achieved functional hearing preservation (average word recognition score [WRS] of 93.%) with 94.3% of patients maintaining a House–Brackmann 1–2 at follow-up. Although gross total resection was achieved in 96% of patients at the time of initial surgery, 14 patients demonstrated recurrent or new tumors in the surgical field on subsequent follow-up, highlighting the need for diligent monitoring of all NF2 patients with serial MRIs.[19]

Because of the high risk of bilateral profound deafness over time, maintenance of hearing in children with NF2 is important for overall long-term quality of life. In a study of pediatric NF2 patients, Slattery and colleagues[20] found that in the majority of patients undergoing middle fossa craniotomy for resection of tumors that were on average 1.1 cm (range 0.4–3.2 cm), hearing could be preserved and even maintained for several years. Factors associated with hearing preservation included fewer NF2-related symptoms, smaller tumor size at the time of operation, better hearing, younger age at operation, and family history of NF-2. In a more recent study of 28 children and young adults ($n = 46$ tumors; mean tumor volume 1.52 cm^3) by Gurgel and colleagues,[21] hearing preservation surgery was associated with an 82% postoperative functional hearing rate, 95% facial function preservation, and 33% reduction in postoperative tumor growth. It should be noted that the majority of patients in this study had deliberate partial resection.[21] At our institution, we favor proactive surgery for children with NF2 (**Fig. 1**).

Taken together, these studies demonstrate favorable long-term hearing prognosis and tumor control in NF2 patients who undergo early proactive hearing preservation surgery for small VSs. Furthermore, by preserving the cochlear nerve, patients still maintain the option for auditory rehabilitative options, such as cochlear implants, when they begin to experience hearing deterioration in the contralateral ear.

Non-hearing preservation surgery

With large VSs or profound hearing loss, total tumor removal via a retrosigmoid or translabyrinthine approach is pursued. At our institution, the translabyrinthine approach is our preferred approach as it minimizes cerebellar retraction and provides maximal exposure of the facial nerve (**Fig. 2**). In addition, the translabyrinthine approach provides a direct line of sight and access to the lateral recess of the fourth ventricle if an auditory brainstem implant is concurrently pursued at the time of initial surgery. Unlike sporadic VSs, gross total resection of medium to large NF2-associated VSs can be challenging as the tumors can be in collision with the seventh or eighth cranial nerves as well as other tumors, such as meningiomas and trigeminal schwannomas. In those cases, priority is placed on minimizing morbidity.

Stereotactic Radiosurgery

Although SRS is a main treatment option for small to medium-sized sporadic VSs, the role for SRS in NF2-associated VSs remains controversial.

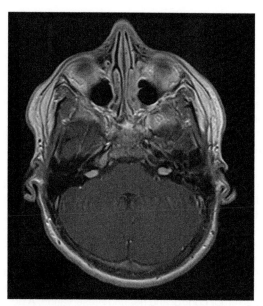

Fig. 1. MRI of a 14-year-old NF2 patient with bilateral VSs who underwent right middle fossa craniotomy. Preoperative axial T1-gadolinium MRI demonstrating bilateral enhancing IAC masses consistent with VSs. IAC, internal auditory canal.

Compared with sporadic VSs, NF2-associated VSs are less responsive to SRS at typical dose levels. In a systematic review of SRS cases for NF-2 associated VSs, the average 5-year local control rate was 75.1% (range 62%–92%; SD 12.1) with a mean hearing preservation rate of 40.1% (range 0%–78%; SD 23.9) and mean facial nerve preservation rate of 92.3% (range 50%–100%, SD 15.5),[22] all lower than reported outcomes for sporadic tumors.[23] Furthermore, because the *NF2* mutation results in loss of the tumor suppressor gene, radiation may accelerate the growth of

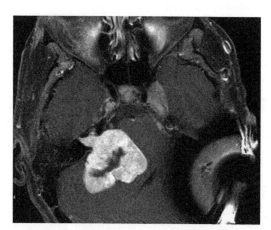

Fig. 2. MRI of a 31-year-old NF2 patient with multiple intracranial tumors who had previously undergone resection of a left-sided VS with ABI placement who presented with declining neurologic status due to right giant VS and underwent right translabyrinthine craniotomy. Preoperative axial T1-gadolinium MRI demonstrating giant vestibular schwannoma causing severe brainstem compression.

other tumors and increase the risk of radiation-induced malignancies, such as glioblastoma and malignant meningiomas. Although the overall 20 year risk for malignant transformation after radiation for all VSs is 25.1 per 100,000 cases and 15.6 per 100,000 cases if NF2 cases are excluded,[24] Baser and colleagues[25] found that radiated NF2 patients had at least a 10-fold risk of malignancy compared with their non-radiated counterparts. Malignant transformation of VSs is also associated with poor prognosis with overall 1-year and 2-year survival rate at 42.3% and 18.6%, respectively.[26] Furthermore, salvage surgery after radiation therapy can be more challenging with more densely adherent nerve-tumor dissection planes, placing the facial nerve and critical neurovascular structures at higher risk for injury.

Medical therapy

To date, there are no FDA-approved pharmacotherapies for NF2. However, with improved knowledge of NF2 tumor pathogenesis, drug development is an area of active research with molecules designed to target vascular angiogenesis, epidermal growth factor family receptors, and cellular signaling pathways involving mitogen-activated protein kinase (MAPK), phosphoinositide 3-kinase (PI3K)/protein kinase B (AKT), and mammalian target of rapamycin (mTOR).

Bevacizumab (Avastin, Roche), a VEGF monoclonal antibody, is the most commonly used medical therapy to treat NF2 patients with growing VSs with encouraging results for local tumor control and hearing preservation. A pooled systematic review and meta-analysis of patients treated with bevacizumab showed partial tumor progression in 41% (95% CI 31–51%), no change in 47% (95% CI 39–55%), and progression in 7% (95% CI 1–15%).[27] In patients with audiometric data, hearing was stable in 69% (95% CI 51–85%) and improved in 20% (95% CI 9–33%).[27] However, there is documented tumor rebound growth after discontinuation of the drug and significant side-effects, such as hypertension, proteinuria, and poor wound healing.[27,28]

Auditory Rehabilitation

For NF2 patients with profound hearing loss, auditory rehabilitation options include cochlear implantation (CI) and auditory brainstem implant (ABI).

The ABI was developed at the House Ear Institute in the 1970s for NF2 patients with bilateral VSs. By bypassing the cochlear nerve and directly stimulating the cochlear nucleus, the ABI can deliver sound perception to NF2 patients with profound hearing loss. In 2000, the US FDA approved the multichannel ABI for NF2 patients 12 years of age or older. Although the retrosigmoid or translabyrinthine approach can be used to place the implant, we favor the translabyrinthine approach as we believe this approach

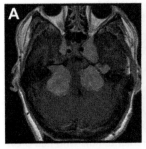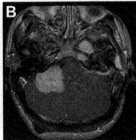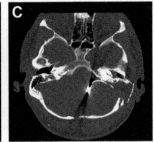

Fig. 3. Radiologic images of a 24-year-old NF2 patient with bilateral VSs. (*A*) Preoperative axial T1-gadolinium MRI demonstrating bilateral large VS. (*B*) Postoperative axial T1-gadolinium MRI following left translabyrinthine craniotomy with ABI placement. (*C*) Postoperative axial CT demonstrating successful placement of left ABI.

provides the most direct access to the cochlear nucleus (**Fig. 3**). The overall audiologic outcomes for ABIs remains mixed with rates of open speech perception ranging from 0% to 41%.[29]

Despite the advances with ABIs, cochlear implants remain the choice of auditory rehabilitation in NF2 patients with an intact cochlea and cochlear nerve. In the English consensus protocol,[30] CI is superior to ABI for NF2 patients with stable VSs or prior radiation treatment. Furthermore, in a large systematic review of all CI cases in NF2 patients, approximately 70% of patients achieved open-set discrimination with nearly all patients reporting improved sound awareness and voice modulation.[31] The long-term hearing outcomes of NF2 patients with CI following VS resection are also excellent with patients achieving up to 96% hearing in noise testing results.[32]

SUMMARY

Management of NF2-associated VSs requires a multidisciplinary team of experienced specialists and must be individually tailored for each patient given the unpredictable nature of the disease. Furthermore, because most of the NF2 patients are at risk for eventual bilateral profound deafness, early proactive resection of small NF2-associated VSs can maintain and even prolong hearing function and should be highly considered in the treatment algorithm.

CLINICS CARE POINTS

- For NF-2 associated VSs, hearing loss is the most common presenting symptom.
- With the high risk of profound deafness over time and associated poor quality of life for NF2 patients, hearing preservation strategies play a larger role for these patients compared to those with sporadic VSs.
- NF2 patients with small intracanilicular VSs with minimal extension into the CPA (<2 cm) are good candidates for attempted hearing preservation with the middle fossa approach.
- Regardless of treatment modality, the ultimate goal in management of NF-2 associated VSs should be to preserve current function while minimizing morbidity.

REFERENCES

1. Evans DG, Howard E, Giblin C, et al. Birth incidence and prevalence of tumor-prone syndromes: estimates from a UK family genetic register service. Am J Med Genet 2010;152a(2):327–32.
2. Evans DGR, Baser ME, O'Reilly B, et al. Management of the patient and family with neurofibromatosis 2: a consensus conference statement. Br J Neurosurg 2005;19(1):5–12.
3. Neary WJ, Hillier VF, Flute T, et al. The relationship between patients' perception of the effects of neurofibromatosis type 2 and the domains of the Short Form-36. Clin Otolaryngol 2010;35(4):291–9.
4. Kontorinis G, Nichani J, Freeman SR, et al. Progress of hearing loss in neurofibromatosis type 2: implications for future management. Eur Arch Otorhinolaryngol 2015;272(11):3143–50.
5. Harris GJ, Plotkin SR, Maccollin M, et al. Three-dimensional volumetrics for tracking vestibular schwannoma growth in neurofibromatosis type II. Neurosurgery 2008;62(6):1314–9 [discussion: 1319-1320].

6. Fisher LM, Doherty JK, Lev MH, et al. Concordance of bilateral vestibular schwannoma growth and hearing changes in neurofibromatosis 2: neurofibromatosis 2 natural history consortium. Otol Neurotol 2009;30(6):835–41.
7. Peyre M, Goutagny S, Bah A, et al. Conservative management of bilateral vestibular schwannomas in neurofibromatosis type 2 patients: hearing and tumor growth results. Neurosurgery 2013;72(6):907–13 [discussion: 914; quiz: 914].
8. Plotkin SR, Merker VL, Muzikansky A, et al. Natural history of vestibular schwannoma growth and hearing decline in newly diagnosed neurofibromatosis type 2 patients. Otol Neurotol 2014;35(1):e50–6.
9. Aboukais R, Zairi F, Bonne NX, et al. Causes of mortality in neurofibromatosis type 2. Br J Neurosurg 2015;29(1):37–40.
10. Bosch MM, Boltshauser E, Harpes P, et al. Ophthalmologic findings and long-term course in patients with neurofibromatosis type 2. Am J Ophthalmol 2006; 141(6):1068–77.e1062.
11. Mautner VF, Lindenau M, Baser ME, et al. The neuroimaging and clinical spectrum of neurofibromatosis 2. Neurosurgery 1996;38(5):880–5 [discussion: 885-886].
12. Dewan R, Pemov A, Kim HJ, et al. Evidence of polyclonality in neurofibromatosis type 2-associated multilobulated vestibular schwannomas. Neuro Oncol 2015; 17(4):566–73.
13. Bernardeschi D, Peyre M, Collin M, et al. Internal auditory canal decompression for hearing maintenance in neurofibromatosis type 2 patients. Neurosurgery 2016;79(3):370–7.
14. Gadre AK, Brackmann DE, Kwartler JA, et al. Middle fossa decompression of the internal auditory canal in acoustic neuroma surgery: a therapeutic alternative. Laryngoscope 1990;100(9):948–52.
15. Slattery WH, Hoa M, Bonne N, et al. Middle fossa decompression for hearing preservation: a review of institutional results and indications. Otol Neurotol 2011;32(6):1017–24.
16. Parry RH. A case of tinnitus and vertigo treated by division of the auditory nerve. Journal of Laryngology, Rhinology, and Otology 1904;19(8):402–6.
17. Hitselberger WE, Hughes RL. Bilateral acoustic tumors and neurofibromatosis. Arch Otolaryngol 1968;88(6):700–11.
18. Brackmann DE, Fayad JN, Slattery WH 3rd, et al. Early proactive management of vestibular schwannomas in neurofibromatosis type 2. Neurosurgery 2001;49(2):274–80 [discussion: 280-273].
19. Friedman RA, Goddard JC, Wilkinson EP, et al. Hearing preservation with the middle cranial fossa approach for neurofibromatosis type 2. Otol Neurotol 2011; 32(9):1530–7.
20. Slattery WH, Fisher LM, Hitselberger W, et al. Hearing preservation surgery for neurofibromatosis Type 2–related vestibular schwannoma in pediatric patients. J Neurosurg 2007;106(4):255–60.
21. Gugel I, Grimm F, Teuber C, et al. Management of NF2-associated vestibular schwannomas in children and young adults: influence of surgery and clinical factors on tumor volume and growth rate. J Neurosurg 2019;24(5):584–92.
22. Chung LK, Nguyen TP, Sheppard JP, et al. A systematic review of radiosurgery versus surgery for neurofibromatosis type 2 vestibular schwannomas. World Neurosurgery 2018;109:47–58.
23. Flickinger JC, Kondziolka D, Niranjan A, et al. Acoustic neuroma radiosurgery with marginal tumor doses of 12 to 13 Gy. Int J Radiat Oncol Biol Phys 2004; 60(1):225–30.

24. Seferis C, Torrens M, Paraskevopoulou C, et al. Malignant transformation in vestibular schwannoma: report of a single case, literature search, and debate: case report. J Neurosurg 2014;121(Suppl_2):160–6.
25. Baser M, Evans D, Jackler R, et al. Neurofibromatosis 2, radiosurgery and malignant nervous system tumours. Br J Cancer 2000;82(4):998.
26. Li J, Wang Q, Zhang M, et al. Malignant transformation in vestibular schwannoma: clinical study with survival analysis. Front Oncol 2021;11:655260.
27. Lu VM, Ravindran K, Graffeo CS, et al. Efficacy and safety of bevacizumab for vestibular schwannoma in neurofibromatosis type 2: a systematic review and meta-analysis of treatment outcomes. Journal of Neuroncology 2019;144(2): 239–48.
28. Blakeley JO, Evans DG, Adler J, et al. Consensus recommendations for current treatments and accelerating clinical trials for patients with neurofibromatosis type 2. Am J Med Genet 2012;158A(1):24–41.
29. Sanna M, Di Lella F, Guida M, et al. Auditory brainstem Implants in NF2 patients: results and review of the literature. Otol Neurotol 2012;33(2):154–64.
30. Tysome JR, Axon PR, Donnelly NP, et al. English consensus protocol evaluating candidacy for auditory brainstem and cochlear implantation in neurofibromatosis type 2. Otol Neurotol 2013;34(9):1743–7.
31. Carlson ML, Breen JT, Driscoll CL, et al. Cochlear implantation in patients with neurofibromatosis type 2: variables affecting auditory performance. Otol Neurotol 2012;33(5):853–62.
32. Neff BA, Wiet RM, Lasak JM, et al. Cochlear implantation in the neurofibromatosis type 2 patient: long-term follow-up. Laryngoscope 2007;117(6):1069–72.

Targeted Therapies in the Treatment of Vestibular Schwannomas: Current State and New Horizons

D. Bradley Welling, MD, PhD[a,b]

KEYWORDS

- Vestibular schwannoma • NF2-related schwannomatosis • Neurofibromatosis type 2
- Pharmacotherapy • Acoustic neuroma • Bevacizumab • Molecular-targeted therapy

KEY POINTS

- There are no FDA-approved drugs for the treatment of vestibular schwannoma (VS).
- Bevacizumab is the most commonly used drug intended to control growth of VSs and preserve or improve hearing.
- Other targeted therapies have shown promise.
- Gene replacement in neurofibromatosis type 2-related schwannomatosis, as it is developed, may avoid tumor formation and improve long-term prognosis.

INTRODUCTION

Vestibular schwannomas (VSs) are tumors of Schwann cell origin which are histologically benign, but clinically significant as hearing loss, facial weakness paralysis, and disequilibrium are common complications. Vestibular nerves, for unknown reasons, are the most likely of the cranial nerves to develop VS, but multiple tumor-forming diseases of the nervous system can occur. Neurofibromatosis type 2 (NF2)-related schwannomatosis (NF2-SWN) occurs rarely with a birth incidence of one in 33,000 and a prevalence of one in 60,000.[1] Sporadic VSs have an incidence of 4 to 20 per 100,000 per year and disease prevalence reaching one in 500 individuals aged 70 years or older.[2] Somatic mutations of the NF2 gene result in unilateral VS. The hallmark of NF2-SWN is bilateral VSs. The loss of tumor suppressor function is also associated with multiple meningiomas, ependymomas, posterior lenticular opacities, and cutaneous schwannoma.[3]

[a] Harvard Department of Otolaryngology Head & Neck Surgery, 243 Charles Street, Boston, MA, USA; [b] Massachusetts Eye and Ear Infirmary and Massachusetts General Hospital
E-mail address: Brad_welling@meei.harvard.edu

Otolaryngol Clin N Am 56 (2023) 543–556
https://doi.org/10.1016/j.otc.2023.02.013

An international consortium recently agreed on new definitions on the minimal clinical and genetic criteria for diagnosing NF2 and SWN which added molecular diagnosis to clarify areas of clinical overlap between NF2 and SWN. The term "neurofibromatosis type 2" was retired to improve diagnostic accuracy and specificity in favor of "NF2-related Schwannomatosis".[4] The new and useful classification schema is depicted in **Fig. 1**.

NF2-SWN is an autosomal-dominant, tumor predisposing syndrome characterized by bi-allelic inactivation of the NF2 gene on chromosome 22q 11.2 resulting in the loss of function of its protein product merlin. Mutation of the tumor suppressor NF2-gene results in the loss of functional merlin with the loss of contact inhibition of Schwann cells. Schwann cells normally form the insulating myelin sheath around.[5,6] Pathogenic variants in the NF2 gene help define NF2-SWN separating it from SWI/SNF (SWitch/Su-crose Non-Fermentable) related, Matrix associated, Actin dependent Regulator of Chromatin, subfamily B member 1 (SMARCB1)-related SWN or Leucine Zipper like Transcription Regulator 1 (LZTR1)-related SWN. Other tumors which are influenced by the loss of the tumor suppressor protein merlin include mesotheliomas, thyroid, breast, prostate, colorectal, hepatic, clear cell renal carcinoma, and melanomas.[7,8]

A review of clinical trials in NF2-SWN is limited by the rarity of the disease and the number of potential participants. Most study designs are single-arm, open-label, single-drug studies focused on VSs treatment.[9] This commentary will discuss (1) clinical trials of targeted pharmacological treatments published, (2) those in ongoing clinical trials, and (3) potential future treatment options. There are no FDA-approved drugs for the treatment of NF2 or VS. It is worth noting that although clinical trials to date have targeted single agents, preclinical studies indicate that all NF2-related tumors are not susceptible to the same treatment pathways and that multidrug mechanisms may be necessary to block key merlin-related pathways.[10] Single drugs which could target all NF2-related tumors would be ideal, but such have not yet been identified.

The measures of clinical success in NF2-SWN are rather different than conventional oncologic trials where tumor regression and disease-free survival are common outcomes. In NF2, tumor regression greater than 20% by volume reduction is the standard,[11] but stabilization of previously growing tumors is also clinically highly relevant (**Fig. 2**).

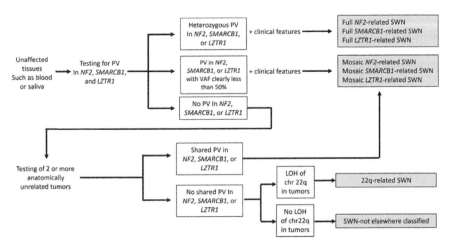

Fig. 1. Schematic of genetic testing strategy for NF2 and SWN. LOH, loss of heterozygosity; NF2, neurofibromatosis type 2; PV, pathogenic variant; SWN, schwannomatosis; VAF, variant allele fraction. (Plotkin et al. Gen in Med 2022 https://doi.org/10.1016/j.gim.2022.05.007 creative commons open access license.[1])

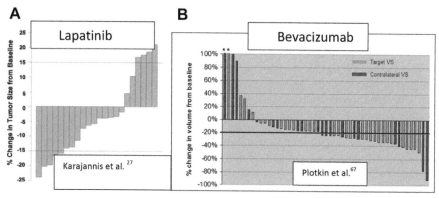

Fig. 2. Waterfall plots of the percentage of change in tumor size from baseline for each evaluable ear on (A) lapatinib where 16 of 21 study subjects exhibited some decrease in tumor size and (B) where 43 of 51 subjects on bevacizumab showed no growth or decrease tumor size. **, indicates greater than 100% growth.

CLINICAL TRIALS COMPLETED
Bevacizumab

Bevacizumab is a humanized Immunoglobulin G1 (IgG1) monoclonal antibody that binds all biologically active isoforms of human vascular endothelial growth factor (VEGF or VEGF-A) with high affinity.[12,13] Plotkin first reported hearing improvement and volumetric reduction of VS by bevacizumab in 2009.[14] Numerous studies since have confirmed these findings.[15–18] Systematic reviews by Lu and colleagues and Shi and colleagues reported NF2-related VS treated with bevacizumab showed 30% to 41% with a favorable radiographic response and a 20% to 32% favorable hearing response. Tumor volume reduction was noted usually in the first 4 to 6 months of treatment. Major complications of bevacizumab included hypertension and proteinuria, menstrual disorders, and hemorrhage. Serious adverse events were reported in 12% to 17% of patients. About one-third of NF2-VS patients may benefit significantly from bevacizumab[19,20] (**Fig. 3**).

Hearing improvement has been reported in multiple studies, particularly in speech recognition scores, in 35% to 50% of patients. There was no change in spatial perception, and tinnitus reduction did not reach statistical significance[21,22]; however, a reduction in tinnitus-related distress was noted.[15] Unfortunately, results with bevacizumab do not show as much improvement in tumor reduction and hearing restoration or preservation in children as in adults.[15,23]

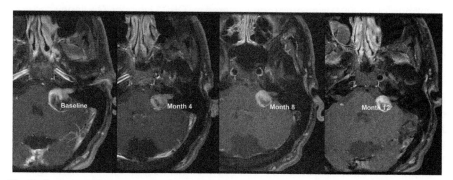

Fig. 3. Radiographic response to bevacizumab. (*Courtesy of* Scott R. Plotkin, MD, PhD.)

Meningiomas, which are associated with NF2-SWN in 50% to 80% of cases, have not shown a durable response to bevacizumab treatment.[24] Spinal ependymoma were shown in two retrospective studies to have beneficial response to bevacizumab.[25,26]

Toxicity associated with bevacizumab includes fatigue, hypertension, proteinuria, hemorrhage, and infection. Proteinuria may persist after cessation of bevacizumab. Age greater than 30 years and induction regimen of 7.5 mg/kg q3 weeks are associated with higher rates of hypertension. Reported dosage ranges from 5 mg/kg intravenous (IV) every 4 weeks to 10 mg/kg every 2 weeks. However, higher dosing was no more effective than standard dose for treatment of patients with NF2 for hearing loss.[15] A progressive sporadic VS has shown sustained tumor shrinkage on bevacizumab,[17] which points to the opening of new treatment options for some sporadic VS or meningioma patients if NF2 can be effectively terminated.

There has been some controversy about potential rebound of tumor growth when a patient has discontinued bevacizumab. It is the authors' observation that tumors generally appear to resume their pretreatment growth rate without an increase in pretreatment growth rate. If surgical treatment becomes necessary, bevacizumab must be stopped at least 6 weeks preoperatively. Increased vascularity in previously bevacizumab-treated VS has been documented in which the VS tumors develop very thin-walled vascular spaces and thin-walled vessels which predispose to bleeding. Therefore, caution is warranted for surgical treatment after long-term bevacizumab treatment (unpublished observation).

Lapatinib

Lapatinib is a dual epidermal growth factor receptor Epidermal Growth Factor Receptor/erb-b2 receptor tyrosine kinase 2 (EGFR/Erb2) inhibitor, a member of the family of drugs that targets the EGFR receptor tyrosine kinases. In a phase II open-label trial of lapatinib in adult and pediatric patients with NF2-associated VS, 4 of 17 patients experienced an objective volumetric response and 4 of 13 patients evaluable for hearing met hearing improvement criteria. Toxicity was generally minor and no permanent dose modifications were required.[27] Although the volumetric tumor reduction and hearing response were not strong, the number of tumors with no growth during the study was rather impressive. Similar stability was seen with patients on bevacizumab (see **Fig. 2**). Stabile, nonprogressive disease is a very useful outcome in NF2 treatments and should not be discounted. In addition, lapatinib showed a growth inhibitory effect on meningiomas in NF2 patients in a small clinical study.[28]

Everolimus

Everolimus (or Rad001) is an orally administered mTORC1 inhibitor. Goutagny and colleagues[29] in a prospective trial of everolimus for progressive VS in NF2 patients showed five of ten patients with decrease in growth rates and resumption of growth after termination of drug.

Karajannis and colleagues reported the results of a separate trial using everolimus in 10 patients with NF2 and progressive VSs. No objective improvement in hearing or imaging response was seen.[30] Subsequently, in a phase 0 presurgical clinical trial, blood levels of everolimus were found to be in a high therapeutic range. The tumor tissue drug concentration was determined. Only partial inhibition of phosphorylated S6 protein (phospho-S6) was found in the treated tumors, indicating incomplete target inhibition compared with control tissues from untreated patients. Everolimus led to the incomplete inhibition of mTORC1 and downstream signaling. The investigators concluded that their data may explain the "limited antitumor effect of everolimus observed in clinical studies for patients with NF2" and that such preclinical surgical studies may influence future preclinical and clinical studies.[31]

Side effects of everolimus include mouth ulcers early in the treatment course, anemia, decreased neutrophil and lymphocyte counts, peripheral edema, hyperglycemia, and pericardial effusion.[32]

Rec-2282

Rec-2282 (formerly AR42) is an oral pan-histone deacetylase inhibitor, which modulates apoptosis inhibitors and cell survival regulators through phosphatidylinositol 3-kinase/protein kinase B (PI3K/Akt) pathway inhibition. Two pilot studies in NF2-related tumors included endpoints of safety, intra-tumoral pharmacokinetics (PK) and pharmacodynamics (PD). The first pilot study was a subset analysis of a phase 1 study of Rec-2282 in solid tumors, including NF2 or sporadic meningiomas. Of 15 tumors (8 VS and 7 meningiomas), volume increased in 40%, stabilized in 53%, and decreased 7%. The annual percent growth rate decreased in 53%, remained static in 20%, and increased in 27%. The dose-limiting toxicities included grade 3 thrombocytopenia and one grade 4 psychosis.[33]

A phase 0 surgical study of Rec-2282 assessed intra-tumoral PK and PD. The drug was administered orally for 3 weeks preoperatively, and blood and tumor sampled at the time of surgery. Four patients with sporadic VS and one patient with meningioma experienced no grade 3/4 toxicities. The expression of phosphorylated-protein kinase B (p-AKT) decreased in three of four VS tissues. All tumors had higher Arno therapeutics compound 42 (AR-42) concentrations than plasma. It was concluded that single-agent Rec-2282 was safe, well-tolerated, and modestly effective in growth suppression in most tumors. It was concentrated in tumor.[34] Further phase 2 studies of Rec-2282 are recruiting for NF2-related meningiomas (ClinicalTrials.gov Identifier NCT05130866).

Other Studies

See **Table 1** for other completed trials with references.

CLINICAL TRIALS IN PROGRESS

See **Table 2**.

Brigatinib

Brigatinib is a reversible dual inhibitor of anaplastic lymphoma kinase (ALK) and EGFR which is Food and Drug Administration (FDA)-approved to treat ALK positive metastatic non-small cell lung cancer.[38] Brigatinib is the first drug in the Innovative Trial for Understanding the Impact of Targeted Therapies in NF2 which is a multisite, phase II, platform-basket trial for testing a new treatment of progressive NF2-associated tumors (ClinicalTrials.gov Identifier NCT04374305). This format allows for ongoing testing of multiple experimental therapies in patients with NF2-SWN. Embedded in the trial are individual drug substudies. The most common adverse reactions ($\geq$25%) with brigatinib were diarrhea, fatigue, nausea, rash, cough, myalgia, headache, hypertension, vomiting, and dyspnea. In preclinical trials, brigatinib caused tumor shrinkage in both NF2-deficient meningioma and schwannoma through the inhibition of multiple tyrosine kinases, but interestingly, not through ALK.[39]

Aspirin

Aspirin (ASA) is a member of the acetylsalicylic acid family with anti-inflammatory, antipyretic, and platelet aggregation inhibition effects. It is classified as a

Table 1
Clinical trials completed

Name	Mechanism	VS Response	Hearing Response	Complications	References
Bevacizumab	VEGF inhibitor	30–41%	20–32%	Hypertension, proteinuria, amenorrhea, hemorrhage	Refs[12-23]
Lapatinib	EGFR, Erb2 inhibition	23%	31%	Rash, diarrhea, fatigue, elevated liver function tests (LFT), headache, nail changes, possible delayed wound healing	Karajannis et al,[27] 2012; Osorio et al,[28] 2018
Everolimus	mTORC1 inhibition	0%	0%	Mouth ulcers, anemia, neutropenia, lymphocytopenia, peripheral edema, hyperglycemia, and pericardial effusion	[29-32]
REC-2282 (formerly AR-42)	Histone deacetylase inhibitor	7%	-	Thrombocytopenia, psychosis	Collier et al,[33] 2021; Welling et al,[34] 2021
Erlotinib	EGFR inhibitor	0%	11% transient	Rash, elevated bilirubin, hair thinning	Plotkin et al,[35] 2010; Bush et al,[36] 2012
Nilotinib	Tyrosine kinase inhibitor	-	-	-	Trial stopped before completion
Tacrolimus	Immunosuppressant	100%	100%	None	Delmas et al,[37] 2020 (case report)

Table 2
Ongoing clinical trials

Name	Mechanism	Study Design	Primary Target	Locations (No Of Sites)	ClinicalTrial.gov (References)
Brigatinib Neratinib	ALK and EGFR inhibitor Selective EGFR, HER2, and HER4 inhibitor	Adaptive basket trial	VS, non-VS, meningioma, ependymoma	CA, FL MD, MA, MN, NY	NCT04374305 Zhang et al,[38] 2016 & Chang et al,[39] 2021
Aspirin	COX2 inhibitor	Randomized controlled Phase 2	Sporadic and NF2 VS	MA, MN, IA, UT, CA, FL	NCT03079999[40-47]
REC-2282	Histone deacetylase inhibitor	Parallel-group, two-staged, phase 2/3, randomized, multicenter study	NF2-related meningiomas	CA(2), DC, FL(2), KS, MA(2), MN(2), NC, NY, TX	NCT05130866 Collier et al,[33] 2021 & Welling et al,[34] 2021
Doxycycline	MMP-14 and VEFG inhibition, decreases NLRP3 formation	Open-label pilot	Cutaneous schwannomas	MA	NCT05521048 Tan et al,[48] 2017 & Ali et al,[49] 2017
Vismodegib GSK2256098 Capivasertib Abemaciclib	Hedgehog inhibitor FAK inhibitor AKT inhibitor CDK inhibitor	Phase 2	Progressive NF2-related meningioma	MA, AL, and 708 sites	NCT02523014
Selumetinib	MEK inhibitor	Phase 2	Hearing VS, other tumors	OH	NCT03095248 Ammoun et al,[50] 2011
Losartan	IL-6/SSTAT3 inhibition Antihypertensive	Phase 2 with proton beam radiotherapy	Hearing	MA	NCT01199978 Wu et al,[51] 2021
Axitinib	VEGFR 1–3 inhibitor	Phase I/II	Not reported	Mucositis, nausea, fatigue, and rash	NCT02129647 Schiller et al,[52] 2009

nonselective cyclooxygenase (COX) inhibitor[40]. Preclinical studies indicate COX-2 pathway is associated with VS growth[41,42] but retrospective clinical studies of the effect of aspirin on VS growth are conflicting.[43–47] As the dose of aspirin and regularity of use were not well controlled and selection bias likely in the retrospective studies, a prospective randomized phase II clinical trial to clarify the effect of ASA on VS growth in NF2 and sporadic VS has been initiated (Clinicaltrials.gov Identifier NCT03079999). The common adverse effects of aspirin are well known and include dyspepsia, nausea, abdominal pain, and platelet inhibition. The low cost, ready access, and known adverse event profile would make it an attractive treatment option if shown to be effective.

Losartan

Losartan is an FDA-approved antihypertensive drug that blocks fibrotic and inflammatory signaling. It was shown in preclinical studies to stabilize the tumor microenvironment in VS by reducing neuroinflammatory interleukin-6/Signal Transducers and Activators of Transcription subgroup 3 (IL-6/SSTAT3) signaling and preventing hearing loss in mouse models. It may also normalize tumor vasculature and increase oxygen delivery and enhance the efficacy of radiation therapy.[51] These data have led to a prospective clinical trial to observe the ability of losartan to preserve hearing in VS patients (ClinicalTrials.gov Identifier NCT01199978).

Axitinib

Axitinib is a second-generation tyrosine kinase inhibitor that works by selectively inhibiting VEGF receptors (VEGFR-1, VEGFR-2, and VEGFR-3). Through this mechanism of action, axitinib blocks angiogenesis, tumor growth, and metastases.[52–54] In a phase I/II open label study, 10 patients were enrolled. Mucositis, nausea, fatigue, and rash were reported side effects with no serious adverse events. The completed results have not been reported (ClinicalTrials.gov Identifier NCT02129647).

Doxycycline

The direct cutaneous schwannoma injection of doxycycline hyclate, a well-known broad-spectrum antibiotic, is under study based on its sclerosing and anticancer properties. It has been shown to suppress numerous cancers in vitro.[48,49] It is currently recruiting for NF2 patients with cutaneous and subcutaneous schwannomas and is the only direct tumor injection delivery study at present (ClinicalTrials.gov Identifier NCT05521048).

Preclinical Studies

There are numerous preclinical studies being conducted targeting various pathways affected by the loss of the Merlin protein. Examples include ponatinib, a novel Breakpoint Cluster Region-Abelson (BCR-ABL) tyrosine kinase inhibitor FDA-approved for leukemia, which promotes G1 cell-cycle arrest of merlin/NF2-deficient human Schwann cell.[55] Fimepinostat (CUDC_907) is a dual inhibitor of histone deacetylase (HDAC) and PI3K which was identified in the Synodos Consortium screening for potentially effective therapeutic agents against schwannomas and meningiomas.[56] Cell viability studies revealed it to be one of the top candidates along with GSK2126458 and Panobinostat.[10] In addition, some single agents with promise are being testing in combined therapies such as lapatinib, nilotinib, and radiation combinations for NF2-associated peripheral schwannoma.[50,57]

FUTURE DIRECTIONS
Repositioning

Drug repositioning identifies FDA-approved drugs through algorithm-based programs which query the human VS transcriptome to identify drugs which may be reappropriated for targeting VS-related growth pathways. As an example, mifepristone, a progestational and glucocorticoid hormone antagonist used for pregnancy termination, was identified as a potential agent but has not yet been reported in clinical trials.[58] Other similarly identified agents may be considered.

Immunotherapy

Tamura and colleagues reported a novel study in which cytotoxic T-lymphocyte activation against VEGF receptors obtained tumor control and hearing results similar to those seen with bevacizumab. Immunotherapy against benign lesions is in its infancy but of great interest. Twenty-three tumors in seven patients showed that shrinkage was seen in four, minimal response in eleven, stable disease in seven, and growth in one cystic tumor. Improved hearing was seen in two of five subjects with no change in the other three. Adverse events included local skin reactions, hypertension, neutropenia and anemia. Grade 3 diverticulitis and grade 5 intracranial hemorrhage were not deemed drug-related.[59]

Naturally Occurring Pharmacotherapeutics

Owing to their antineoplastic, antioxidant, and anti-inflammatory properties, the selected natural compounds could be useful as a primary therapy or as an adjuvant therapy before or following surgery and/or radiation for patients with NF2-SWN. Patients often take dietary supplements for health enhancement purposes. For example, sulforane, an element in broccoli, has shown in vitro evidence of VS tumor suppression.[60] A thorough review of the multiple compounds under study in NF was recently published by Amaravathi and colleagues.[61]

Bacteriotherapy

A novel approach to NF2-associated tumor control is via direct intratumoral injection of *Salmonella typhimurium*, an inactivated bacteria in a preclinical mouse schwannoma tumor model. Following bacterial injection, the mice were treated with injection of enrofloxacin which significantly decreased the growth of schwannoma tumors in mice compared with phosphate buffered saline (PBS)-treated controls.[62]

Gene Therapy

Gene therapy to restore the NF2 gene to merlin deficient cells is of great interest, but still in the preclinical realm. Impressive success has been demonstrated in a gene therapy for spinal muscular atrophy[63] and Duchenne muscular dystrophy.[64] The direct retinal injection of gene replacement with RPE65 has also shown vision restoration in Leber congenital amaurosis.[65] Disease processes such as NF2-SWN with single gene mutations offer good targets for gene replacement therapy applications. Cautious progress is being made with consideration for avoidance of complications. Adeno-associated virus (AAV) vectors are largely being used for in vivo studies as AAVs evoke a more mild course of innate immunity. They also reduce the likelihood of oncogenesis accompanying retroviral vectors.

Prabhakar and colleagues recently demonstrated schwannoma shrinkage after direct tumor injection with AAV1-NF2, which expresses the merlin protein by decreasing the activation of the mammalian Target of Rapamycin Complex 1 (mTORC1) pathway.[66] In vivo, a single injection of AAV1-merlin directly into human

NF2-null Schwann cells derived tumors growing in the sciatic nerve of nude mice led to regression of tumor over a 10-week period. A decrease in dividing cells and an increase in apoptosis were demonstrated when compared with vehicle. Central nervous system AAV vector optimization in nonhuman primates is progressing. Selected adenoviral vector capsids from a library have shown intrathecal injection in cynomolgus monkeys to transduce spinal cord, brain, and Schwann cells. Beharry and colleagues demonstrated higher efficiency of transduction into spinal cord and Schwann cells with an AAV-F and higher dorsal root ganglion cell transduction with AAV-9. Intrathecal injection of AAV-9 to transduce brain and spinal cord has been less affected by preexisting antibodies than vectors administered systemically.[67] Such groundwork may open the avenue to intrathecal human NF2-gene delivery.

Progress is being made toward medical and gene intervention in NF2-SWN striking at the source of the neoplastic proliferation of schwannoma cells rather than solely at the resulting tumors with their attendant comorbidities. It is likely that multiple target inhibition using combination of small molecule therapies may be more potent than single agents have been. Immunotherapy is largely unexplored for benign lesions but holds some promise. However, gene replacement, when it can be accomplished safely and effectively, seems the most satisfying long-term solution for this devastating disease.

CLINICS CARE POINTS

- Small molecule inhibitors of growth of NF2-associated VS are yet in their infancy except bevacizumab.
- Unfortunately the testing of the majority of the drugs discussed do not meet the bar for evidence-based pearls except as stated in the Key Points for bevacizumab.

FINANCIAL DISCLOSURES

D.B. Welling is a consultant for Skylark Bio, Inc; Mulberry Therapeutics; Recursion; Salubritas Therapeutics, LLC; and NF2 Bio. Recursion controls the rights to REC-2282 which is discussed. Dr D.B. Welling solely wrote this review, from conceptualization and visualization, up to and including all writing from original draft, through review, and editing.

ACKNOWLEDGMENTS

There is no data acquisition involved, nor funding source for this article.

REFERENCES

1. Evans DG, Howard E, Giblin C, et al. Birth incidence and prevalence of tumor-prone syndromes: estimates from a UK family genetic register service. Am J Med Genet 2010;152A(2):327–32.
2. Carlson ML, Link MJ. Vestibular Schwannomas. N Engl J Med 2021;384(14):1335–48.
3. Petrilli AM, Fernández-Valle C. Role of Merlin/NF2 inactivation in tumor biology. Oncogene 2016;35(5):537–48.
4. Plotkin SR, Messiaen L, Legius E, et al. Updated diagnostic criteria and nomenclature for neurofibromatosis type 2 and schwannomatosis: an international consensus recommendation. Genet Med 2022;24(9):1967–77.

5. Rouleau GA, Merel P, Lutchman M, et al. Alteration in a new gene encoding a putative membrane-organizing protein causes neuro-fibromatosis type 2. Nature 1993;363(6429):515–21.

6. Trofatter JA, MacCollin MM, Rutter JL, et al. A novel moesin-, ezrin-, radixin-like gene is a candidate for the neurofibromatosis 2 tumor suppressor. Cell 1993; 72(5):791–800, published correction appears in Cell. 1993 Nov 19;75(4):826.

7. Jhanwar SC, Xu XL, Elahi AH, et al. Cancer genomics of lung cancer including malignant mesothelioma: a brief overview of current status and future prospects. Adv Biol Regul 2020;78:100723.

8. Stamenkovic I, Yu Q. Merlin, a "magic" linker between extracellular cues and intracellular signaling pathways that regulate cell motility, proliferation, and survival. Curr Protein Pept Sci 2010;11(6):471–84.

9. Dhaenens BAE, Ferner RE, Evans DG, et al. Lessons learned from drug trials in neurofibromatosis: a systematic review. Eur J Med Genet 2021;64(9):104281.

10. Synodos for NF2 Consortium, Allaway R, Angus SP, et al. Traditional and systems biology based drug discovery for the rare tumor syndrome neurofibromatosis type 2. PLoS One 2018;13(6):e0197350.

11. Dombi E, Ardern-Holmes SL, Babovic-Vuksanovic D, et al. Recommendations for imaging tumor response in neurofibromatosis clinical trials. Neurology 2013; 81(21 Suppl 1):S33–40.

12. Wong HK, Lahdenranta J, Kamoun WS, et al. Anti-vascular endothelial growth factor therapies as a novel therapeutic approach to treating neurofibromatosis-related tumors. Cancer Res 2010;70(9):3483–93.

13. London NR, Gurgel RK. The role of vascular endothelial growth factor and vascular stability in diseases of the ear. Laryngoscope 2014;124(8):E340–6.

14. Plotkin SR, Stemmer-Rachamimov AO, Barker FG 2nd, et al. Hearing improvement after bevacizumab in patients with neurofibromatosis type 2. N Engl J Med 2009;361(4):358–67.

15. Plotkin SR, Duda DG, Muzikansky A, et al. Multicenter, prospective, phase ii and biomarker study of high-dose bevacizumab as induction therapy in patients with neurofibromatosis type 2 and progressive vestibular schwannoma. J Clin Oncol 2019;37(35):3446–54, published correction appears in J Clin Oncol. 2020 Feb 20;38(6):656.

16. Huang V, Bergner AL, Halpin C, et al. Improvement in patient-reported hearing after treatment with bevacizumab in people with neurofibromatosis type 2. Otol Neurotol 2018;39(5):632–8.

17. Karajannis MA, Hagiwara M, Schreyer M, et al. Sustained imaging response and hearing preservation with low-dose bevacizumab in sporadic vestibular schwannoma. Neuro Oncol 2019;21(6):822–4.

18. Fujii M, Ichikawa M, Iwatate K, et al. Bevacizumab Therapy of neurofibromatosis type 2 associated vestibular schwannoma in Japanese patients. Neurol Med-Chir 2020;60(2):75–82.

19. Shi J, Lu D, Gu R, et al. Reliability and toxicity of bevacizumab for neurofibromatosis type 2-related vestibular schwannomas: A systematic review and meta-analysis. Am J Otolaryngol 2021;42(6):103148.

20. Lu VM, Ravindran K, Graffeo CS, et al. Efficacy and safety of bevacizumab for vestibular schwannoma in neurofibromatosis type 2: a systematic review and meta-analysis of treatment outcomes. J Neuro Oncol 2019;144(2):239–48.

21. Blakeley JO, Ye X, Duda DG, et al. Efficacy and biomarker study of bevacizumab for hearing loss resulting from neurofibromatosis type 2-associated vestibular schwannomas. J Clin Oncol 2016;34(14):1669–75.

22. Sverak P, Adams ME, Haines SJ, et al. Bevacizumab for hearing preservation in neurofibromatosis type 2: emphasis on patient-reported outcomes and toxicities. Otolaryngol Head Neck Surg 2019;160(3):526–32.

23. Renzi S, Michaeli O, Salvador H, et al. Bevacizumab for NF2-associated vestibular schwannomas of childhood and adolescence. Pediatr Blood Cancer 2020; 67(5):e28228.

24. Nunes FP, Merker VL, Jennings D, et al. Bevacizumab treatment for meningiomas in NF2: a retrospective analysis of 15 patients. PLoS One 2013;8(3):e59941.

25. Farschtschi S, Merker VL, Wolf D, et al. Bevacizumab treatment for symptomatic spinal ependymomas in neurofibromatosis type 2. Acta Neurol Scand 2016; 133(6):475–80.

26. Kalamarides M, Essayed W, Lejeune JP, et al. Spinal ependymomas in NF2: a surgical disease. J Neuro Oncol 2018;136(3):605–11.

27. Karajannis MA, Legault G, Hagiwara M, et al. Phase II trial of lapatinib in adult and pediatric patients with neurofibromatosis type 2 and progressive vestibular schwannomas. Neuro Oncol 2012;14(9):1163–70.

28. Osorio DS, Hu J, Mitchell C, et al. Effect of lapatinib on meningioma growth in adults with neurofibromatosis type 2. J Neuro Oncol 2018;139(3):749–55.

29. Goutagny S, Giovannini M, Kalamarides M. A 4-year phase II study of everolimus in NF2 patients with growing vestibular schwannomas. J Neuro Oncol 2017; 133(2):443–5.

30. Karajannis MA, Legault G, Hagiwara M, et al. Phase II study of everolimus in children and adults with neurofibromatosis type 2 and progressive vestibular schwannomas. Neuro Oncol 2014;16(2):292–7.

31. Karajannis MA, Mauguen A, Maloku E, et al. Phase 0 clinical trial of everolimus in patients with vestibular schwannoma or meningioma. Mol Cancer Ther 2021; 20(9):1584–91.

32. Devarakonda S, Pellini B, Verghese L, et al. A phase II study of everolimus in patients with advanced solid malignancies with *TSC1, TSC2, NF1, NF2* or *STK11* mutations. J Thorac Dis 2021;13(7):4054–62.

33. Collier KA, Valencia H, Newton H, et al. A phase 1 trial of the histone deacetylase inhibitor AR-42 in patients with neurofibromatosis type 2-associated tumors and advanced solid malignancies. Cancer Chemother Pharmacol 2021;87(5): 599–611.

34. Welling DB, Collier KA, Burns SS, et al. Early phase clinical studies of AR-42, a histone deacetylase inhibitor, for neurofibromatosis type 2-associated vestibular schwannomas and meningiomas. Laryngoscope Investig Otolaryngol 2021; 6(5):1008–19.

35. Plotkin SR, Halpin C, McKenna MJ, et al. Erlotinib for progressive vestibular schwannoma in neurofibromatosis 2 patients. Otol Neurotol 2010;31(7):1135–43.

36. Bush ML, Burns SS, Oblinger J, et al. Treatment of vestibular schwannoma cells with ErbB inhibitors. Otol Neurotol 2012;33(2):244–57.

37. Delmas J, Varoquaux A, Troude L, et al. Incidental effect of long-term tacrolimus treatment on sporadic vestibular schwannoma volume shrinkage and clinical improvement. Otol Neurotol 2020;41(1):e89–93.

38. Zhang S, Anjum R, Squillace R, et al. The Potent ALK Inhibitor Brigatinib (AP26113) Overcomes Mechanisms of Resistance to First- and Second-Generation ALK Inhibitors in Preclinical Models. Clin Cancer Res 2016;22(22): 5527–38.

39. Chang LS, Oblinger JL, Smith AE, et al. Brigatinib causes tumor shrinkage in both NF2-deficient meningioma and schwannoma through inhibition of multiple tyrosine kinases but not ALK. PLoS One 2021;16(7):e0252048.

40. Ornelas A, Zacharias-Millward N, Menter DG, et al. Beyond COX-1: the effects of aspirin on platelet biology and potential mechanisms of chemoprevention. Cancer Metastasis Rev 2017;36(2):289–303.

41. Dilwali S, Kao SY, Fujita T, et al. Nonsteroidal anti-inflammatory medications are cytostatic against human vestibular schwannomas. Transl Res 2015;166(1):1–11.

42. Schulz A, Büttner R, Hagel C, et al. The importance of nerve microenvironment for schwannoma development. Acta Neuropathol 2016;132(2):289–307.

43. Kandathil CK, Dilwali S, Wu CC, et al. Aspirin intake correlates with halted growth of sporadic vestibular schwannoma in vivo. Otol Neurotol 2014;35(2):353–7.

44. Kandathil CK, Cunnane ME, McKenna MJ, et al. Correlation between aspirin intake and reduced growth of human vestibular schwannoma: volumetric analysis. Otol Neurotol 2016;37(9):1428–34.

45. Hunter JB, O'Connell BP, Wanna GB, et al. Vestibular schwannoma growth with aspirin and other nonsteroidal anti-inflammatory drugs. Otol Neurotol 2017; 38(8):1158–64.

46. Marinelli JP, Lees KA, Tombers NM, et al. Impact of aspirin and other NSAID use on volumetric and linear growth in vestibular schwannoma. Otolaryngol Head Neck Surg 2019;160(6):1081–6.

47. MacKeith S, Wasson J, Baker C, et al. Aspirin does not prevent growth of vestibular schwannomas: a case-control study. Laryngoscope 2018;128(9):2139–44.

48. Tan Q, Yan X, Song L, et al. Induction of mitochondrial dysfunction and oxidative damage by antibiotic drug doxycycline enhances the responsiveness of glioblastoma to chemotherapy. Med Sci Monit 2017;23:4117–25.

49. Ali I, Alfarouk KO, Reshkin SJ, et al. Doxycycline as potential anti-cancer agent. Anti Cancer Agents Med Chem 2017;17(12):1617–23.

50. Ammoun S, Schmid MC, Triner J, et al. Nilotinib alone or in combination with selumetinib is a drug candidate for neurofibromatosis type 2. Neuro Oncol 2011; 13(7):759–66.

51. Wu L, Vasilijic S, Sun Y, et al. Losartan prevents tumor-induced hearing loss and augments radiation efficacy in NF2 schwannoma rodent models. Sci Transl Med 2021;13(602):eabd4816.

52. Schiller JH, Larson T, Ou SH, et al. Efficacy and safety of axitinib in patients with advanced non-small-cell lung cancer: results from a phase II study. J Clin Oncol 2009;27(23):3836–41.

53. Zhao Y, Liu P, Zhang N, et al. Targeting the cMET pathway augments radiation response without adverse effect on hearing in NF2 schwannoma models. Proc Natl Acad Sci U S A 2018;115(9):E2077–84 (Crizotinib).

54. Troutman S, Moleirinho S, Kota S, et al. Crizotinib inhibits NF2-associated schwannoma through inhibition of focal adhesion kinase 1. Oncotarget 2016; 7(34):54515–25.

55. Petrilli AM, Garcia J, Bott M, et al. Ponatinib promotes a G1 cell-cycle arrest of merlin/NF2-deficient human schwann cells. Oncotarget 2017;8(19):31666–81.

56. Huegel J, Dinh CT, Martinelli M, et al. CUDC907, a dual phosphoinositide-3 kinase/histone deacetylase inhibitor, promotes apoptosis of NF2 Schwannoma cells. Oncotarget 2022;13:890–904.

57. Paldor I, Abbadi S, Bonne N, et al. The efficacy of lapatinib and nilotinib in combination with radiation therapy in a model of NF2 associated peripheral schwannoma. J Neuro Oncol 2017;135(1):47–56.

58. Sagers JE, Brown AS, Vasilijic S, et al. Computational repositioning and preclinical validation of mifepristone for human vestibular schwannoma. Sci Rep 2018; 8(1):5437, published correction appears in Sci Rep. 2018 Nov 23;8(1):17449.
59. Tamura R, Fujioka M, Morimoto Y, et al. A VEGF receptor vaccine demonstrates preliminary efficacy in neurofibromatosis type 2. Nat Commun 2019;10(1):: 5758. https://doi.org/10.1038/s41467-019-13640, published correction appears in Nat Commun. 2020 Apr 21;11(1):2028.
60. Kim BG, Fujita T, Stankovic KM, et al. Sulforaphane, a natural component of broccoli, inhibits vestibular schwannoma growth in vitro and in vivo. Sci Rep 2016;6: 36215. https://doi.org/10.1038/srep36215.
61. Amaravathi A, Oblinger JL, Welling DB, et al. Neurofibromatosis: Molecular Pathogenesis and Natural Compounds as Potential Treatments. Front Oncol 2021;11: 698192. https://doi.org/10.3389/fonc.2021.698192.
62. Ahmed SG, Brenner GJ. Effect of antibiotic treatment on attenuated salmonella typhimurium VNP20009 mediated schwannoma growth control. Anticancer Res 2023;43(1):1–6.
63. Mendell JR, Al-Zaidy S, Shell R, et al. Single-dose gene-replacement therapy for spinal muscular atrophy. N Engl J Med 2017;377(18):1713–22.
64. Asher DR, Thapa K, Dharia SD, et al. Clinical development on the frontier: gene therapy for duchenne muscular dystrophy. Expert Opin Biol Ther 2020;20(3): 263–74.
65. Aguirre GD, Cideciyan AV, Dufour VL, et al. Gene therapy reforms photoreceptor structure and restores vision in NPHP5-associated Leber congenital amaurosis. Mol Ther 2021;29(8):2456–68, published correction appears in Mol Ther. 2021 Dec 1;29(12):3528.
66. Prabhakar S, Beauchamp RL, Cheah PS, et al. Gene replacement therapy in a schwannoma mouse model of neurofibromatosis type 2. Mol Ther Methods Clin Dev 2022;26:169–80.
67. Beharry A, Gong Y, Kim JC, et al. The AAV9 variant capsid AAV-f mediates widespread transgene expression in nonhuman primate spinal cord after intrathecal administration. Hum Gene Ther 2022;33(1–2):61–75.

Salvage Management of Vestibular Schwannoma

Emily Kay-Rivest, MD, MSc[a,b],*, John Thomas Roland Jr, MD[b,1]

KEYWORDS

- Vestibular schwannomas • Microsurgery • Stereotactic radiosurgery
- Treatment failures • Revisions • Functional outcomes

KEY POINTS

- Treatment failures can occur after both microsurgery (MS) and stereotactic radiosurgery (SRS) for vestibular schwannoma (VS).
- SRS is the most favored second treatment modality following subtotal VS resection and SRS does not prevent recovery of post-operative facial nerve weakness.
- Salvage MS can be considered after primary MS or SRS, but may be surgically challenging, and usually is reserved for tumors that are quickly growing or symptomatic.
- Repeat SRS is a possibility and may be considered in asymptomatic, smaller tumors. The long-term adverse event profile of re-irradiation still requires future research.

INTRODUCTION

The current management of vestibular schwannomas (VS) includes observation, microsurgery (MS), and stereotactic radiosurgery (SRS) or radiotherapy. Treatment failures can occur with any primary treatment modality. In the case of microsurgical failures, recurrence should be distinguished from residual tumor. A recurrence consists of a newly discovered tumor after gross-total resection (GTR) or continued growth after incomplete removal. In contrast, residual tumor is described as the persistence of tumor after a near-total (NRT) or subtotal resection (STR) (**Fig. 1** for examples of each). Microsurgery failures may be treated with observation, revision surgery, and radiotherapy.

The use of radiation for VS can include fractionated radiation therapy, fractionated stereotactic radiotherapy (FSRT), and most commonly SRS. SRS has been used for over 30 years to manage VS and has an excellent safety and side effect profile. It

a Division of Otology and Neurotology, Department of Otolaryngology–Head and Neck Surgery, McGill University, Montreal, Quebec, Canada; b Division of Otology and Neurotology, Department of Otolaryngology–Head and Neck Surgery, New York University, New York, NY, USA
1 Present address: 550 First Avenue, Suite 7 Q, New York, NY 10016.
* Corresponding author. 3755 Chemin de la Cote-Sainte-Catherine, Montreal, H3T 1E2, Quebec.
E-mail address: Emily.kay-rivest@mcgill.ca

Otolaryngol Clin N Am 56 (2023) 557–565
https://doi.org/10.1016/j.otc.2023.02.014

A Gross total resection.

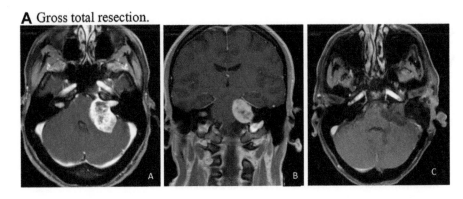

B Near total resection.

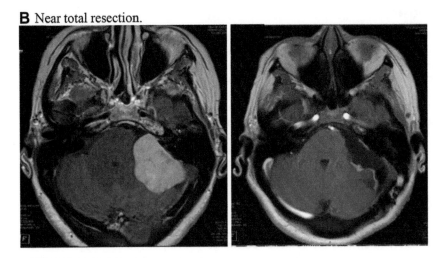

C Subtotal resection.

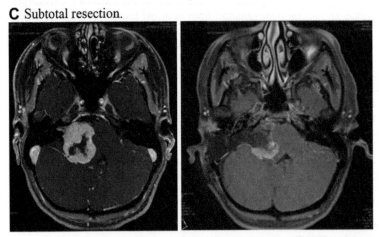

Fig. 1. (*A*) GTR. Images of a patient with NF2 who had remote left VS surgery via a RS approach. A revision surgery was performed via a translabyrinthine and transcochlear approach. Panels A and B show axial and coronal views of a left VS before revision surgery. Panel C shows GTR after revision surgery. (*B*) Near-total resection. Example of a near-total resection of a left cerebello-pontine angle meningioma. (*C*) Subtotal resection. Example of a subtotal resection of a right VS.

can be used as a primary treatment in certain patient populations, including older patients, those unfit for surgery, and commonly in small-sized to medium-sized tumors.
Nonetheless, failures after radiosurgery may also occur. It is important to differentiate
treatment failure from the expected transient volume increase that may occur
following treatment, usually in the first months after SRS. For this reason, multiple
consecutive scans following irradiation should be performed before determining a
treatment failure.

SURGICAL FAILURES

Recurrent disease after GTR of VS is uncommon.[1–3] Recurrences can occur along the
facial nerve, cochlear, or vestibular nerves when preserved, or in the fundus of the internal auditory canal (IAC). For all three surgical approaches, the rates of recurrence
are low, although the rate is thought to be lowest following the translabyrinthine (TL)
approach.[1,2,4,5] Indeed, the TL allows for excellent visualization along the length of
the IAC, which may not always be true for other approaches. In the retrosigmoid
(RS) approach, although recurrence rates are also low,[1,6,7] the dissection of the fundus
of the IAC may be partially blind and lead to slightly higher rates of recurrence
compared with the TL approach. Finally, the middle fossa (MF) approach may have
a slight increased likelihood of recurrent disease, possibly related to its infrequent
use.[8] Because the RS and MF approaches are commonly used for hearing preservation surgery, incomplete tumor removal from the nerve to preserve its function may account for a slightly higher recurrence rate in these cases.

Certain reports suggest that recurrences may occur several years after the original
resection.[9] Our institution's protocol requires patients to undergo an MRI 4 months after surgery, and then yearly for 5 years, with an additional scan at the 10-year mark.
Certain groups may even prolong this follow-up to 15 years. Imaging should include
a gadolinium-enhanced MRI, with fat-suppressed sequences to allow for differentiation between the abdominal fat used to fill the surgical defect or fibrous scar tissue.
Usually, a recurrence will appear as an enhancing, nodular lesion.

RESECTION FOLLOWED BY RADIOSURGERY

GTR is achieved in a majority of patients after microsurgery for VS. Nonetheless, a
small number of patients have a residual disease and an even smaller number experience recurrent tumors. When the residual disease is left behind after subtotal resection, the overall tumor progression rate is estimated at 20%.[10]

Gadolinium-enhanced MRI is used to monitor residual tumors postoperatively
because often these will be asymptomatic. The rate of regrowth varies widely in the
literature. Bloch and colleagues found a regrowth rate of 3% in their near-total resection (NTR) and 32% in their STR cohorts.[11] However, regrowth rates as low as 0% for
NTR and 18% for STR[12] and as high as 52% and 63% for NRT and STR, respectively[13]
have been described. This speaks of the importance of continued follow-up of residual
disease.

Interval Between Surgery and Adjuvant radiation

The first question is when to begin considering adjuvant irradiation. Usually, the decision is made after two or more MRIs indicating progressive growth. Pollock and colleagues found an interval between surgery and tumor recurrence of 57 months in
patients with previous complete resection. In subtotally resected tumors, the median
interval to radiosurgery due to tumor progression was 37 months.[10] If there is clear residual tumor after resection, many centers will schedule elective radiosurgery within 3

to 6 months after recovery. We feel that documenting the growth of the residual tumor before initiating SRS is best.

Tumor Control Rates

Reports of SRS have revealed excellent tumor control results after primary microsurgical residual in the range of approximately 95%.[14] Furthermore, a recent systematic review revealed tumor control rates after surgery and subsequent SRS were 93.9%.[15] Pollock and colleagues reviewed a cohort of 76 patients who underwent SRS following microsurgery.[10] In 28 patients (36% of tumors), tumor size decreased following SRS and remained unchanged in 45 patients (58% of tumors). Five tumors (6% of the cohort) had tumor progression after the radiosurgery at a median interval of 31 months. Among these patients, four required repeat surgery and one was re-irradiated. Interestingly, two patients required a salvage surgery due to new symptoms of hydrocephalus and ataxia, without evidence of tumor growth. Upon retrospective reflection, their group questioned whether observation and treatment with corticosteroid or a ventriculo-peritoneal (VP) shunt may have precluded the need for surgery.

Facial Nerve Outcomes

New facial weakness with current SRS doses is rare. Brokinkel and colleagues reviewed six studies comprising a total of 159 patients.[16] They found that 82.8% of patients maintained a facial function of house-Brackmann (HB) 1 to 2 after surgery, which subsequently stayed stable in 94% of those patients after adjuvant SRS. Moreover, 17 patients showed progressive recovery of facial nerve function as compared to the immediate post-operative period.

Other Functional Outcomes

Varying rates of trigeminal neuropathy are reported following secondary SRS, with an incidence reaching up to 29%.[17] This is highly dependent on trigeminal nerve compression by the tumor at the time of SRS. Pollock and colleagues found that 14% of patients developed new trigeminal symptoms,[10] however, 50% of their cohort already had prior fifth nerve symptoms.

Complications

Other adverse events may occur following SRS after MS which include ataxia, vestibulopathies, hydrocephalus, and lower cranial nerve dysfunctions. These side effects are rare, occurring usually in less than 5% of patients. **Table 1** is a summary of our institutional review of all salvage modalities with a focus on the interval between treatments, rates of GTR, and complications.

RESECTION FOLLOWED BY RESECTION

A repeat resection is a feasible option for both recurrent and residual VS, although SRS is more commonly employed. Revision microsurgery may be necessary if there is compression of the brainstem, in patients who strongly prefer surgery, or in individuals with intractable trigeminal neuralgia, which may improve after nerve decompression.[18]

If the previous resection involved extensive dissection of the facial nerve, there may be increased adhesions and scarring, and therefore, increased risk of injury at the second surgery. Although in most cases, an intact plane between the facial nerve and recurrent tumor exists, this may not always be the case. There is no consensus on the best approach for repeat MS. Some groups will advocate using the same approach,[7] whereas others suggest that an alternate approach may allow dissection

Table 1 Institutional summary of outcomes after second intervention for vestibular schwannoma treatment				
	MS Then SRS **n = 61**	**MS Then MS** **n = 9**	**SRS Then MS** **n = 7**	**SRS Then SRS** **n = 7**
Interval between 1st and 2nd intervention in months (median, range)	34 (1–336)	49 (9–225)	42 (30–59)	60 (21–70)
GTR after salvage MS	—	5 (56%)	3 (43%)	—
Facial function				
No change	51 (84%)	1 (11%)	5 (71%)	7 (100%)
Deteriorated	2 (3%)	7 (78%)	2 (29%)	0 (0%)
Improved	8 (13%)	1 (11%)	0 (0%)	0 (0%)
Trigeminal nerve deficit	2 (3%)	1 (11%)	0 (0%)	1 (14%)
Facial spasms	2 (3%)	0 (0%)	0 (0%)	1 (14%)
Complications				
CSF leak	0 (0%)	2 (22%)	1 (14%)	0 (0%)
Other CN deficit	0 (0%)	1 (11%)	0 (0%)	0 (0%)
Stroke	0 (0%)	0 (0%)	0 (0%)	0 (0%)
Wound infection	0 (0%)	0 (0%)	0 (0%)	0 (0%)
Meningitis	0 (0%)	0 (0%)	1 (14%)	0 (0%)
Hydrocephalus	0 (0%)	1 (11%)	0 (0%)	1 (14%)

Abbreviations: CN, cranial nerve; CSF, cerebrospinal fluid; GTR, gross-total resection; MS, microsurgery; SRS, stereotactic radiosurgery.

through healthy tissue devoid of scarring.[5,19] We strongly recommend a different approach for revision microsurgery.

Interval Between Surgery and Repeat Surgery

Among the few studies that report outcomes of repeat MS after recurrence of disease, the mean time to second surgery was 73 months.[1,2,5,7,19] Among these patients, the same approach for resection was used in 90% of cases.

Facial Nerve Outcomes

Facial nerve outcomes vary significantly throughout the literature following the second surgery. In general, the rates of *favorable* facial nerve function after repeat MS are often less than 50%. The cohort described above by Samii and colleagues found that 48% of patients who underwent MS followed by repeat MS maintained favorable facial nerve function (HB grades I to II) in the immediate post-operative period. At 1-year post-op, this had improved to 64.7%.

Complications

As mentioned above, in the unique situation where resection is repeated, we are often faced with symptomatic patients. For this reason, some of the complications caused by the enlarging tumor may in fact resolve after surgery. In Samii's cohort, it was reported that gait disturbances improved in 12 of 14 patients, dizziness improved in 7 of 10 patients, swallowing issues improved in 4 of 7 patients, and finally, trigeminal function improved in 3 of 5 patients.[7] Given the small number of reported patients, it is difficult to say whether surgical complications occur more frequently after the second surgery.

RADIOSURGERY FAILURES

As described above, SRS is a good alternative to MS in the treatment of VS and affords high rates of tumor control. The rates of facial and auditory neuropathies are believed to be comparable to MS rates. Overall, the need for further intervention following SRS is approximately 3% to 5%. However, given the increasing number of tumors treated with SRS, a certain number of failures do occur and can be addressed with resection or re-irradiation.

One must differentiate treatment failure from the known tumor expansion that occurs initially after SRS. Nagano and colleagues described a transient expansion in as many as 75% of patients. It is thought that an initial volume increase is a common phenomenon and will usually be followed by slight regression as time passes.[20] Neurologic deficits may not necessarily be linked to tumor growth following SRS but may be a result of the radiation itself. During this time, a course of corticosteroids is recommended, rather than immediately resorting to salvage surgery. Radiation-induced neuropathies are thought to resolve within 3 to 12 months in more than half the cases.[21] Intervention following SRS should only occur if there is sustained tumor growth on serial imaging: usually, two or more MRIs or if a patient is symptomatic from mass effect.

RADIOSURGERY FOLLOWED BY REPEAT RADIOSURGERY

Salvage SRS after previous treatment remains an option for tumors that progress after initial SRS. Although relatively few cases are reported in the literature, there appears to be promising evidence regarding retreatment, with high efficacy and low levels of toxicity. Most groups will advocate for waiting a minimum of 2 to 3 years before a treatment failure is confirmed. Following this, the decision must be made between salvage MS and re-irradiation. If there is any clinical or radiologic evidence of brainstem compression, MS is the preferred approach. Patient age, co-morbidities, as well as individual preferences, may also play into the decision-making process.

Interval Between Initial and Repeat Radiosurgery

The interval of time between initial and re-irradiation is quite similar across the literature, ranging from 43 to 63 months.[17,22–27] At our center, the mean interval of time was 60 months, which is comparable to current literature. Patients are therefore being followed for the regular 2-year interval, and then progressive growth is noted over approximately 3 more years before the decision is made to repeat SRS.

Tumor Control Rates

From the small number of patients reported to date, control rates vary from 85% to 100%, with a mean follow-up of 49 months.[17,22–27] Despite certain patients with progressive growth, some may still be monitored with serial imaging. Only two reported cases in the current literature required additional intervention after re-irradiation. Indeed, if a second dose of SRS fails, surgical resection remains the only option and may be challenging.

Facial Nerve Outcomes

The incidence of worsened facial nerve function on follow-up is low but not nonexistent. Fu and colleagues found that in their cohort of repeat SRS, 3 out of 38 had new onset facial palsies. Liscak and colleagues had 1 out of 24 patients with new facial palsy after the second dose of radiation.[17] Overall, the literature suggests that when treating a tumor margin dose of 10 to 13 Gy, at a median follow-up of 66 months, new permanent facial nerve weakness was found in 0% and 25% of patients.[17,22–27] In our cohort of patients who underwent repeat SRS, none had worsened facial nerve function, although one patient developed facial spasms after their second SRS.[18]

Other Functional Outcomes

Many patients undergoing re-irradiation were noted to have trigeminal nerve dysfunction. This is because many have a larger tumor with trigeminal nerve compression. Within the literature reviewed, although patients received almost uniformly the same dose of radiation, certain groups had much higher numbers of trigeminal nerve dysfunctions. In their review of 24 patients, Liscak and colleagues reported seven new cases of facial numbness.[17] On the other hand, Lonneville and colleagues reported on 25 similar patients, and no cases of new facial numbness were described.[26] Very little is known about the incidence of facial pain following re-irradiation.

Complications

Overall, neurologic side effects are more prevalent after retreatment of any kind. One complication that can occur both after primary SRS and re-irradiation is cerebellar edema. Most patients may experience transient edema without symptoms, whereas a small number of patients report headaches. Most series containing over 25 patients reported usually had one patient with evidence of cerebellar edema. Overall, within the 126 patients reported in the literature to date, only one required a ventriculo-periotoneal shunt.[17] In general, a small amount of symptomatic cerebellar edema can be managed with a course of steroids with usually leads to resolution.

RADIOSURGERY FOLLOWED BY SALVAGE RESECTION

Centers that treat large volumes of VS will often report that salvage resection after SRS tends to be more tenuous, with lower rates of GTR and poorer facial nerve outcomes. Surgeries have also been reported to be longer, with reports of 1.5 hours of increased surgical time on average.[28]

A large group of patients who underwent SRS followed by MS was reviewed and combined patients from the University of Pittsburgh Medical Center and the Mayo Clinic. Overall, 452 patients were found to have adequate imaging and follow-up (NF-2 patients were excluded).[21] They noted 13 patients (2.9%) who required delayed surgical resection after SRS. The facial nerve was preserved in 10 of 13 patients. Surgeons were questioned and reported increased difficulty of resection in 8 of 13 patients. This was thought to be related to tumor fibrosis, loss of an arachnoidal plane, or a combination of the two. In terms of histopathology, 12 cases had typical schwannoma features whereas one was considered malignant.

Overall, salvage microsurgery after SRS is challenging. To improve the rates of facial nerve preservation, less than GTR might be strongly considered.

SUMMARY

Both MS and SRS have very low rates of failure. Repeat SRS carries a low adverse event profile, although few cases are reported to date and long-term follow-up is required. It should be considered in smaller tumors that are growing but asymptomatic. On the other hand, salvage MS following SRS is usually surgically challenging. It is often reserved for symptomatic patients and rapidly growing tumors. Nonetheless, good facial nerve outcomes are achievable. Finally, revision MS is an option following failed MS, although is reserved for specific cases as adjuvant SRS is usually the mainstay of treatment.

CLINICS CARE POINTS

- Treatment failures from both microsurgery and SRS for VS are rare occurences.
- Facial nerve outcomes are excellent in patients who undergo MS followed by SRS, and SRS does not preclude recovery of post-operative weakness.
- Salvage MS following previous MS and SRS can be surgically challenging and is usually reserved for symptomatic patients with rapidly growing tumors.
- Our group suggests a different surgical approach for repeat microsurgical intervention.
- Treatment failure following SRS should not be confused with the known tumor expansion that occurs initially after treatment.
- Re-irradiation carries a low adverse event profile, although further research is needed to better understand long-term outcomes.

DISCLOSURE

No relevant disclosures.

REFERENCES

1. Ahmad RARL, Sivalingam S, Topsakal V, et al. Rate of recurrent vestibular schwannoma after total removal via different surgical approaches. Ann Otol Rhinol Laryngol 2012;121(3):156–61.
2. Shelton C. Unilateral acoustic tumors: how often do they recur after translabyrinthine removal? Laryngoscope 1995;105(9):958–66.
3. Hong B, Krauss JK, Bremer M, et al. Vestibular schwannoma microsurgery for recurrent tumors after radiation therapy or previous surgical resection. Otol Neurotol 2014;35(1):171–81.
4. Glasscock ME 3rd, Kveton JF, Jackson CG, et al. A systematic approach to the surgical management of acoustic neuroma. Laryngoscope 1986;96(10):1088–94.
5. Freeman SRM, Ramsden RT, Saeed SR, et al. Revision surgery for residual or recurrent vestibular schwannoma. Otol Neurotol 2007;28(8):1076–82.
6. Mazzoni A, Calabrese V, Moschini L. Residual and recurrent acoustic neuroma in hearing preservation procedures: neuroradiologic and surgical findings. Skull Base Surg 1996;6(2):105–12.
7. Samii M, Metwali H, Gerganov V. Microsurgical management of vestibular schwannoma after failed previous surgery. J Neurosurg 2016;125(5):1198–203.
8. Sughrue ME, Kaur R, Rutkowski MJ, et al. Extent of resection and the long-term durability of vestibular schwannoma surgery. J Neurosurg 2011;114(5):1218–23.
9. Jacob JT, Carlson ML, Driscoll CL, et al. Volumetric analysis of tumor control following subtotal and near-total resection of vestibular schwannoma. Laryngoscope 2016;126(8):1877–82.
10. Pollock BE, Lunsford LD, Flickinger JC, et al. Vestibular schwannoma management: Part I. Failed microsurgery and the role of delayed stereotactic radiosurgery. J Neurosurg 1998;89(6):944–8.

11. Bloch DC, Oghalai JS, Jackler RK, et al. The fate of the tumor remnant after less-than-complete acoustic neuroma resection. Otolaryngol Head Neck Surg 2004; 130(1):104–12.
12. Chen Z, Prasad SC, Di Lella F, et al. The behavior of residual tumors and facial nerve outcomes after incomplete excision of vestibular schwannomas. J Neurosurg 2014;120(6):1278–87.
13. Fukuda M, Oishi M, Hiraishi T, et al. Clinicopathological factors related to regrowth of vestibular schwannoma after incomplete resection. J Neurosurg 2011;114(5):1224–31.
14. Pollock BE, Link MJ. Vestibular schwannoma radiosurgery after previous surgical resection or stereotactic radiosurgery. Prog Neurol Surg 2008;21:163–8.
15. Starnoni D, Daniel RT, Tuleasca C, et al. Systematic review and meta-analysis of the technique of subtotal resection and stereotactic radiosurgery for large vestibular schwannomas: a "nerve-centered" approach. Neurosurg Focus 2018; 44(3):E4.
16. Brokinkel B, Sauerland C, Holling M, et al. Gamma Knife radiosurgery following subtotal resection of vestibular schwannoma. J Clin Neurosci 2014;21(12): 2077–82.
17. Liscak R, Vladyka V, Urgosik D, et al. Repeated treatment of vestibular schwannomas after gamma knife radiosurgery. Acta neurochirurgica 2009;151(4):317.
18. Kay-Rivest E, Golfinos JG, McMenomey SO, et al. Outcomes of Salvage Resection and Radiosurgery Following Failed Primary Treatment of Vestibular Schwannomas. Otolaryngol Head Neck Surg 2022;166(5):957–63.
19. Roche P-H, Khalil M, Thomassin J-M. Microsurgical removal of vestibular schwannomas after failed previous microsurgery. Modern Management of Acoustic Neuroma 2008;21:158–62. Karger Publishers.
20. Nagano O, Higuchi Y, Serizawa T, et al. Transient expansion of vestibular schwannoma following stereotactic radiosurgery. J Neurosurg 2008;109(5):811–6.
21. Pollock BE, Lunsford LD, Kondziolka D, et al. Vestibular schwannoma management: Part II. Failed radiosurgery and the role of delayed microsurgery. J Neurosurg 1998;89(6):949–55.
22. Dewan S, Norén G. Retreatment of vestibular schwannomas with Gamma Knife surgery. J Neurosurg 2008;109(Supplement):144–8.
23. Fu VX, Verheul JB, Beute GN, et al. Retreatment of vestibular schwannoma with Gamma Knife radiosurgery: clinical outcome, tumor control, and review of literature. J Neurosurg 2018;129(1):137–45.
24. Hafez RFA, Morgan MS, Fahmy OM, et al. Outcomes of Gamma Knife Surgery retreatment for growing vestibular schwannoma and review of the literature. Clin Neurol Neurosurg 2020;198:106171.
25. Kano H, Kondziolka D, Niranjan A, et al. Repeat stereotactic radiosurgery for acoustic neuromas. Int J Radiat Oncol Biol Phys 2010;76(2):520–7.
26. Lonneville S, Delbrouck C, Renier C, et al. Repeat Gamma Knife surgery for vestibular schwannomas. Surg Neurol Int 2015;6:153.
27. Yomo S, Arkha Y, Delsanti C, et al. Repeat gamma knife surgery for regrowth of vestibular schwannomas. Neurosurgery 2009;64(1):48–55.
28. Limb CJ, Long DM, Niparko JK. Acoustic neuromas after failed radiation therapy: challenges of surgical salvage. Laryngoscope 2005;115(1):93–8.

Management of Complications in Vestibular Schwannoma Surgery

Joe Walter Kutz Jr, MD[a,*], Donald Tan, MD[b],
Jacob B. Hunter, MD[b], Samuel Barnett, MD[c],
Brandon Isaacson, MD[a]

KEYWORDS

- Vestibular schwannoma • Complications • Facial nerve paralysis • Meningitis
- Cerebrospinal fluid leak

KEY POINTS

- Facial nerve injury, cerebrospinal fluid leakage, and meningitis are the 3 main complications of surgery for vestibular schwannoma that need to be discussed with every patient.
- Optimal facial nerve outcomes take precedence over complete tumor removal. If the facial nerve is severely adherent to the tumor, near-total resection should be considered. The small remnant tumor rarely enlarges, and if the remnant does enlarge, it can be treated with radiosurgery.
- Although severe vascular injuries and complications are rare, surgeons need to be able to control intraoperative bleeding, as well as recognize and treat postoperative vascular complications.

INTRODUCTION

In the early twentieth century, vestibular schwannoma surgery was associated with high morbidity and mortality rates—many patients presented with life-threatening brainstem compression secondary to giant tumors. The goal of surgery in the early years of surgical management was to relieve pressure from the brainstem and prevent hydrocephalus—hearing preservation and facial nerve outcomes were secondary. In addition, the surgical approach was typically through a midline occipital craniotomy, and the lack of imaging made the anatomy and tumor characteristics unknown.

[a] Departments of Otolaryngology and Neurological Surgery, The University of Texas Southwestern Medical Center, 2001 Inwood Road, Dallas TX 75390, USA; [b] The University of Texas Southwestern Medical Center, 2001 Inwood Road, Dallas TX 75390, USA; [c] Departments of Neurological Surgery and Otolaryngology, The University of Texas Southwestern Medical Center, 2001 Inwood Road, Dallas TX 75390, USA
* Corresponding author. 2100 Inwood Road, Dallas, TX 75390-9035.
E-mail address: walter.kutz@utsouthwestern.edu

Otolaryngol Clin N Am 56 (2023) 567–576
https://doi.org/10.1016/j.otc.2023.02.015
0030-6665/23/© 2023 Elsevier Inc. All rights reserved.

The introduction of the surgical microscope and the refinement of advanced skull base approaches resulted in improved visualization and less brain retraction. Current surgical techniques and standardized intraoperative cranial nerve monitoring have advanced to the point that mortality is rare. In appropriate patients, facial nerve and hearing preservation is the rule and not the exception. However, despite advances in surgical technique, complications still occur. This article will focus on the management of complications in vestibular schwannoma surgery.

Vascular Injuries

Venous injury can occur during the surgical approach or tumor dissection. Venous structures most commonly at risk include the sigmoid sinus, superior petrosal sinus, and petrosal veins.

Injury to the sigmoid sinus usually occurs either when drilling, either by direct injury with the burr, damage from the shaft of the burr, or when removing bone over the sigmoid sinus. Another common area of injury is where the emissary vein enters the posterior aspect of the sigmoid sinus. The emissary vein is usually ligated with a suture or a vascular clip if more exposure to the retrosigmoid dura is required. The superior petrosal sinus is also at risk for injury during translabyrinthine and middle fossa approaches. Bleeding from the superior petrosal sinus can often be controlled with bipolar cautery, suture, vascular clip ligation, or gentle pressure with gelfoam. In addition, extreme caution with drilling needs is necessary when utilizing cotton pledgets or oxidized cellulose gauze because the rotating burr can catch the fibers and traumatize surrounding soft tissues.

Despite careful dissection, injury to the sigmoid sinus occurs. Minor injuries often result in brisk bleeding; applying thrombin-soaked absorbable gelfoam will stop even medium-sized vessel defects. The sinus rarely requires ligation or extraluminal occlusion with oxidized cellulose gauze if a significant tear occurs. In a recent retrospective study, the authors reported a major sinus injury in 2.9%, most of which originated at the mastoid emissary vein entry into the sigmoid sinus, with the authors suggesting that reconstruction without hemostatic agents could maintain long-term patency.[1]

Exposure of the sigmoid sinus and jugular bulb, even without intraoperative trauma, can result in postoperative cerebral venous sinus thrombosis, with reports ranging from 5% to 38.9%.[2] A study by Shew and colleagues showed an incidence of dural venous thrombosis of 17.3% with either a retrosigmoid or translabyrinthine approach.[3] A recent study showed cerebral venous thrombosis occurred in 38.9% of patients and identified the following risk factors: surgical exposure of the sigmoid sinus and jugular bulb, surgical decompression and or manipulation of the sigmoid sinus, mastoid obliteration at the end of the case, and heat conduction from the operative microscope or drill.[4] Preoperative determination of a dominant or absent contralateral venous drainage system using the MRI could raise suspicion for a complication of dural sinus thrombosis. Gerges and colleagues found that a shorter internal auditory canal distance to the sigmoid sinus and a more acute petrous angle are 2 anatomic variables associated with thrombosis formation following a translabyrinthine approach.[5]

Thrombosis is associated with increased rates of cerebrospinal fluid (CSF) leakage, which is more common with increased venous sinus pressure and resulting CSF reabsorption.[2,4] In a single institutional study, Shew and colleagues reported a 3-fold increase in odds of CSF leakage after controlling for the surgical approach in those patients with thrombosis, with no correlation between thrombus formation and age, body-mass index, or tumor size.[3] Treatment remains inconsistent given the risk of anticoagulation immediately after surgery, with the potential development of intracranial hemorrhagic complications; however, most dural venous sinus thromboses resolve with time. For example, Krystkiewicz and colleagues showed 58% of dural venous thrombosis resolved within 1 year.[6] Brahimaj and colleagues reported dural venous thrombosis in 22 of 63 patients with postoperative vestibular schwannoma (VS) resection, all were asymptomatic, and none was treated with anticoagulation.[7] If a patient develops hydrocephalus from dural venous thrombosis, anticoagulation could be considered but this would be a rare scenario and may result in complications from the anticoagulation.[8]

In addition to increased CSF leak rates, occlusion or thrombosis of the sigmoid sinus may result in the propagation of thrombus proximally to involve the inferior anastomotic vein, also known as the vein of Labbe. The vein of Labbe travels from the middle or posterolateral aspect of the Sylvian fissure and drains into the anterior transverse sinus. Because the vein of Labbe may be the only venous outflow for the temporal lobe, a catastrophic venous infarct could occur if it is injured or occluded. The middle fossa craniotomy approach has a higher incidence of temporal lobe infarcts because of the prolonged retraction of the temporal lobe.

Additional vessels at risk for injury include the anterior inferior cerebellar artery (AICA), the most vulnerable artery during surgery for vestibular schwannoma (**Fig. 1**). It most commonly originates from the basilar artery, typically splitting in the cerebellopontine angle into rostral and caudal branches, the former typically following the vestibulocochlear and facial nerves, often forming a loop at the internal auditory meatus.[9] Reisser and colleagues demonstrated that the AICA could enter the internal auditory canal in 26% of people, and it can also become embedded in the bone or dura adjacent to the IAC in 1% to 6% of people.[10,11] Bauer and colleagues recently described the case of an aberrant AICA within the petrous portion of the temporal bone during a translabyrinthine approach, which was not visible on retrospectively reviewing the preoperative imaging.[12] However, arterial anatomic variations can often be detected on preoperative MRI with 3D-Fast Imaging Employing Steady-state Acquisition (FIESTA) sequencing.[11] In a recent single-institutional review over 15 years with 591 vestibular schwannoma resections, Rayan and colleagues reported on 8

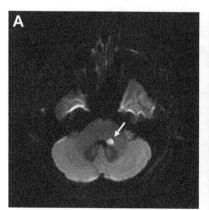 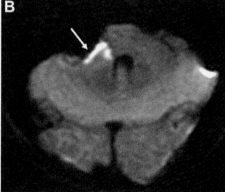

Fig. 1. (*A*) Diffusion-weighting imaging demonstrating a small acute infarct in the left middle cerebellar peduncle secondary to a distal AICA injury suffered during translabyrinthine resection of an acoustic neuroma. (*B*) Right distal AICA infarct. The (*arrow*) represents the infarct.

documented operative vascular injuries (1.4%), AICA in 4 patients (0.7%), PICA in 1 patient (0.2%), and petrosal venous complex branches in 3 patients (0.5%).[13] In their series, only 4 patients demonstrated clinical cerebrovascular complications, with radiographic findings of middle cerebellar peduncle T2 changes and areas of ence-phalomalacia in 2 of the patients.[13] The authors did not find a significant difference in vascular complications based on their surgical approach.[13] Similarly, Sade and col-leagues compared vascular complications between surgical approaches in 413 VS procedures during 24 years, reporting that vascular complication incidences were similar for both the translabyrinthine and retrosigmoid approaches.[14] Distal AICA injury results in ischemia to the middle cerebellar peduncle, which causes dysmetria, ataxia, motor weakness, dysarthria, and dysdiadochokinesia.[15] Fortunately, most patients have satisfactory recovery from AICA injuries.

Venous air embolism is a rare complication that occurs more frequently when sur-gery is performed in a sitting or semisitting position as opposed to a supine position.[16] Although the semisitting position has the advantages of reduced bleeding, lower intra-cranial pressure, and possible bimanual microsurgical dissection, rates of venous air embolism during surgery in the semisitting position range from 1.6% to 76%.[17] Several studies have compared the outcomes of semisitting and supine positioning in posterior cranial fossa surgery,[17–19] with data being mixed on improved facial nerve outcomes[17,20] but most studies cautioned about a higher chance of air emboli in the semisitting position. If the sigmoid is opened, air can enter the sinus and travel to the heart where it can create an air embolism. Initial findings include unexplained hypoten-sion, tachycardia, and decreased end-tidal carbon dioxide. An air embolism is treated by laying the patient in a left decubitus position with their head down, which can pre-vent air from entering the pulmonary arteries. Other important maneuvers include stopping nitrous oxide, increasing oxygen to 100%, positive pressure ventilation, va-sopressors, and possible air aspiration through catheterization to the right heart.

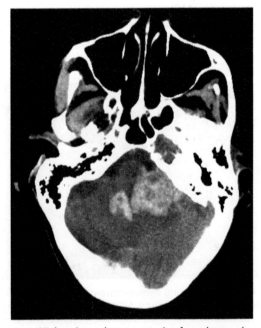

Fig. 2. Axial noncontrast CT showing a large posterior fossa hemorrhage.

A feared complication of any intracranial surgery is intracranial hemorrhage (**Fig. 2**). Meticulous hemostasis is essential but a postoperative hemorrhage may still occur. A computed tomography (CT) scan can be obtained 6 to 8 hours after surgery but neuro-intensive critical care monitoring with hourly neurologic checks for at least 24 hours is best to monitor for signs of intracranial hemorrhage. If a patient is rapidly decompensating, reopening the craniotomy site at the bedside can be a life-saving maneuver, as well as considering an external ventricular drain. Return to the operating room would then allow identification and control of the offending vessel.

Stroke is an uncommon but potentially devastating complication of posterior fossa surgery. A brainstem stroke may result from injury to a vessel during a translabyrinthine or retrosigmoid approach. Signs of a brainstem stroke include vertigo, cranial nerve symptoms, and crossed or uncrossed corticospinal tract findings.[21] Khan and colleagues recently published a large single-institutional experience of more than 400 vestibular schwannoma surgeries during 20 years and reported only 1 brainstem stroke (0.24%).[22]

Cranial Nerve Injuries

The facial nerve is always at risk during vestibular schwannoma surgery, with preservation of the facial nerve being the primary goal of surgery, even beyond complete tumor removal. Successful facial nerve preservation is best achieved by direct visualization as early in the dissection as possible. In both translabyrinthine and middle fossa approaches, the distal facial nerve is identified before tumor dissection begins. The proximal facial nerve, because it exits the brainstem, is found after tumor debulking. Tumor removal commences with both ends of the nerve identified.

Despite identification and careful dissection, facial nerve injury can occur. The mechanisms of injury include transection, heat from cautery, stretch injury, or a compromised blood supply. If the nerve is no longer in continuity at the end of the dissection, the nerve should be grafted if possible. Direct neurorrhaphy can occasionally be performed if the nerve is transposed from the labyrinthine, tympanic, and mastoid segments and delivered to the cerebellopontine angle. A cable graft using the greater auricular nerve or the sural nerve is more often required. The greater auricular nerve is often used because it is in the operative field.

Nerve repair is performed by approximating the epineurium using a 9 to 0 or 10 to 0 nylon suture; however, placing a suture in the cerebellopontine angle (CPA) is difficult. Another easier and equally successful method to repair the nerve is to accurately reapproximate the nerve endings and secure them with fibrin glue.[23] The neurorrhaphy is wrapped in fascia or other soft tissue. Another option is to use neurogenic tubules, which provide a conduit for axonal regeneration.[24]

Deciding on the best management of thermal or stretch injuries can be more difficult because many of these injuries will recover without treatment. Determining the injured segment's ability to transduce a stimulus can guide treatment. Neff and colleagues demonstrated with a regression analysis of 74 patients that stimulus thresholds of 0.05 mA or less and a response amplitude greater than 240 μV predicted House-Brackmann Grade I and II outcomes with 98% (56/57) probability.[25] If no transduction occurs through the injured area, sectioning and grafting the injured segment should be considered.

Injury to other cranial nerves is less common. Trigeminal nerve injury is uncommon, is seen in large tumors, and most often occurs with cautery. Abducens nerve injury results in paralytic strabismus, resulting in diplopia with lateral gaze. The diplopia typically resolves over time if the injury is due to stretching the nerve. Rarely, a patient may need strabismus surgery or botulinum toxin injection to correct the diplopia.[26]

The supratrochlear nerve is a small nerve that runs along the tentorium and is rarely injured during surgery for vestibular schwannoma. A supracochlear nerve injury will result in more subtle symptoms such as difficulty walking down stairs and diplopia when looking down. Injury to the lower cranial nerves is uncommon and can be seen with large tumors. Patients may develop hoarseness, stridor, dysphasia, and aspiration. Intraoperative treatment is limited if an injury occurs to the lower cranial nerves; however, identifying that an injury may have happened is important to prevent aspiration in the postoperative period.

Postoperative Complications

CSF leakage is common after any skull base procedure if the dura is violated. The estimated rates of a CSF leak after surgery for vestibular schwannoma range from 0% to 30%. However, it is challenging to compare series due to differences in techniques used to close the craniotomy and surgical site.[27] The most common pathway for a CSF leak is via the middle ear through the Eustachian tube, with resulting clear rhinorrhea. If a CSF leak is suspected, the patient can be asked to tilt their head downward for a few minutes. If a CSF leak is present, clear fluid can be seen coming from the ipsilateral nostril. If the leak occurs within the first few days after surgery, a lumbar drain trial is performed by draining 20 cc of CSF every 4 hours for 3 to 4 days. If the patient continues to leak after a lumbar drain trial, the external auditory canal is closed in a blind sac fashion, and the eustachian tube is tightly packed with muscle, followed by bone wax. Transnasal eustachian tube closure has been described but this approach is less successful than direct packing via the middle ear.[28]

CSF can also leak through the incision. Meticulous closure of the craniotomy incision in layers usually prevents a CSF leak through the incision; however, if a patient develops elevated CSF pressure, a leak may still occur. An active incisional leak can be closed by oversewing the leaking area with a large silk or polypropylene suture. Cyanoacrylate tissue adhesive can also be used to treat small wound leaks successfully. If the wound continues to leak, a lumbar drain trial can be performed. Rarely will a patient require exploration and reclosure of the incision.

A pseudomeningocele can develop behind an intact closure with elevated CSF pressure, most often after a translabyrinthine approach in the setting of a large tumor (**Fig. 3**). Adequate fat packing and minimal periosteal elevation can sometimes prevent a pseudomeningocele. If a pseudomeningocele occurs, a CSF leak can develop through the incision. Treatment is usually conservative with the placement of a tight head wrap. Needle aspiration of the fluid is possible; however, this could result in contamination of the CSF space resulting in meningitis, and the CSF often recollects. Mehendale and colleagues retrospectively reviewed 375 patients who underwent neurotologic procedures at a single institution, identifying 17 patients who developed pseudomeningoceles, with a formation rate of 4.5%, with 14 (82.3%) spontaneously resolving with pressure dressing, bed rest, and lumbar spinal drainage.[29] Pseudomeningoceles may also be present for weeks but typically resolve spontaneously. Higgins and colleagues retrospectively reviewed 9 patients who underwent translabyrinthine resections for VS who developed headaches, CSF leaks, or pseudomeningoceles and were subsequently referred for sigmoid sinus stenting.[30] The headache improved or resolved in 5 patients, 1 of 2 CSF leaks resolved, and 2 patients had resolution of symptomatic pseudomeningoceles, leading the authors to suggest these symptoms are the result of increased intracranial pressure caused by acquired venous outflow obstructions.[30]

Bacterial meningitis is a potentially life-threatening complication that may occur after surgery for a VS. The incidence of meningitis is likely underestimated. Huang

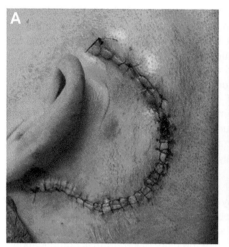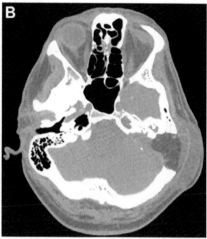

Fig. 3. (A) Left pseudomeningocele 6 weeks postoperatively from a left translabyrinthine craniectomy, (B) which presented with an incisional leak 10 days postoperatively, with the incisional reinforced with a mattress suture before application of cyanoacrylate tissue adhesive and a head wrap.

reported a higher than expected 5.5% to 9.85% rate of meningitis after vestibular schwannoma surgery.[31] It is essential to identify bacterial meningitis early and start treatment as soon as possible because it can result in significant morbidity and death. Patients should be aware of signs of meningitis at discharge, including worsening headaches, fever, myalgia, neck stiffness, and photophobia. Patients with these signs and symptoms should be seen urgently. A lumbar puncture is performed, and broad-spectrum antibiotics are started. If a delay in the lumbar puncture is expected, broad-spectrum antibiotics should be started as soon as possible. However, CSF sterilization may occur within the first 2 hours of administration of antibiotics for meningococci and within 4 hours for pneumococci.[32] Patients with suspected postoperative meningitis are started on broad-spectrum antibiotics such as vancomycin, cefepime, and metronidazole. The antibiotic regimen is often adjusted once cultures and sensitivities become available. Treating bacterial meningitis takes a minimum of 2 weeks and can often be 4 to 6 weeks, depending on the pathogen. Infectious disease is consulted to guide antimicrobial treatment.

Aseptic meningitis is a clinical entity that mimics bacterial meningitis and can create uncertainty in the diagnosis and management of bacterial meningitis. Aseptic meningitis, also referred to as chemical meningitis, represents inflammation of the meninges with negative bacterial CSF culture. The presenting symptoms mimic bacterial meningitis—namely headache, fever, malaise, and meningismus. The CSF characteristics may also mimic bacterial meningitis with leukocytosis, elevated protein, but rarely, low glucose.[33] Aseptic meningitis may have a variety of infectious and noninfectious causes but in the postoperative context it is thought to be caused by delayed inflammation in response to blood, bone dust, surgical products, manipulation, or viral infection.[34] Aseptic meningitis differs from bacterial meningitis in that it typically follows a benign course, does not require broad-spectrum antibiotics, and instead responds to systemic steroid treatment. Few studies have aimed to identify characteristics that can distinguish aseptic from bacterial meningitis early in the clinical course. Sanchez and colleagues suggest that patients without wound infections, focal neurologic changes, or high fevers (>102°F [39°C]) who exhibit a mild CSF leukocytosis less than 2000 cells/μL, a normal CSF glucose when serum glucose is within normal limits, and only mild elevation of serum white blood cell (WBC) counts (<12,000 cells/μL) could be considered for steroid therapy without antibiotics while CSF cultures are pending.[35]

Hydrocephalus is another complication seen most with large tumors. The symptoms of hydrocephalus are related to intracranial hypertension and include headache, nausea and vomiting, depressed level of consciousness, and papilledema.[36] A CT scan can confirm hydrocephalus. Treatment includes medical management with acetazolamide or topiramate, placement of a lumbar drain, and placement of a ventriculoperitoneal shunt. In one study determining the incidence of communicating hydrocephalus following VS treatment, only 1 of the 146 patients developed communicating hydrocephalus.[37]

Seizures are uncommon after vestibular schwannoma surgery and would be more common after a middle fossa craniotomy approach. The middle fossa craniotomy approach requires prolonged temporal lobe retraction, which increases the risk of intracranial complications. Intermittent relaxation of the retractor and the removal of the retractor as soon as possible will decrease the risks of intracranial complications. Antiepileptics are not routinely used after surgery for vestibular schwannoma. In a recent single-institutional review assessing the surgical risks for older patients, analyzing 67 middle cranial fossa approaches for VS resection in patients, with 16 patients aged older than 60 years, they reported no seizures in either cohort.[38]

SUMMARY

Safe techniques for removing vestibular schwannoma have advanced significantly since the early twentieth century. However, surgeons must continue recognizing the potential for intraoperative and postoperative complications. Prioritizing facial nerve outcomes over complete tumor resection is the modern paradigm and has resulted in better facial nerve outcomes. It is also essential to discuss potential complications with patients during the preoperative visit. If a complication occurs, it must be recognized, and the surgeon understands management to ensure the best outcome possible.

DECLARATION OF INTERESTS

None.

REFERENCES

1. Matsushima K, Kohno M, Tanaka Y, et al. Management of sigmoid sinus injury: retrospective study of 450 consecutive surgeries in the cerebellopontine angle and intrapetrous region. Oper Neurosurg (Hagerstown) 2020;19(6):721–9.

2. Benjamin CG, Sen RD, Golfinos JG, et al. Postoperative cerebral venous sinus thrombosis in the setting of surgery adjacent to the major dural venous sinuses. J Neurosurg 2018;1–7. https://doi.org/10.3171/2018.4.JNS18308.

3. Shew M, Kavookjian H, Dahlstrom K, et al. Incidence and risk factors for sigmoid venous thrombosis following CPA tumor resection. Otol Neurotol 2018;39(5): e376–80.

4. Guazzo E, Panizza B, Lomas A, et al. Cerebral venous sinus thrombosis after translabyrinthine vestibular schwannoma-a prospective study and suggested management paradigm. Otol Neurotol 2020;41(2):e273–9.

5. Gerges C, Malloy P, Rabah N, et al. Functional outcomes and postoperative cerebral venous sinus thrombosis after translabyrinthine approach for vestibular schwannoma resection: a radiographic demonstration of anatomic predictors. J Neurol Surg B Skull Base 2022;83(Suppl 2):e89–95.

6. Krystkiewicz K, Wrona D, Tosik M, et al. Dural sinus thrombosis after resection of vestibular schwannoma using suboccipital retrosigmoid approach-thrombosis classification and management proposal. Neurosurg Rev 2022;45(3):2211–9.

7. Brahimaj BC, Beer-Furlan A, Crawford F, et al. Dural venous sinus thrombosis after vestibular schwannoma surgery: the anticoagulation dilemma. J Neurol Surg B Skull Base 2021;82(Suppl 3):e3–8.

8. Abou-Al-Shaar H, Gozal YM, Alzhrani G, et al. Cerebral venous sinus thrombosis after vestibular schwannoma surgery: a call for evidence-based management guidelines. Neurosurg Focus 2018;45(1):E4.

9. Kim HN, Kim YH, Park IY, et al. Variability of the surgical anatomy of the neurovascular complex of the cerebellopontine angle. Ann Otol Rhinol Laryngol 1990;99(4 Pt 1):288–96.

10. Reisser C, Schuknecht HF. The anterior inferior cerebellar artery in the internal auditory canal. Laryngoscope 1991;101(7 Pt 1):761–6.

11. Warren DT, Warren MD, Malfair D, et al. An incidence of anteroinferior cerebellar artery/posteroinferior cerebellar artery anatomic variants penetrating the subarcuate fossa dura: operative technique and identification with 3-dimensional fast imaging employing steady-state acquisition magnetic resonance imaging. Neurosurgery 2010;66(6 Suppl Operative):199–203 [discussion: 204].

12. Bauer AM, Angster K, Schuman AD, et al. Aberrant AICA injury during translabyrinthine approach. Otol Neurotol 2020;41(10):1423–6.

13. Rayan T, Helal A, Graffeo CS, et al. Cerebrovascular complications of vestibular schwannoma surgery. J Neurol Surg B Skull Base 2022;83(Suppl 2):e443–8.

14. Sade B, Mohr G, Dufour JJ. Vascular complications of vestibular schwannoma surgery: a comparison of the suboccipital retrosigmoid and translabyrinthine approaches. J Neurosurg 2006;105(2):200–4.

15. Hegarty JL, Jackler RK, Rigby PL, et al. Distal anterior inferior cerebellar artery syndrome after acoustic neuroma surgery. Otol Neurotol 2002;23(4):560–71.

16. Ture H, Harput MV, Bekiroglu N, et al. Effect of the degree of head elevation on the incidence and severity of venous air embolism in cranial neurosurgical procedures with patients in the semisitting position. J Neurosurg 2018;128(5): 1560–9.

17. Scheller C, Rampp S, Tatagiba M, et al. A critical comparison between the semisitting and the supine positioning in vestibular schwannoma surgery: subgroup analysis of a randomized, multicenter trial. J Neurosurg 2019;3:1–8.

18. Konrad FM, Mayer AS, Serna-Higuita LM, et al. Occurrence and severity of venous air embolism during neurosurgical procedures: semisitting versus supine position. World Neurosurg 2022;163:e335–40.

19. Al-Afif S, Elkayekh H, Omer M, et al. Analysis of risk factors for venous air embolism in the semisitting position and its impact on outcome in a consecutive series of 740 patients. J Neurosurg 2021;5:1–8.

20. Song G, Liu D, Wu X, et al. Outcomes after semisitting and lateral positioning in large vestibular schwannoma surgery: A single-center comparison. Clin Neurol Neurosurg 2021;207:106768.

21. Ortiz de Mendivil A, Alcala-Galiano A, Ochoa M, et al. Brainstem stroke: anatomy, clinical and radiological findings. Semin Ultrasound CT MR 2013;34(2):131–41.

22. Khan NR, Elarjani T, Jamshidi AM, et al. Microsurgical management of vestibular schwannoma (acoustic neuroma): facial nerve outcomes, radiographic analysis, complications, and long-term follow-up in a series of 420 surgeries. World Neurosurg 2022. https://doi.org/10.1016/j.wneu.2022.09.125.
23. Bacciu A, Falcioni M, Pasanisi E, et al. Intracranial facial nerve grafting after removal of vestibular schwannoma. Am J Otolaryngol 2009;30(2):83–8.
24. Rbia N, Bulstra LF, Saffari TM, et al. Collagen Nerve Conduits and Processed Nerve Allografts for the Reconstruction of Digital Nerve Gaps: A Single-Institution Case Series and Review of the Literature. World Neurosurg 2019; 127:e1176–84.
25. Neff BA, Ting J, Dickinson SL, et al. Facial nerve monitoring parameters as a predictor of postoperative facial nerve outcomes after vestibular schwannoma resection. Otol Neurotol 2005;26(4):728–32.
26. Bagheri A, Babsharif B, Abrishami M, et al. Outcomes of surgical and nonsurgical treatment for sixth nerve palsy. J Ophthalmic Vis Res 2010;5(1):32–7.
27. Hoffmann J, Goadsby PJ. Update on intracranial hypertension and hypotension. Curr Opin Neuro 2013;26(3):240–7.
28. Lucke-Wold B, Brown EC, Cetas JS, et al. Minimally invasive endoscopic repair of refractory lateral skull base cerebrospinal fluid rhinorrhea: case report and review of the literature. Neurosurg Focus 2018;44(3):E8.
29. Mehendale NH, Samy RN, Roland PS. Management of pseudomeningocele following neurotologic procedures. Otolaryngol Head Neck Surg 2004;131(3): 253–62.
30. Higgins JN, Macfarlane R, Axon PR, et al. Headache, Cerebrospinal Fluid Leaks, and Pseudomeningoceles after Resection of Vestibular Schwannomas: Efficacy of Venous Sinus Stenting Suggests Cranial Venous Outflow Compromise as a Unifying Pathophysiological Mechanism. J Neurol Surg B Skull Base 2019; 80(6):640–7.
31. Huang B, Ren Y, Wang C, et al. Risk factors for postoperative meningitis after microsurgery for vestibular schwannoma. PLoS One 2019;14(7):e0217253.
32. Kanegaye JT, Soliemanzadeh P, Bradley JS. Lumbar puncture in pediatric bacterial meningitis: defining the time interval for recovery of cerebrospinal fluid pathogens after parenteral antibiotic pretreatment. Pediatrics 2001;108(5):1169–74.
33. Carmel PW, Fraser RA, Stein BM. Aseptic meningitis following posterior fossa surgery in children. J Neurosurg 1974;41(1):44–8.
34. JACKSON IJ. Aseptic hemogenic meningitis; an experimental study of aseptic meningeal reactions due to blood and its breakdown products. Arch Neurol Psychiatry 1949;62(5):572–89.
35. Sanchez GB, Kaylie DM, O'Malley MR, et al. Chemical meningitis following cerebellopontine angle tumor surgery. Otolaryngol Head Neck Surg 2008;138(3): 368–73.
36. Prabhuraj AR, Sadashiva N, Kumar S, et al. Hydrocephalus Associated with Large Vestibular Schwannoma: Management Options and Factors Predicting Requirement of Cerebrospinal Fluid Diversion after Primary Surgery. J Neurosci Rural Pract 2017;8(Suppl 1):S27–32.
37. Jeon CJ, Kong DS, Nam DH, et al. Communicating hydrocephalus associated with surgery or radiosurgery for vestibular schwannoma. J Clin Neurosci 2010; 17(7):862–4.
38. Kohlberg GD, Lipschitz N, Raghavan AM, et al. Middle Cranial Fossa Approach to Vestibular Schwannoma Resection in the Older Patient Population. Otol Neurotol 2021;42(1):e75–81.

Quality of Life in Sporadic Vestibular Schwannoma

John P. Marinelli, MD[a,b], Christine M. Lohse, MS[c], Michael J. Link, MD[b,d],
Matthew L. Carlson, MD[b,d],*

KEYWORDS

- Quality of life • Decisional regret • Observation • Wait-and-scan
- Conservative management • Microsurgery • Radiosurgery • Treatment

KEY POINTS

- Greater disease detection has shifted the patient demographic toward smaller tumors diagnosed in older patients with fewer symptoms.
- No treatment modality confers a global advantage over another for all patients.
- Observation, even if temporary, before definitive treatment, appears to offer improved patient satisfaction for those with small tumors on a population level.
- The Vestibular Schwannoma Quality of Life Index represents a new disease-specific QoL instrument that addresses prior limitations and includes unique patient-driven metrics.

THE GROWING CENTRALITY OF QUALITY OF LIFE IN SPORADIC VESTIBULAR SCHWANNOMA

The last century has witnessed a dramatic evolution in the management of sporadic vestibular schwannoma.[1] Whereas skull base surgeons of the early twentieth century were hailed for reducing mortality rates below 20%,[2,3] the twenty-first century has been increasingly characterized by maximal preservation of function over radical tumor extirpation.[4] The advent and general availability of MRI, along with the widespread adoption of screening protocols for asymmetrical sensorineural hearing loss, have resulted in a major epidemiologic shift in the vestibular schwannoma patient demographic.[5–7] Population-based data demonstrate that patients are now diagnosed on average 10 years older than in the pre-MRI era with the majority harboring tumors

Funding: No external funding sources.
[a] Department of Otolaryngology–Head and Neck Surgery, San Antonio Uniformed Services Health Education Consortium, JBSA, TX, USA; [b] Department of Otolaryngology–Head and Neck Surgery, Mayo Clinic, Rochester, MN, USA; [c] Department of Quantitative Health Sciences, Mayo Clinic, Rochester, MN, USA; [d] Department of Neurologic Surgery, Mayo Clinic, Rochester, MN, USA
* Corresponding author. Department of Otolaryngology–Head and Neck Surgery, Mayo Clinic, 200 1st Street Southwest, Rochester, MN 55905.
E-mail address: carlson.matthew@mayo.edu

Otolaryngol Clin N Am 56 (2023) 577–586
https://doi.org/10.1016/j.otc.2023.02.016
0030-6665/23/© 2023 Elsevier Inc. All rights reserved.

confined to the internal auditory canal, often with minimal associated symptoms.[8] Notably, this epidemiologic evolution has transpired in the backdrop of rising global incidence rates of sporadic vestibular schwannoma to a rate nearly five-fold that of 30 years prior.[9] As a result of greater detection rates, population-based data suggest that more sporadic vestibular schwannomas are treated today per capita than ever before,[10] even though the rising incidence appears largely attributable to screening protocols and incidental discovery of tumors on MRI rather than a true biological shift of more tumor development per capita. In this way, many patients with sporadic vestibular schwannoma who would have previously lived their whole lives without knowledge of their tumor are now being diagnosed and treated at increasing rates (**Fig. 1**).

In the wake of this epidemiologic evolution, a growing appreciation for the centrality of quality of life (QoL) in sporadic vestibular schwannoma has transpired. Over the past decade, two novel disease-specific QoL instruments have been developed for

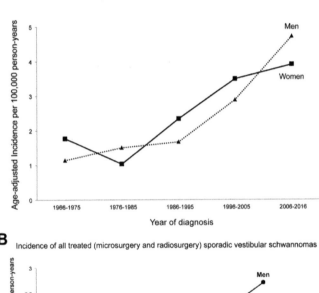

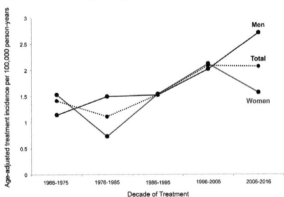

Fig. 1. (A) Rising incidence rates of sporadic vestibular schwannoma over the past half-century; (B) Concomitant rising incidence of treated cases with either microsurgery or radiosurgery over the same period. (*From* Marinelli JP, Grossardt BR, Lohse CM, Carlson ML. Is Improved Detection of Vestibular Schwannoma Leading to Overtreatment of the Disease? Otol Neurotol 2019; 40:847-850.)

sporadic vestibular schwannoma: the Penn Acoustic Neuroma Quality of Life (PAN-QOL) Scale developed by Shaffer and colleagues in 2010,[11] and more recently, the Mayo Clinic Vestibular Schwannoma Quality of Life (VSQOL) Index developed by Carlson and colleagues in 2022.[12] In the current article, the two available disease-specific QoL instruments will be reviewed. Subsequently, published data over the last decade will be leveraged to explore the influence of diagnosis and treatment on QoL in sporadic vestibular schwannoma.

OVERVIEW OF DISEASE-SPECIFIC QUALITY OF LIFE INSTRUMENTS IN VESTIBULAR SCHWANNOMA

i. PANQOL Scale

The PANQOL Scale, developed by Shaffer and colleagues in 2010, represents the first disease-specific QoL instrument for sporadic vestibular schwannoma and has been the focus of most recent large QoL investigations over the last decade.[11] The PANQOL Scale consists of 26 items with five possible responses to each item. Contrary to generic QoL indices, the PANQOL Scale includes vestibular schwannoma-specific domains including facial function, balance, and hearing, as well as more generalized domains including pain, anxiety, energy, and general health. Domain scores are calculated by taking the average of responses to the items within each domain, and an overall QoL score is obtained by taking an equally-weighted average across the seven domains. Similar to many generic QoL measures, scores range from 0 to 100, with higher scores suggesting better QoL. The PANQOL Scale has been successfully demonstrated to better differentiate patients with sporadic vestibular schwannoma from non-tumor controls compared with generic QoL instruments. Originally validated within the United States, the PANQOL Scale has subsequently been validated in Japanese,[13] French,[14] Spanish,[15] Hindi,[16] and Dutch.[17]

ii. Mayo Clinic VSQOL Index

The Mayo Clinic VSQOL Index, published by Carlson and colleagues in 2022, represents the most recently developed disease-specific QoL instrument for sporadic vestibular schwannoma.[12] The motivation behind the development of a new disease-specific QoL instrument extended from several observations. In light of the controversy regarding optimal management for patients with small-to-medium-sized sporadic vestibular schwannoma, investigations into QoL using the PANQOL Scale have failed to meaningfully differentiate QoL outcomes across management modalities. Whether these findings result from a true absence of a QoL benefit of one management modality over another versus insufficient sensitivity of the PANQOL Scale to detect these differences remains unknown. Second, although a wide variety of pain-related sequelae (eg, headache, trigeminal-related pain, nuchal pain) significantly drive QoL in vestibular schwannoma, the PANQOL Scale only incorporates a single item in this domain, "I have problems with head pain on the side of my acoustic neuroma tumor." Finally, clinical and research experience over time has revealed that many patients with sporadic vestibular schwannoma experience difficulty with cognition and decisional regret—a reality highlighted by over 1500 patients with vestibular schwannoma undergoing a national longitudinal study of QoL who provided input into the design of the VSQOL Index. Importantly, assessments of cognitive function, decisional regret, and occupation status are largely absent in previous QoL instruments but are represented in the VSQOL Index. For these reasons, and in combination with multiple key stakeholders including the Acoustic Neuroma Association, patients, and specialists in patient-reported outcome measure development, the Mayo Clinic VSQOL Index was developed.

The VSQOL Index itself contains 40 items grouped into eight categories including Hearing Problems; Dizziness and Imbalance; Pain, Discomfort, and Tinnitus; Problems with Face or Eyes; Impact on Physical, Emotional, and Social Well-Being; Difficulty with Thinking and Memory; Satisfaction or Regret; and Impact on Employment. The first seven categories related to the impact of vestibular schwannoma on QoL are comprised of items with five possible responses, and domain scores are calculated as the average of responses to the items within each domain. A global QoL score is calculated by taking an equally-weighted average of the domain scores. The Satisfaction or Regret domain score is not included in the global QoL score and is instead reported separately. As with previous instruments, domain and overall QoL scores range from 0 to 100, with higher scores denoting a better QoL.

Internal validation of the VSQOL Index showed strong intraclass correlations, with every domain exceeding the reliability benchmark for group analysis. Moreover, specific domains showed strong convergent validity with other widely available survey instruments. For example, the dizziness and imbalance domain showed strong correlation with the Dizziness Handicap Inventory. Uniquely, the decisional Satisfaction or Regret domain showed limited correlation with every other studied QoL instrument, including the PANQOL Scale, suggesting that this domain is poorly captured by previous instruments. Interestingly, the items surrounding the impact on employment collectively demonstrated significant correlation with each domain of the Index (all $P < .01$), suggesting that these items bear notable prognostic information.

QUALITY OF LIFE OUTCOMES
Overview

Significant controversy exists surrounding the management of small-to-medium-sized vestibular schwannoma. As no single treatment modality has been shown to harbor a global treatment advantage in all cases, the study of QoL becomes paramount. Instead of unilateral advantages by a single treatment strategy, specific symptoms appear to constitute the largest drivers of QoL, with ongoing dizziness and headache being the strongest predictors of poorer long-term QoL.[18] Hearing function and facial nerve status also influence QoL,[19] but many of these less tangible (dizziness, headache) metrics appear to exhibit greater influence on QoL outcomes. When compared with non-tumor controls, simply the diagnosis of vestibular schwannoma seems to reduce QoL more than any individual treatment modality (**Fig. 2**).[20,21]

Minimal Clinically Important Difference

Fundamental to accurately interpreting the QoL literature is the concept of a Minimal Clinically Important Difference (MCID). Not all statistically detectable differences are clinically relevant. The MCID represents the smallest difference in QoL scores that a patient or provider perceives as important enough to affect management decisions. As the frequency and magnitude of studies examining QoL in vestibular schwannoma increase, so does the likelihood of detecting statistically significant differences in outcomes (ie, either through the increased statistical power to detect a difference in a single study with a large sample size or through meta-analysis of multiple smaller studies). For this reason, recent work defined the MCID in the context of the PANQOL Scale.[22,23] The MCID (interquartile range) was 11 (10–12) for the total score. Among the specific domains, the MCID was 6 (5–8) for Hearing, 16 (14–19) for Balance, 20 (no interquartile range) for Facial, 11 (10–13) for Pain, 13 (10–17) for Energy, 11 (5–22) for Anxiety, and 15 (11–19) for General (**Fig. 3**).

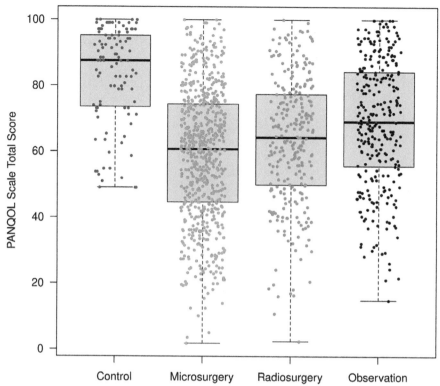

Fig. 2. Comparative global QoL across management modalities compared with control patients without vestibular schwannoma using the PANQOL Scale. (*Data from* Chweya CM, Tombers NM, Lohse CM, Link MJ, Carlson ML. Disease-Specific Quality of Life in Vestibular Schwannoma: A National Cross-sectional Study Comparing Microsurgery, Radiosurgery, and Observation. Otolaryngol Head Neck Surg 2021; 164:639-644.)

Prospective Disease-Specific Quality of Life Data

Several large prospective studies have investigated QoL outcomes, most of which are regarding patients with small-to-medium-sized vestibular schwannoma. Carlson and colleagues studied 244 patients with sporadic vestibular schwannoma, including 78 (32%) who elected observation, 118 (48%) microsurgery, and 48 (20%) radiosurgery.[24] At an average follow-up duration of 2.1 years, the study found minimal change in QoL after treatment (about a 1-point change or less for all three treatment modalities; recall MCID for the total score of the PANQOL Scale is 11). Even after adjusting for baseline features including tumor size and patient age, there was no significant difference in the facial function, general health, balance, hearing loss, energy, and pain domains or the total score. The only significant difference surrounded post-treatment anxiety, where those undergoing microsurgery had an 11-point improvement compared with 1.5 ($P =.73$) and 5.3 ($P =.31$) for observation and radiosurgery, respectively ($P =.002$ for difference; recall MCID for the anxiety domain score of the PANQOL Scale is 11).[24] This finding likely extends from the psychological benefit of having a "cure" following gross total resection, whereas in both observation and radiosurgery, the patient knows they still have a "brain tumor" that has to be monitored. This claim is substantiated by other prospective QoL data that show patients who

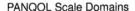

PANQOL Scale Domains

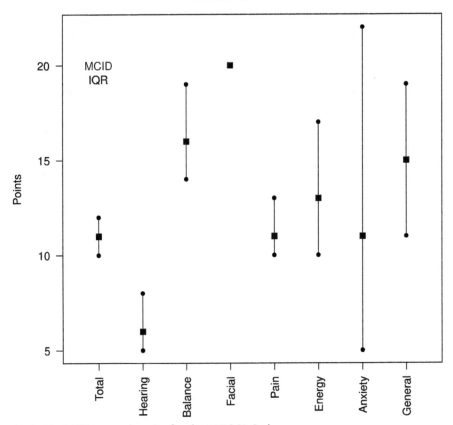

Fig. 3. The MCID across domains for the PANQOL Scale.

underwent gross total resection harbor improved QoL compared with those who did not.[25] Notwithstanding improvements for a subset of patients who benefit from no longer having a "brain tumor," QoL research from the originating institution of the PANQOL Scale has suggested that anxiety scores actually decline (ie, get worse) over time in patients undergoing microsurgery compared with radiosurgery or observation.[26] Whether or not this finding is attributable to the subset of patients who underwent less than gross total resection remains to be determined.

Cross-Sectional Disease-Specific Quality of Life Data

Large cross-sectional studies using the PANQOL Scale corroborate the general trends observed by the more recent prospective data. In 2015, a large international study of 642 respondents (n = 247 for radiosurgery, 148 for observation, 144 for microsurgery, and 103 for non-tumor controls) showed overall that simply the diagnosis of vestibular schwannoma portended poorer QoL compared with non-tumor controls more so than any individual treatment modality.[20] However, both radiosurgery and observation exhibited better QoL in certain domains, with those who underwent microsurgery having worse scores in the PANQOL Scale facial and pain domains, achieving both statistical significance and surpassing the MCID for these domains. Microsurgery was also statistically significantly worse in the balance domain and the total score, but these differences did not surpass the MCID thresholds.[20] These observations are corroborated by both a national survey of the Acoustic Neuroma Association[21] as well as a recent longitudinal cross-sectional study performed between 2014 and 2020 from the Netherlands that showed no treatment modality offered an advantage in QoL assessed by the PANQOL Scale (no domain surpassed the MCID).[27]

A 2014 study by Robinett and colleagues that reported outcomes through 10 years of follow-up similarly showed that microsurgery displayed decreased QoL assessed by the PANQOL Scale total score compared with radiosurgery or observation; however, this association was apparent only through the first 5 years of follow-up and was attenuated during the second half of the follow-up period.[28] Interestingly, this study also found that patients undergoing radiosurgery had statistically significantly better PANQOL Scale total scores than observation, but this association was also attenuated after 10 years of follow-up. Notably, the significantly improved QoL through years 0 to 5 of radiosurgery compared with the other two modalities surpassed the MCID for total score on the PANQOL Scale. Nonetheless, the authors ultimately concluded that long-term (>5 years) QoL is comparable across the three treatment modalities.[28]

Disease-Specific Quality of Life Among Those with Small Vestibular Schwannoma

Although many prior investigations include patients with small tumors, few studies have included *only* patients with small tumors. In light of the evolution toward a growing proportion of patients diagnosed with small tumors in recent years (indeed, recent population-based data suggest this is the most common subgroup),[6] this question has become increasingly relevant. A recent joint investigation by the Acoustic Neuroma Association and Mayo Clinic examining 346 patients with small tumors suggested that, overall, 89% of patients were satisfied with the treatment pathway they chose.[29] Interestingly, observation management with serial imaging harbored the highest satisfaction rates at 96%, whereas both radiosurgery and microsurgery were significantly lower at 86% and 85%, respectively ($P < .001$).[29] This pattern was also observed among patients undergoing upfront treatment, with those undergoing exclusive observation reporting the highest satisfaction at 96%, followed by those who were initially observed but eventually required treatment (88%), and lastly by those who underwent upfront treatment with either microsurgery or radiosurgery (81%; $P = .001$ for difference among the three groups).[29]

These data are corroborated by prior cross-sectional data that demonstrated an initial period of observation (≥ 6 months) improves QoL—particularly the anxiety domain of the PANQOL Scale—in the short term following diagnosis.[30] Similarly, QoL investigations from the Netherlands showed that patients with small vestibular schwannoma who were observed ≥ 6 months experienced better disease-specific QoL assessed by the PANQOL Scale, compared with those who underwent active management.[31]

It is possible that patient perceptions surrounding decisional regret may influence these trends. Because diagnosis is often associated with significant anxiety and a temporary reduction in QoL, a period of observation allows patients to come to terms with their diagnosis and potentially make a more informed decision. What is more, when tumor growth or symptom progression occurs, patients may be more accepting of the need for definitive intervention whereas those treated upfront with minimal or no symptoms may experience regret if they experience negative sequelae from the treatment. Because the element of decisional regret is uniquely included in the recent Mayo Clinic VSQOL Index, one of the primary interests of future research surrounding the

VSQOL Index will be to determine if this domain significantly influences QoL outcomes across treatment modalities.[12]

SUMMARY

The focus of management in sporadic vestibular schwannoma has dramatically evolved over the last 100 years. Whereas the early twentieth century was characterized by mortality reduction, the early twenty-first century is being increasingly characterized by the optimization of QoL in the setting of "chronic disease management." The centrality of QoL is being underscored by an ongoing epidemiologic shift toward an older patient demographic that is being diagnosed with smaller tumors and often with few associated symptoms. Over the last decade, two disease-specific QoL instruments have been developed for sporadic vestibular schwannoma: the PANQOL Scale in 2010, and more recently, the Mayo Clinic VSQOL Index in 2022. Especially for small-to-medium-sized vestibular schwannoma, QoL data underscore the importance of shared decision-making with patients, recognizing that no management modality consistently confers a global advantage over another. Even when individual studies demonstrate statistically significant differences in certain domains, these differences generally do not exceed the MCID. The current article examines the growing centrality of QoL in vestibular schwannoma management while leveraging available disease-specific instruments to highlight the importance of individualized management of sporadic vestibular schwannoma in the modern era.

CLINICS CARE POINTS

- No single treatment modality has been demonstrated to confer a global advantage for all patients.
- In Population-based data suggest more vestibular schwannomas are treated today than ever before, suggesting some degree of overtreatment may be present.
- An initial period of observation with serial imaging appears to improve patient satisfaction likely through minimizing decisional regret surrounding treatment.

ACKNOWLEDGMENTS

The views expressed herein are those of the authors and do not reflect the official policy or position of Brooke Army Medical Center, the U.S. Army Medical Department, the U.S. Army Office of the Surgeon General, the Department of the Army, the Department of the Air Force, or the Department of Defense or the U.S. Government.

CONFLICTS OF INTEREST

No authors have relevant conflicts of interest to disclose.

REFERENCES

1. Carlson ML, Link MJ. Vestibular Schwannomas. N Engl J Med 2021;384:1335–48.
2. Cushing H. Tumors of the nervus acusticus and the syndrome of the cerebello-pontile ange. Philadelphia and London: W.B. Saunders Company; 1917.
3. Ramsden RT. The bloody angle: 100 years of acoustic neuroma surgery. J R Soc Med 1995;88:464P–8P.

4. Carlson ML, Habermann EB, Wagie AE, et al. The Changing Landscape of Vestibular Schwannoma Management in the United States–A Shift Toward Conservatism. Otolaryngol Head Neck Surg 2015;153:440–6.

5. Marinelli JP, Grossardt BR, Lohse CM, et al. Prevalence of Sporadic Vestibular Schwannoma: Reconciling Temporal Bone, Radiologic, and Population-based Studies. Otol Neurotol 2019;40:384–90.

6. Marinelli JP, Lohse CM, Carlson ML. Incidence of Vestibular Schwannoma over the Past Half-Century: A Population-Based Study of Olmsted County, Minnesota. Otolaryngol Head Neck Surg 2018;159:717–23.

7. Reznitsky M, Petersen M, West N, et al. Epidemiology Of Vestibular Schwannomas - Prospective 40-Year Data From An Unselected National Cohort. Clin Epidemiol 2019;11:981–6.

8. Marinelli JP, Beeler CJ, Carlson ML, et al. Global incidence of sporadic vestibular schwannoma: a systematic review. Otolaryngol Head Neck Surg 2022;167(2): 209–14.

9. Marinelli JP, Lohse CM, Grossardt BR, et al. Rising Incidence of Sporadic Vestibular Schwannoma: True Biological Shift Versus Simply Greater Detection. Otol Neurotol 2020;41:813–47.

10. Marinelli JP, Grossardt BR, Lohse CM, et al. Is Improved Detection of Vestibular Schwannoma Leading to Overtreatment of the Disease? Otol Neurotol 2019;40: 847–50.

11. Shaffer BT, Cohen MS, Bigelow DC, et al. Validation of a disease-specific quality-of-life instrument for acoustic neuroma: the Penn Acoustic Neuroma Quality-of-Life Scale. Laryngoscope 2010;120:1646–54.

12. Carlson ML, Lohse CM, Link MJ, et al. Development and validation of a new disease-specific quality of life instrument for sporadic vestibular schwannoma: the Mayo Clinic Vestibular Schwannoma Quality of Life Index. J Neurosurg 2022;1–11.

13. Nishiyama T, Oishi N, Kojima T, et al. Validation and multidimensional analysis of the japanese penn acoustic neuroma quality-of-life scale. Laryngoscope 2020; 130:2885–90.

14. Oddon PA, Montava M, Salburgo F, et al. Conservative treatment of vestibular schwannoma: growth and Penn Acoustic Neuroma Quality of Life scale in French language. Acta Otorhinolaryngol Ital 2017;37:320–7.

15. Medina MD, Carrillo A, Polo R, et al. Validation of the Penn Acoustic Neuroma Quality-of-Life Scale (PANQOL) for Spanish-Speaking Patients. Otolaryngol Head Neck Surg 2017;156:728–34.

16. Pattankar S, Churi O, Misra BK. Validation of the Penn Acoustic Neuroma Quality of Life (PANQOL) Scale for Hindi-Speaking Patients Recently Diagnosed with Vestibular Schwannoma. Neurol India 2022;70:978–82.

17. van Leeuwen BM, Herruer JM, Putter H, et al. Validating the Penn Acoustic Neuroma Quality Of Life Scale in a sample of Dutch patients recently diagnosed with vestibular schwannoma. Otol Neurotol 2013;34:952–7.

18. Carlson ML, Tveiten OV, Driscoll CL, et al. What drives quality of life in patients with sporadic vestibular schwannoma? Laryngoscope 2015;125:1697–702.

19. Peris-Celda M, Graffeo CS, Perry A, et al. Beyond the ABCs: Hearing Loss and Quality of Life in Vestibular Schwannoma. Mayo Clin Proc 2020;95:2420–8.

20. Carlson ML, Tveiten OV, Driscoll CL, et al. Long-term quality of life in patients with vestibular schwannoma: an international multicenter cross-sectional study comparing microsurgery, stereotactic radiosurgery, observation, and nontumor controls. J Neurosurg 2015;122:833–42.

21. Chweya CM, Tombers NM, Lohse CM, et al. Disease-Specific Quality of Life in Vestibular Schwannoma: A National Cross-sectional Study Comparing Microsurgery, Radiosurgery, and Observation. Otolaryngol Head Neck Surg 2021;164:639–44.
22. Carlson ML, Tveiten OV, Yost KJ, et al. The Minimal Clinically Important Difference in Vestibular Schwannoma Quality-of-Life Assessment: An Important Step beyond P <.05. Otolaryngol Head Neck Surg 2015;153:202–8.
23. Kerezoudis P, Yost KJ, Tombers NM, et al. Defining the Minimal Clinically Important Difference for Patients With Vestibular Schwannoma: Are all Quality-of-Life Scores Significant? Neurosurgery 2019;85:779–85.
24. Carlson ML, Barnes JH, Nassiri A, et al. Prospective Study of Disease-Specific Quality-of-Life in Sporadic Vestibular Schwannoma Comparing Observation, Radiosurgery, and Microsurgery. Otol Neurotol 2021;42:e199–208.
25. Link MJ, Lund-Johansen M, Lohse CM, et al. Quality of Life in Patients with Vestibular Schwannomas Following Gross Total or Less than Gross Total Microsurgical Resection: Should We be Taking the Entire Tumor Out? Neurosurgery 2018;82:541–7.
26. Miller LE, Brant JA, Naples JG, et al. Quality of Life in Vestibular Schwannoma Patients: A Longitudinal Study. Otol Neurotol 2020;41:e256–61.
27. Neve OM, Jansen JC, Koot RW, et al. Long-term quality of life of vestibular schwannoma patients: a longitudinal analysis. Otolaryngol Head Neck Surg 2023;168(2):210–7.
28. Robinett ZN, Walz PC, Miles-Markley B, et al. Comparison of Long-term Quality-of-Life Outcomes in Vestibular Schwannoma Patients. Otolaryngol Head Neck Surg 2014;150:1024–32.
29. Nassiri AM, Lohse CM, Tombers NM, et al. Comparing Patient Satisfaction After Upfront Treatment Versus Wait-and-Scan for Small Sporadic Vestibular Schwannoma. Otol Neurotol 2022;44(1):e42–7.
30. Carlson ML, Tombers NM, Kerezoudis P, et al. Quality of Life Within the First 6 Months of Vestibular Schwannoma Diagnosis With Implications for Patient Counseling. Otol Neurotol 2018;39:e1129–36.
31. Soulier G, van Leeuwen BM, Putter H, et al. Quality of Life in 807 Patients with Vestibular Schwannoma: Comparing Treatment Modalities. Otolaryngol Head Neck Surg 2017;157:92–8.

Cochlear Implantation in Sporadic Vestibular Schwannoma and Neurofibromatosis Type II

Fiona McClenaghan, MBBS, FRCS (ORL-HNS)[a,b],
Simon Freeman, MB ChB, MPhil, FRCS (ORL-HNS)[a,b],
Simon Lloyd, MBBS, MPhil(Oxon), FRCS(ORL-HNS)[a],
Emma Stapleton, MB ChB, FRCS (ORL-HNS)[b,*]

KEYWORDS

- Cochlear implantation • Hearing rehabilitation • Vestibular schwannoma
- Neurofibromatosis type 2

KEY POINTS

- Cochlear implant (CI) offers significantly better hearing outcomes than auditory brainstem implantation (ABI) in appropriately selected patients with vestibular schwannoma (VS).
- CI has a role in single-sided deafness because of the natural history or treatment of VS.
- Neither treatment modality nor the cause of VS (NF2 related or sporadic) seem to have a significant effect on hearing outcomes with CI.

INTRODUCTION

Vestibular schwannoma (VS) is the most common tumor of the cerebellopontine angle (CPA) with an incidence of approximately 1 in 100,000.[1] The most common presenting symptom of VS is unilateral hearing loss, seen in 80% of patients.[2] Regardless of choice of therapeutic intervention or observation, at a decade after initial presentation, less than one-quarter of patients who initially present with serviceable hearing maintain a pure tone average (PTA) less than 50 dB or word recognition score

a Department of ENT, Salford Royal Hospital, Stott Road, Manchester M6 8HD, UK;
b Department of Otolaryngology, The Richard Ramsden Centre for Hearing Implants, Peter Mount Building, Manchester Royal Infirmary, Oxford Road, Manchester M13 9WL, UK
* Corresponding author. Department of Otolaryngology, The Richard Ramsden Centre for Hearing Implants, Peter Mount Building, Manchester Royal Infirmary, Oxford Road, Manchester M13 9WL, UK.
E-mail address: Emma.stapleton@mft.nhs.uk

Otolaryngol Clin N Am 56 (2023) 587–598
https://doi.org/10.1016/j.otc.2023.02.017
0030-6665/23/© 2023 Elsevier Inc. All rights reserved.

(WRS) greater than 50%.[3] Hearing preservation has been shown to be an independent determinant of quality of life in VS, with WRS being the most reliable predictor of hearing-related quality of life.[4,5]

Hearing preservation in VS is dependent on the functionality of the cochlear nerve. Cochlear implantation (CI) is considered if the cochlear nerve remains anatomically intact with a present fluid signal in the cochlea.[6] Patients within this category therefore may have an untreated tumor, a previously irradiated tumor, a failed attempt at hearing preservation surgery with a functioning cochlear nerve, or intentional nonhearing preservation tumor resection with cochlear nerve preservation. Developments in electrophysiologic testing aim to confirm neural function and to predict functional outcome with CI.[7] Historically CI was assumed to be contraindicated in patients with VS because of the neural component of hearing loss.[8] However, it is now well-recognized that for patients with an intact cochlear nerve, CI offers superior hearing outcomes to auditory brainstem implantation (ABI) and the opportunity to attain open set hearing discrimination.[9,10]

SPORADIC VERSUS NEUROFIBROMATOSIS TYPE 2 VESTIBULAR SCHWANNOMA

Most patients with VS experience a decline in hearing in the affected ear regardless of whether observation, radiation, or surgery is selected as the primary treatment modality. Commonly single-sided deafness has been accepted as a consequence of disease progression or intervention in sporadic tumors. Rehabilitation options have previously been limited to contralateral rerouting of sound aids or bone conduction devices (active or passive), with no attempt to provide auditory input to the effected ear.[11] However, studies of CI in nontumor-related single-sided deafness have shown significant benefits in spatial perception, sound localization, speech intelligibility, and quality of life in patients with a contralateral hearing ear.[12] Some patients struggle to integrate the signal from their CI with their natural hearing; however, this is not universal, and trends show improvement over time.[13] CI is a feasible method of hearing rehabilitation in selected cases of sporadic VS regardless of the hearing status of the contralateral ear and is increasingly being used.

Hearing rehabilitation in neurofibromatosis type 2 (NF2), or sporadic VS in the only hearing ear, is a greater challenge because of the threat of bilateral hearing loss, from either natural course of disease or treatment, often at a young age.[14] Because of this, the traditional approach has been to wait for hearing loss to occur before surgical resection, to preserve auditory function for as long as possible. The resulting larger tumor confers a higher risk at surgery, including facial nerve palsy and intracranial complications, in addition to loss of candidature for hearing preservation surgery.[15,16] A move toward earlier intervention in smaller tumors, with the aim of cochlear nerve preservation for CI, can reduce these additional surgical risks. In the case of NF2, a successful unilateral CI may also impact decision making for a contralateral VS, with surgical treatment in an ear with residual hearing considered in the knowledge that the patient will continue to function from an audiologic perspective.[17]

ABI remains an option for cases where cochlear nerve preservation is not possible. ABI stimulates the cochlear nucleus directly in the brainstem to restore hearing sensation. Although recent studies have reported improved hearing outcomes with ABI in patients with NF2, a higher proportion of patients achieve functional open set speech recognition, environmental sound awareness, voice modulation, and lip reading with CI when compared with ABI.[15,18–22] It remains rare to achieve open set speech discrimination that enables use of the telephone with ABI.[23] CI is therefore the pre-served hearing rehabilitation option where possible.

VESTIBULAR SCHWANNOMA TREATMENT OPTIONS

Because preservation of the cochlear nerve is crucial for the functionality of CI, several recent reviews have focused on the feasibility and success of CI in view of the chosen treatment modality.[8,14,15,17,22,24–27] The generally accepted treatment options for spo-radic VS are observation with serial imaging, stereotactic radiotherapy, or surgery, with medical treatment with bevacizumab being an additional option in NF2.[28] The use of CI in conjunction with observation, bevacizumab, or following radiotherapy is a straightforward proposition, because the cochlear nerve is anatomically intact and most patients will benefit, although there remains some uncertainty because the nerve is not always functionally intact. Unfortunately, electrophysiologic testing in these sit-uations shows poor diagnostic accuracy and so most authors propose proceeding directly to implantation where appropriate.[24]

Tumors treated with radiotherapy have been postulated to have poorer outcomes with CI than observed tumors.[29,30] However, Borsetto and colleagues[22] found that hearing outcomes were comparable post-CI regardless of whether tumor stability had been achieved by radiosurgery or as part of the natural course of the disease and this is supported by the recent 15-year review of CI in patients with NF2 in the United Kingdom. Schlacter and colleagues[8] also found that irradiated VS had no worse speech discrimination scores when compared with observed tumors, with mean postoperative constant-nucleus-consonant word scores of 45.4% for observed VS and 43.4% for irradiated VS. This observation may be partially explained by the mechanism of action of radiotherapy in VS, acting to cause vascular injury to deprive the tumor of blood supply, rather than directly damaging tumor cells.[31] It has further been postulated that radiation-induced injury to the cochlea occurs at the level of the stria vascularis, and so can be bypassed by a CI.[8]

For patients who have not undergone ipsilateral tumor removal, the possibility of future tumor regrowth, which may affect cochlear nerve function resulting in decreased hearing performance, must be considered.[15] This is of greater concern in the NF2 group in which VS demonstrate a less predictable growth pattern[17] and show a less predictable response to radiotherapy.[32] The use of bevacizumab, a vascular endothelial growth factor receptor antagonist, may ameliorate this variable by stabilizing tumor growth in an implanted ear; however, tumor growth control is seen in only 50% to 70% of cases, with a significant risk of regrowth on stopping treat-ment.[33] The difficulty of predicting which NF2-related tumors will grow and at what rate remains a significant problem. Long-term follow-up data (>10 years) on CI in NF2 is sparse; however, it is likely that in the long-term, a subset of patients with NF2 will lose benefit from CI because of tumor regrowth and will require ABI for hearing rehabilitation.[26,27]

Surgery

Although recent trends in management have favored less invasive treatment options, the need for surgical intervention remains in many patients. Although it is possible to preserve hearing in select cases, with increasing tumor size the cochlear nerve be-comes harder to preserve, with best outcomes in tumors less than 1 cm. Routine cochlear nerve preservation is challenging because the sensory cochlear nerve is more friable than the motor facial nerve and so more vulnerable to mechanical or ther-mal injury.[34] Although hearing preservation is technically challenging, high-volume centers have reported good results in sporadic VS.[35,36] Wilkinson and colleagues[37] found postoperative dead ears in 29% of middle fossa and 41% of retrosigmoid approaches. If the hearing is lost but the cochlear nerve is anatomically and functionally intact, then a CI is considered. Transcanal microscopic endoscopic-assisted resection of VS with simultaneous CI has also been described. Although not yet common practice, the approach allows for preservation of the cochlear nerve function without morbidity associated with open approaches.[38]

The situation is more complex in NF2 because of the multifocal origin of the tumors.[39] The tumors almost inevitably extend to the fundus of the internal auditory canal (IAC), meaning a retrosigmoid hearing preservation attempt will leave residual tumor. A middle fossa approach is made for small tumors, but the results are poorer than in sporadic VS.[40] An alternative approach is the translabyrinthine; although functional hearing is lost, the cochlear nerve can be preserved to enable successful CI with the added benefit that the cochlea is readily accessible.

Electrophysiology

If a CI is to be considered after surgical resection, confirmation of an anatomically and functionally intact nerve is required. Postoperatively promontorial stimulation remains the most commonly performed method of testing[10,41–43] with a positive test shown to be predictive of good CI hearing outcomes at 100 and 200 Hz.[44] The sensitivity and specificity of promontory testing has been questioned, with several reports of CI failure, despite reassuring results[19,45] and good hearing outcomes with poor integrity testing.[10]

Electrical auditory brainstem response testing is used intraoperatively to confirm cochlear nerve function. The stimulating electrode is placed at the round window niche or within the cochlea with the recording electrodes placed on the scalp. Although hearing preservation surgery uses sound stimulation with recording electrodes optimally either on the cochlear nerve (measuring the cochlear nerve action potential) or on the brainstem in the foramen of Luschka (measuring the dorsal cochlear nucleus action potential), the near-field effect when using electrical stimulation tends to cause substantial artefact, making these recording sites less useful. A robust electrical auditory brainstem response, however, has been shown to correlate with a good auditory outcome from CI.[15,46,47]

The question of whether to place an implant at the time of surgery or at a secondary procedure is of particular consequence with translabyrinthine tumor removal. Ossification of the cochlea has been reported postsurgery, with the percentage of completely patent cochleae decreasing from 75% to 38% in 6 to 12 months after surgery.[48] The use of a placeholder electrode in patients for planned future CI or of an inactive sleeper electrode to be activated in the event of contralateral hearing loss have also been described to circumvent the risk of cochlear ossification.[11,15,19] Additionally, there is evidence that spiral ganglion cells may deteriorate after surgery, leading to poorer hearing outcomes.[49] Despite this, successful implantation has been reported using perimodiolar electrodes at up to 14 months posttranslabyrinthine surgery.[50]

HEARING OUTCOMES

Postimplant hearing outcomes are reported through various measures in the literature, making meaningful comparisons between studies, and thus metanalysis, challenging to achieve (**Table 1**).

Table 1
Comparative postimplant hearing outcomes in published studies

			Treatment Modality				Tumor Type			Postimplant Hearing Outcomes								
	Studies	Patients	Observation	Radiotherapy	Surgery	Multiple/Other	Sporadic	NF2	Hearing Status (dB)	SRS (%)	WRS (%)	BKBq (%)	BKBn (%)	HINT (%)	CUNY (%)	PAT (dB)	AzBio (%)	CNC (%)
Bartindale et al,[51] 2019	15	45	—	—	45	—	45	—	28.8	56 ± 27.6	—	—	—	—	—	28.8 ± 8.3	75.0 ± 14.3	—
Borsetto et al,[22] 2020	12	50	29	—	—	—	1	28	33 ± 20	43 ± 33	45 ± 32	57 ± 40	—	68 ± 27	—	—	—	—
			21	—	—	—	4	17	39 ± 9	71 ± 31	43 ± 25	64 ± 31	—	96	86 ± 15	—	—	53
West et al,[24] 2020	29	86	—	—	86	—	53	33	—	57	58	—	—	—	—	—	—	—
Tadokoro et al,[14] 2021	32	132	24	34	74	—	39	—	25 (IQR, 2.5)	60 (IQR, 41.5)	—	—	—	—	—	72 (IQR, 50)	—	37 (IQR, 29)
								91	35 (IQR, 27)	46 (IQR, 60)	—	—	—	—	—	70 (IQR, 7.25)	—	60 (IQR, 32)
Smith et al,[26] 2022	—	64	20	17	13	14	—	64	—	—	—	45.8 (0–100)	41.6 (0–88)	—	60.9 (0–100)	—	—	—
North et al,[17] 2016	—	13	—	—	7	—	—	7	—	—	—	94 (69–100)	68 (30–98)	—	95 (89–100)	—	—	—
			6	—	—	—	—	6	—	—	—	85 (26–100)	64 (0–84)	—	98.5 (76–100)	—	—	—
Lloyd et al,[15] 2014	—	6	—	—	6	—	—	6	—	—	—	64	42	—	97	—	—	—
Sanna et al,[45] 2016	—	13	—	—	13	—	—	—	—	83	73	—	—	—	—	—	—	—
Schlacter et al,[8] 2022	—	99	53	—	—	—	—	—	—	—	—	—	—	—	—	—	55.9 (SD, 28.4)	45.4 (SD, 24.2)
			—	46	—	—	—	—	—	—	—	—	—	—	—	—	62.5 (SD, 34.8)	43.6 (SD, 21.0)

Abbreviations: AzBio, Arizona biomedical sentence recognition; BKBn, Bamford-Kowal-Bench sentence test in noise; BKBq, Bamford-Kowal-Bench sentence test in quiet; CNC, consonant-nucleus-consonant word recognition; CUNY, City University New York sentence test; HINT, hearing in noise test; IQR, interquartile range; PAT, photo articulation test; SD, standard deviation; SRS, speech recognition score.

In their systematic review of prior radiotherapy treatment versus observation on auditory outcome after CI, Borsetto and colleagues[22] found that, despite limited comparable data sets, both cohorts achieved similar average post-CI PTA and WRS of 33 ± 20 dB and 45 ± 32% for the postradiotherapy cohort and 39 ± 9 dB with 43 ± 25% for observational cohort. This finding is supported in the review by Schlacter and colleagues[8] of CI in retrocochlear pathology finding postoperative constant-nucleus-consonant scores of 45.4% (standard deviation, 24.2) for observed and 43.6% (standard deviation, 21.0) for previously irradiated VS. Smith and colleagues[26] similarly found no difference in audiometric outcome between treatment modalities with mean audiometric scores at 9 to 12 months of City University New York sentence test (CUNY) (60.9%), Bamford-Kowal-Bench sentence test in quiet (BKBq) (45.8%), and BKBn, Bamford-Kowal-Bench sentence test in noise (BKBn) (41.6%). The lowest incidence of nonbenefit was found in patients who received no treatment (5.6%) or radiotherapy (5.9%).[26]

Reported auditory outcomes after surgical resection are more varied. Bartindale and colleagues[51] in their metanalysis of 15 studies of surgically resected sporadic VS found an average post-CI hearing threshold of 28.8 dB with speech recognition score 56 ± 27.6%. West and coworkers[24] in a larger metanalysis of 29 studies of sporadic (n = 53) and NF2-related (n = 33) VS similarly found an average speech recognition score of 57% with WRS of 58%. Sanna and colleagues,[45] in a study of 13 patients with sporadic VS simultaneously implanted after modified translabyrinthine tumor resection found a PTA average of 56 dB with 80% mean speech recognition. BKB in quiet scores in the published literature after surgical resection vary from 45.8% to 94%,[15,17,26] BKB in noise 41.6% to 68%,[15,17,26] and CUNY scores from 60.9% to 98.5%.[15,17,26]

The interpretation of audiometric outcomes after surgical resection is compounded by differences in surgical approach and the tendency for larger tumors to fall within the surgical treatment group. The largest metanalysis in the literature by West and colleagues[24] of 29 studies with 86 patients, found good and comparable postoperative outcomes regardless of surgical approach; however, most patients (n = 64) underwent tumor excision via the translabyrinthine approach. Lloyd and colleagues[15] in a pooled analysis of 37 patients having undergone cochlear nerve–preserving surgery with complete resection of VS and CI found that 68% achieved some degree of open set speech discrimination subdivided by surgical approach with 100% via the translabyrinthine approach, 60% via middle fossa approach, and 50% via retrosigmoid approach.

Although the biology of NF2 and sporadic tumors is different, postimplant outcomes have been found to be similar in NF2-associated and sporadic VS in several studies.[8,14,22,24] Both Schlacter and colleagues[8] and West and colleagues[24] in their metanalyses found that NF2 association did not significantly impact postoperative word discrimination scores. Tadokoro and colleagues[14] also found comparable average Arizona biomedical sentence recognition scores for NF2-associated tumors (72%; interquartile range, 50) and sporadic VS (70%; interquartile range, 7.25), but more variation was seen in postimplantation PTA averages and word recognition sores, averaging of 25 dB and 60% for sporadic VS versus 35 dB and 46% for NF2-associated tumors. Despite this they concluded that most CI recipients functioned in the high-to-intermediate performer category regardless of tumor association.

Larger tumor size has been found to be predictive of poorer hearing outcome in several sudies.[14,24,27] West and coworkers[24] finding that smaller tumor size (7 mm in high-performance group) was an independent predictor of good postoperative outcome, in addition to good preoperative hearing (AAO-HNS group A or B).[24] Deep and colleagues[27] have also reported that tumors 1.5 cm or less had better speech understanding after CI. For tumors greater than 1.5 cm, patients who underwent microsurgery had a lower rate of open-set speech understanding compared with those treated with radiation or observation. In our unit translabyrinthine cochlear nerve–

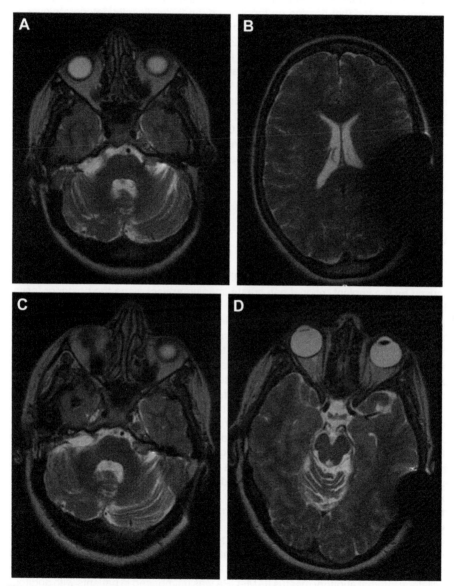

Fig. 1. Comparative MRI scans with and without magnet removal (all scans are of one patient, preremoval and postremoval of ABI magnet). (*A*) MRI artifact at level of IAM with left-sided ABI, magnet in situ. Area of maximal distortion of image on same scan, left ABI with magnet removed. (*B*) Area of maximal artifact on MRI with left-sided ABI, magnet in situ (same scan as *A*). (*C*) MRI artifact at level of IAM with left-sided ABI, magnet removed. Level of distortion at level of IAM with ABI + magnet in situ. (*D*) Area of maximal artifact on MRI with left-sided ABI, magnet removed (same scan as *C*).

preserving surgery is only considered if the CPA component of the tumor is 10 mm or less, because the cochlear nerve is difficult to preserve beyond this size.[15]

Long-term hearing outcomes for CI in VS are lacking in the literature. Smith and colleagues[26] reported a deterioration of 12.9% using CUNY sentences over a median follow-up of 3.6 years in patients with NF2-associated tumors. Neff and colleagues,[10] however, reported that hearing performance did not significantly deteriorate over an extended postoperative follow-up, with maximum follow-up of 93 months. In view of the less predictable growth pattern of NF2-assiociated VS, the proportion of patients with NF2 who will potentially lose benefit from CI caused by tumor regrowth and will require ABI for hearing rehabilitation remains to be determined.[27]

Overall outcomes for CI in patients with VS show favorable results with observed or irradiated tumors, sporadic and NF2-related, but outcomes after tumor resection are more variable with a greater chance of no benefit.[17,26,27] Despite poorer outcomes in patients with VS than seen in the general CI population, (Lloyd SK, Trudel M, Rutherford S, Behr R. Hearing rehabilitation in patients with a vestibular schwannoma. 2023 Unpublished) a CI should always be considered in a stable or resected tumor with cochlear nerve preservation because it will almost always outperform an ABI.[8,10,52]

MRI

The presence of a magnet within auditory implants requires consideration, especially in the NF2 population, who will require life-long MRI surveillance. Signal distortion caused by the implant magnet can create imaging artifact along the posterior fossa, limiting the ability to closely monitor a VS.[51] There is also the risk of magnet displacement or demagnetization during MRI scanning. These risks are minimized with the use of head wrapping[53] and devices with self-aligning magnets, able to orientate to the magnetic field of the scanner, creating less torque and so decreasing risk of displacement.[17,54] However, despite these measures, pain or discomfort during MRI scanning, magnet polarity reversal, and compromised diagnosis of ipsilateral brain lesions caused by magnet artifact are still reported.[55]

An alternative approach is to remove the magnet and replace it with a nonmagnetic spacer before MRI scanning. The artifact reduction after magnet removal has been shown to improve the image quality and diagnostic usefulness of lesions affecting the ipsilateral brainstem, CPA, and parieto-occipital lobe at 1.5 and 3 T in a cadaveric study.[56] However, the practical experience in our unit has demonstrated little difference (**Fig. 1**). Magnet removal is performed as a local anesthetic procedure in adult patients; however, the risks of removing the magnet (namely implant damage or introduction of infection) must be weighed against the risks of image distortion caused by artifact or pain during scanning.

Advancements in scanning protocols for patients with CI to reduce artifact and allow visualization of the ipsilateral CPA have negated the need for routine magnet removal in our unit. Walton and colleagues[57] found that in 85% of MRI brains the view of the ipsilateral internal auditory meatus (IAM)-CPA was unimpaired in patients with auditory implants with magnet in situ in 100% of axial three-dimensional inversion recovery prepared fast spoiled gradient echo scans, 88.9% of 2-mm coronal T1-weighted of the IAM-CPA scans, and 76.9% of 2-mm axial T1-weighted of the IAM-CPA scans. MRI scanning without magnet removal is therefore reasonably safe with MRI conditional models and with appropriate sequences image quality is not significantly impaired.

SUMMARY

The priorities of treatment in VS, as highlighted by Bartindale and colleagues,[52] are in order of importance to preserve life, facial function, and hearing, and to minimize other complications. Hearing preservation must remain a key factor in decision making for patients with VS. Schlacter and colleagues[8] in their metanalysis have reported that 82% of patients demonstrated improvement in speech perception scores after CI. The same proportion were regular daily users (as defined as more than 8 hours per day). Similarly, Smith and colleagues[26] reported that 84.9% of recipients remained regular daily CI users after a median follow-up of 3.6 years.

Although uncertainty remains regarding long-term hearing outcomes, CI offers significantly better outcomes than ABI.[8,10,17,51] CI also offers clear benefits in single-sided deafness.[12] Neither the primary treatment modality nor the cause of the tumor (NF2 related or sporadic) seems to have a significant effect on outcome. CI in VS serves to offer patients, with a functioning cochlear nerve, the possibility of open set speech discrimination with consequent positive impact on quality of life.

CLINICS CARE POINTS

- The priorities of VS treatment, in order of importance, are to preserve life, facial function, and hearing, and to minimise complications.
- Hearing restoration with cochlear implants in VS may be less predictable than in patients without VS.
- A meta-analysis reports that 82% of patients with VS and ipsilateral cochlear implant demonstrated improvement in speech perception.
- Neither the primary treatment modality for the VS, nor its aetiology (NF2 or sporadic) affects outcome.
- The presence of a magnet within an auditory implant presents challenges for future MRI scanning.
- Removal of implant magnet prior to MRI scanning is an option to reduce metal artifact.
- MRI scanning without magnet removal is safe in MRI conditional implants, and may cause minimal artifact with appropriate imaging sequences.

DISCLOSURE

The authors have nothing to disclose.

REFERENCES

1. Propp JM, McCarthy BJ, Davis FG, et al. Descriptive epidemiology of vestibular schwannomas. Neuro Oncol 2006;8(1):1–11.
2. Foley RW, Shirazi S, Maweni RM, et al. Signs and symptoms of acoustic neuroma at initial presentation: an exploratory analysis. Cureus 2017;9(11):e1846.
3. Carlson ML, Link MJ, Wanna GB, et al. Management of sporadic vestibular schwannoma. Otolaryngol Clin North Am 2015;48(3):407–22.
4. Peris-Celda M, Graffeo CS, Perry A, et al. Beyond the ABCs: hearing loss and quality of life in vestibular schwannoma. Mayo Clin Proc 2020;95(11):2420–8.

5. Cosetti MK, Golfinos JG, Roland JT Jr. Quality of life (QoL) assessment in patients with neurofibromatosis type 2 (NF2). Otolaryngol Head Neck Surg 2015;153(4): 599–605.

6. Patel EJ, Deep NL, Friedmann DR, et al. Cochlear implantation in sporadic vestibular schwannoma and other retrocochlear pathology: a case series. Otol Neurotol 2021;42(4):e425–32.

7. Miyazaki H, Caye-Thomasen P. Intraoperative auditory system monitoring. Adv Otorhinolaryngol 2018;81:123–32. https://doi.org/10.1159/000485577.

8. Schlacter JA, Kay-Rivest E, Nicholson J, et al. Cochlear implantation outcomes in patients with retrocochlear pathology: a systematic review and pooled analysis. Otol Neurotol 2022;43(9):980–6.

9. Hoffman RA, Kohan D, Cohen NL. Cochlear implants in the management of bilateral acoustic neuromas. Am J Otol 1992;13(6):525–8.

10. Neff BA, Wiet RM, Lasak JM, et al. Cochlear implantation in the neurofibromatosis type 2 patient: long-term follow-up. Laryngoscope 2007;117(6):1069–72.

11. Hassepass F, Arndt S, Aschendorff A, et al. Cochlear implantation for hearing rehabilitation in single-sided deafness after translabyrinthine vestibular schwannoma surgery. Eur Arch Oto-Rhino-Laryngol 2016;273(9):2373–83.

12. Vlastarakos PV, Nazos K, Tavoulari EF, et al. Cochlear implantation for single-sided deafness: the outcomes. An evidence-based approach. Eur Arch Oto-Rhino-Laryngol 2014;271(8):2119–26.

13. Galvin JJ 3rd, Fu QJ, Wilkinson EP, et al. Benefits of cochlear implantation for single-sided deafness: data from the House Clinic-University of Southern California-University of California, Los Angeles clinical trial. Ear Hear 2019; 40(4):766–81.

14. Tadokoro K, Bartindale MR, El-Kouri N, et al. Cochlear implantation in vestibular schwannoma: a systematic literature review. J Neurol Surg B Skull Base 2021; 82(6):643–51.

15. Lloyd SK, Glynn FJ, Rutherford SA, et al. Ipsilateral cochlear implantation after cochlear nerve preserving vestibular schwannoma surgery in patients with neurofibromatosis type 2. Otol Neurotol 2014;35(1):43–51.

16. Moffat DA, Lloyd SK, Macfarlane R, et al. Outcome of translabyrinthine surgery for vestibular schwannoma in neurofibromatosis type 2. Br J Neurosurg 2013; 27(4):446–53.

17. North HJ, Mawman D, O'Driscoll M, et al. Outcomes of cochlear implantation in patients with neurofibromatosis type 2. Cochlear Implants Int 2016;17(4):172–7.

18. Colletti L, Shannon R, Colletti V. Auditory brainstem implants for neurofibromatosis type 2. Curr Opin Otolaryngol Head Neck Surg 2012;20(5):353–7.

19. Carlson ML, Breen JT, Driscoll CL, et al. Cochlear implantation in patients with neurofibromatosis type 2: variables affecting auditory performance. Otol Neurotol 2012;33(5):853–62.

20. Roehm PC, Mallen-St Clair J, Jethanamest D, et al. Auditory rehabilitation of patients with neurofibromatosis type 2 by using cochlear implants. J Neurosurg 2011;115(4):827–34.

21. Behr R, Colletti V, Matthies C, et al. New outcomes with auditory brainstem implants in NF2 patients. Otol Neurotol 2014;35(10):1844–51.

22. Borsetto D, Hammond-Kenny A, Tysome JR, et al. Hearing rehabilitation outcomes in cochlear implant recipients with vestibular schwannoma in observation or radiotherapy groups: a systematic review. Cochlear Implants Int 2020; 21(1):9–17.

23. Matthies C, Brill S, Kaga K, et al. Auditory brainstem implantation improves speech recognition in neurofibromatosis type II patients. ORL J Otorhinolaryngol Relat Spec 2013;75(5):282–95.

24. West N, Sass H, Cayé-Thomasen P. Sporadic and NF2-associated vestibular schwannoma surgery and simultaneous cochlear implantation: a comparative systematic review. Eur Arch Oto-Rhino-Laryngol 2020;277(2):333–42.

25. Urban MJ, Moore DM, Kwarta K, et al. Ipsilateral cochlear implantation in the presence of observed and irradiated vestibular schwannomas. Ann Otol Rhinol Laryngol 2020;129(12):1229–38.

26. Smith ME, Edmiston R, Trudel M, et al. Cochlear implantation in neurofibromatosis type 2: experience from the UK neurofibromatosis type 2 service. Otol Neurotol 2022;43(5):538–46.

27. Deep NL, Patel EJ, Shapiro WH, et al. Cochlear implant outcomes in neurofibromatosis type 2: implications for management. Otol Neurotol 2021;42(4):540–8.

28. Doherty JK, Friedman RA. Controversies in building a management algorithm for vestibular schwannomas. Curr Opin Otolaryngol Head Neck Surg 2006;14(5):305–13.

29. Mukherjee P, Ramsden JD, Donnelly N, et al. Cochlear implants to treat deafness caused by vestibular schwannomas. Otol Neurotol 2013;34(7):1291–8.

30. Lassaletta L, Aristegui M, Medina M, et al. Ipsilateral cochlear implantation in patients with sporadic vestibular schwannoma in the only or best hearing ear and in patients with NF2. Eur Arch Oto-Rhino-Laryngol 2016;273(1):27–35.

31. Wackym PA, Runge-Samuelson CL, Nash JJ, et al. Gamma knife surgery of vestibular schwannomas: volumetric dosimetry correlations to hearing loss suggest stria vascularis devascularization as the mechanism of early hearing loss. Otol Neurotol 2010;31(9):1480–7.

32. Mallory GW, Pollock BE, Foote RL, et al. Stereotactic radiosurgery for neurofibromatosis 2-associated vestibular schwannomas: toward dose optimization for tumor control and functional outcomes. Neurosurgery 2014;74(3):292–301.

33. Plotkin SR, Merker VL, Halpin C, et al. Bevacizumab for progressive vestibular schwannoma in neurofibromatosis type 2: a retrospective review of 31 patients. Otol Neurotol 2012;33(6):1046–52.

34. Pisa J, Sulkers J, Butler JB, et al. Stereotactic radiosurgery does not appear to impact cochlear implant performance in patients with neurofibromatosis type II. J Radiosurg SBRT 2017;5(1):63–71.

35. Buchman CA, Chen DA, Flannagan P, et al. The learning curve for acoustic tumor surgery. Laryngoscope 1996;106(11):1406–11.

36. Mangham CA Jr. Retrosigmoid versus middle fossa surgery for small vestibular schwannomas. Laryngoscope 2004;114(8):1455–61.

37. Wilkinson EP, Roberts DS, Cassis A, et al. Hearing outcomes after middle fossa or retrosigmoid craniotomy for vestibular schwannoma tumors. J Neurol Surg B Skull Base 2016;77(4):333–40.

38. Marchioni D, Veronese S, Carner M, et al. Hearing restoration during vestibular schwannoma surgery with transcanal approach: anatomical and functional preliminary report. Otol Neurotol 2018;39(10):1304–10.

39. Evans DG, Stivaros SM. Multifocality in neurofibromatosis type 2. Neuro Oncol 2015;17(4):481–2.

40. Saliba J, Friedman RA, Cueva RA. Hearing preservation in vestibular schwannoma surgery. J Neurol Surg B Skull Base 2019;80(2):149–55.

41. Di Lella F, Merkus P, Di Trapani G, et al. Vestibular schwannoma in the only hearing ear: role of cochlear implants. Ann Otol Rhinol Laryngol 2013;122(2):91–9.

42. Bento RF, Monteiro TA, Bittencourt AG, et al. Retrolabyrinthine approach for cochlear nerve preservation in neurofibromatosis type 2 and simultaneous cochlear implantation. Int Arch Otorhinolaryngol 2013;17(3):351–5.

43. Tran Ba Huy P, Kania R, Frachet B, et al. Auditory rehabilitation with cochlear implantation in patients with neurofibromatosis type 2. Acta Otolaryngol 2009; 129(9):971–5.

44. Alfelasi M, Piron JP, Mathiolon C, et al. The transtympanic promontory stimulation test in patients with auditory deprivation: correlations with electrical dynamics of cochlear implant and speech perception. Eur Arch Oto-Rhino-Laryngol 2013; 270(6):1809–15.

45. Sanna M, Medina MD, Macak A, et al. Vestibular schwannoma resection with ipsilateral simultaneous cochlear implantation in patients with normal contralateral hearing. Audiol Neuro Otol 2016;21(5):286–95.

46. Lassaletta L, Polak M, Huesers J, et al. Usefulness of electrical auditory brainstem responses to assess the functionality of the cochlear nerve using an intracochlear test electrode. Otol Neurotol 2017;38(10):e413–20.

47. Lundin K, Stillesjö F, Rask-Andersen H. Prognostic value of electrically evoked auditory brainstem responses in cochlear implantation. Cochlear Implants Int 2015;16(5):254–61.

48. Carswell V, Crowther JA, Locke R, et al. Cochlear patency following translabyrinthine vestibular schwannoma resection: implications for hearing rehabilitation. J Laryngol Otol 2019;133(7):560–5.

49. Belal A. Is cochlear implantation possible after acoustic tumor removal? Otol Neurotol 2001;22(4):497–500.

50. Facer GW, Facer ML, Fowler CM, et al. Cochlear implantation after labyrinthectomy. Am J Otol 2000;21(3):336–40.

51. Bartindale MR, Tadokoro KS, Kircher ML. Cochlear implantation in sporadic vestibular schwannoma: a systematic literature review. J Neurol Surg B Skull Base 2019;80(6):632–9.

52. Vincenti V, Pasanisi E, Guida M, et al. Hearing rehabilitation in neurofibromatosis type 2 patients: cochlear versus auditory brainstem implantation. Audiol Neuro Otol 2008;13(4):273–80.

53. British Cochlear Implant Group (BCIG) How to do a headwrap. British Cochlear Implant Group. Available at: https://www.bcig.org.uk/mri-scanning-radiologists/ 7-how-to-do-a-head-wrap/. Accessed October 28, 2022.

54. Wackym PA, Michel MA, Prost RW, et al. Effect of magnetic resonance imaging on internal magnet strength in Med-El Combi 40+ cochlear implants. Laryngoscope 2004;114(8):1355–61.

55. Kim BG, Kim JW, Park JJ, et al. Adverse events and discomfort during magnetic resonance imaging in cochlear implant recipients. JAMA Otolaryngol Head Neck Surg 2015;141(1):45–52.

56. Wagner F, Wimmer W, Leidolt L, et al. Significant artifact reduction at 1.5T and 3T MRI by the use of a cochlear implant with removable magnet: an experimental human cadaver study. PLoS One 2015;10(7):e0132483.

57. Walton J, Donnelly NP, Tam YC, et al. MRI without magnet removal in neurofibromatosis type 2 patients with cochlear and auditory brainstem implants. Otol Neurotol 2014;35(5):821–5.

Advances in Facial Reanimation

Vusala Snyder, MD[a],*, Ariel S. Frost, MD[b], Peter J. Ciolek, MD[b]

KEYWORDS

- Facial paralysis • Cross-facial nerve graft • Midface • Nerve transfer

KEY POINTS

- Patients with facial paralysis experience a wide variety of negative physical, psychological, and social outcomes.
- Successful outcomes of facial rehabilitation are predicated on appropriate patient selection and preoperative planning.
- Early reconstructive techniques include primary repair, nerve grafts, and nerve transfers.
- Delayed reconstructive techniques include regional muscle transfer and free tissue transfers.
- Static procedures are also an acceptable option for temporary facial paralysis when nerve recovery is expected.

INTRODUCTION

Facial nerve paralysis is a debilitating clinical entity that presents as a complete or incomplete loss of facial nerve function. The etiology of facial nerve palsy and sequelae varies tremendously. The most common cause of facial paralysis is Bell's palsy, followed by malignant or benign tumors, iatrogenic insults, trauma, virus-associated paralysis, and congenital etiologies.[1–7]

Patients with facial paralysis experience a wide variety of negative physical, psychological, and social outcomes. Noticeable facial asymmetry and inability to practice the complex use of facial muscles to express emotion negatively affects social interactions and quality of life.[1–3] In addition, the physical consequences, such as paralytic lagophthalmos, eyelid retraction, nasal valve collapse, and paralysis of orbicularis oris muscle, lead to exposure keratopathy, ectropion, nasal obstruction, oral incompetence, and swallowing and articulation deficits.[4,5]

[a] Department of Otolaryngology, University of Pittsburgh, 203 Lothrop Street Suite 500, Pittsburgh, PA 15213, USA; [b] Facial Plastic and Reconstructive Surgery, Head and Neck Institute, Cleveland Clinic, 9500 Euclid Avenue A71, Cleveland, OH 44195, USA
* Corresponding author.
E-mail address: snyderv3@upmc.edu

Otolaryngol Clin N Am 56 (2023) 599–609
https://doi.org/10.1016/j.otc.2023.02.020
oto.theclinics.com

Successful outcomes of facial rehabilitation are predicated on appropriate patient selection and preoperative planning. The etiology, timeline, and extent of facial paralysis, viability of facial musculature, and the patient's overall health and expectations are the most important considerations in surgical planning.[6] Etiology is an indicator of prognosis and reversibility of paralysis. The duration of paralysis is an indicator of the viability of existing facial muscles and motor endplates, which are necessary for potential reinnervation.[4,7] This is not applicable to patients with congenital paralysis or those with long-standing facial paralysis, as the muscles are developmentally absent or irreversibly atrophied.[4,7] Patients with acquired facial paralysis who fail to demonstrate any functional recovery by 6 months can be considered for a reinnervation procedure, before complete muscle and motor endplate atrophy ensues. Although no treatment can guarantee a complete recovery and reestablishment of complex facial function, the goal is to optimize symmetry and function of the face.

Early Reconstructive Techniques

Direct repair
In the setting of known facial nerve discontinuity, tension-free primary anastomosis of nerve segments provides the best functional outcomes.[8,9] To optimize the number of regenerating axons, primary coaptation of the injured nerve should be performed within the first few days of injury or at the time of anticipated facial nerve resection.[9] Epineural repair is considered easier and faster than fascicular repair and is generally favored.[10] Fascicular repair could provide a more discrete anatomic anastomosis, albeit at the cost of potential internal disruption of the nerve and its vascular supply.[11] Various sutureless techniques have been developed for peripheral nerve repair, such as gluing, grafting, and laser welding.[12] The limitations of a tension-free, primary end-to-end repair include a wide neuronal gap or an absent nerve stump.

Nerve grafts
Nonvascularized interposition grafts are the most common method of bridging a nerve defect to ensure tension-free anastomosis of the nerve stumps for axonal regeneration. Options for donor nerve grafts are sural nerve, great auricular nerve, medial and lateral antebrachial nerve, and motor nerve to vastus lateralis. Motor nerve grafts are superior to sensory nerve grafts due to higher motor neuron regeneration and survival; however, their harvest may lead to significant side effects.[13] Caliber of the injured nerve, length of the defect, and donor site morbidity must be considered for selecting the ideal autologous nerve graft. For facial nerve injuries with a greater than 6 cm nerve gap and an associated soft tissue defect, a vascularized nerve graft can be considered in lieu of a conventional nonvascularized nerve graft.[14] The limitations of autologous nerve grafts are double anastomosis site and presence of both proximal and distal nerve stumps.

Nerve transfers
This procedure involves anastomosis of a functional donor nerve to an injured recipient nerve for an end-organ function restoration. This approach is indicated in cases of a denervated facial nerve main trunk with present distal branches and viable motor endplates. The success of nerve transfer procedures declines with longer duration of paralysis and should be performed as early as possible, ideally within the first 12 months; however, successful nerve transfer have been described up to 24 months following denervation in adults.[15–17] Facial nerve function in patients with HB grade V or VI after CPA tumor resection is predicted to remain poor if there is no improvement over the first 6 postoperative months.[15] Even in the setting of unclear anatomic continuity, early (6 months vs 1 year) reanimation surgery in these patients with poor

predicted functional outcomes leads to improved reinnervation and better functional outcomes.[15] The most used nerves for transfers are hypoglossal, masseteric, and cross-facial nerve transfers. Current trends favor multiple nerve grafts due to the difference in basal firing rate of hypoglossal nerve (better for tone) and masseteric nerve (better for targeted excursion).[6,7,11,13]

Hypoglossal nerve transfers. The original hypoglossal nerve transfer technique consisted of sacrificing the entire hypoglossal nerve and anastomosing with the main trunk of the facial nerve. This approach resulted in hemi-tongue atrophy and significant morbidity including dysarthria, dysphagia, non-discrete facial movement, hypertonicity, and synkinesis.[18] Various modifications have been developed including the use of interposition grafts, splitting and mobilizing a segment of the hypoglossal nerve for anastomosis, and intratemporal mobilization of the facial nerve for anastomosis. Duration for the return of function is 9 to 12 months, with only 41% of the patients achieving good movement.[19,20] Hypoglossal nerve transfer can produce good resting tone but poor volitional movement and often severe synkinesis.

Masseteric nerve transfers. Smile restoration via masseteric nerve transfer procedure involves anastomosis of an ipsilateral motor branch of the third division of the trigeminal cranial nerve to a distal branch of the facial nerve. It has become a frequently favored option due to its proximity, size match, relative ease of dissection, and low donor site morbidity.[21,22] Given its rich motor input, masseteric nerve transfers can be used for anastomosis to the main trunk or to a midface branch of the facial nerve. Recent studies reported an average of 4.95 months to first movement following masseteric nerve transfer.[23] Time to recovery was quicker in patients undergoing coaptation of the masseteric nerve to a midface branch of the facial nerve versus to the main trunk.[23,24] Limitations include non-spontaneous smile, inadequate tone and symmetry at rest, and masseter muscle atrophy and weakness without significant interference with oral intake.[25]

Cross-facial nerve grafts. When the proximal nerve stump is unavailable, the contralateral unaffected facial nerve can provide motor axons to stimulate intentional and spontaneous movement on the affected side. The cross-facial nerve graft (CFNG) involves coaptation of the contralateral facial nerve branch to the affected cut distal nerve with an interposition nerve graft. The variability of outcomes and long wait time for reinnervation has led to the use of CFNG as an adjunct to other nerve transfer procedures. CFNG procedures may be combined with "babysitter" procedures where a hypoglossal or masseteric nerve transfer is performed concurrently with the first stage of the CFNG to deliver neural input to the affected face.[26] In the second stage, the distal CFNG is anastomosed to recipient branches on the paralyzed side distal to the original nerve transfer.

Traditionally, in a two-stage approach, the donor facial nerve is anastomosed to the proximal end of the nerve graft, which is then positioned in the paralyzed face without a distal coaptation for 6 to 8 months.[21] In the second stage, the distal end of the graft is anastomosed with the recipient injured facial nerve. Advantage of the two-stage approach is a potential spontaneous recovery of the affected nerve, given no manipulation of it at the time of the first stage.

In recent years, interest in the single-stage CFNG has increased to reduce the number of surgeries required. Benefits of the single-stage CFNG are neurotropic stimulation from the distal anastomosis and limiting aberrant regeneration into the distal end of the graft.[21] Direct comparisons of two-stage and single-stage CFNGs are not currently available. The limitations of CFNG include weakening of the uninvolved side and lack of power, making this procedure less common unless used as a neural source for a gracilis free muscle transfer.[26]

Delayed Reconstructive Techniques

Muscle transfers

Contiguous regional muscle transposition is recommended for dynamic restoration in cases of partial, complete, and bilateral facial paralysis. When cable grafting is not available, a muscle transposition is an effective and reliable method for providing timely and acceptable results.[4]

Temporalis is the most commonly used muscle to reanimate a permanent irreversible paralysis. The vascular supply and innervation of this muscle enables adequate arc of rotation without a significant risk of necrosis or denervation.[27]

Temporalis muscle transfer. The temporalis muscle transfer is the most used regional muscle transfer for dynamic restoration of facial paralysis. In the original temporalis muscle transposition, a strip of muscle was elevated from the cranium and rotated inferiorly over the zygoma to reach the oral commissure.[28] Although the upward vector of this rotation was favorable, it resulted in a donor site depression and midface bulk. Various modifications of the temporalis transfer have been developed to minimize morbidity and optimize outcomes. Split fascial graft extensions to the upper and lower lip allow the temporalis muscle to pull the philtrum and lower lip back to midline.[29] To mitigate the risk of temporal fossa depression and midface fullness over the zygoma, the temporalis tendon can be detached from the coronoid process and mobilized down to the oral commissure (orthodromic temporalis tendon transfer). This technique can be performed via a preauricular transzygomatic, transoral, or a transbuccal approach via a nasolabial fold incision.[30–32]

Muscle transfers provide no spontaneous movements; therefore, the role of retraining and biofeedback cannot be overstated.

Free tissue transfers

Free tissue transfer is the gold-standard technique for patients with permanent facial paralysis (flaccid or synkinetic) or unsatisfactory results from nerve transfers. The latissimus dorsi, gracilis, extensor brevis, and the serratus anterior are the most frequently used muscles for dynamic reanimation.

Latissimus dorsi. The latissimus dorsi free tissue transfer was initially described as a two-stage approach for restoration of facial symmetry, tone, and expression. A modified, single-stage technique has since been developed to provide appropriate contraction during smiling.[33] Conventionally, the flap was harvested with the patient in prone or lateral decubitus position, which did not allow for a two-team approach. It has not gained popularity despite modifications such as axillary approach, given limitations such as donor site morbidity, flap bulk, and availability of other options.[34,35]

Gracilis. Gracilis free tissue transfer provides a reliable neurovascular pedicle and remains the gold standard for restoration of oral commissure.[13] Numerous studies demonstrate success of rehabilitation in adult and pediatric patients, yet expanded array of techniques exist regarding surgical technique.

Choice of Innervating Nerve

Chuang and colleagues evaluated rehabilitation outcomes following a gracilis free tissue transfer innervated by either CFNG, spinal accessory nerve, or masseter nerve. Although the most natural and spontaneous smile outcomes were seen with CFNG, higher rates of successful oral commissure excursion were seen with masseteric nerve innervation.[36,37]

The choice of CFNG versus masseteric innervation is patient-dependent, with the tradeoff of a spontaneous smile versus a bite-activated smile, respectively.

Single Versus Two-Staged Approaches

CFNG innervation of a free gracilis muscle transfer is traditionally a 2-stage procedure over 6 to 9 months, to allow for adequate neural regeneration across the nerve graft, but can be performed in a single stage depending on patient preference. Conventional two-staged free gracilis transfer innervated by CFNG continues to be favored due to yielding better symmetry at rest.[38]

Dual Innervation Approaches

To improve oral commissure excursion and spontaneous smile outcomes, dual innervation of the gracilis with the masseteric nerve and the CFNG was developed.[39] Several coaptation patterns and modifications have been described since 2012. One such modification was a novel single-stage gracilis free tissue transferred with dual innervation by the masseteric nerve anastomosed end-to-end to an obturator nerve and a CFNG coapted end-to-side distal to the masseteric neurorrhaphy.[39] Several studies have demonstrated successful spontaneous smile restoration with additive desirable excursion with teeth clenching.[39,40] Most of the facial nerve experts favor a single-stage gracilis free tissue transfer dually innervated via end-to-end masseteric and end-to-side CFNG coaptations.[37,41]

Other neurorrhaphy patterns for neural supply to a gracilis free transfer exist, but are beyond the scope of this article.

Multivector Approaches

A genuine (Duchenne) smile results from multivector and multi-zonal activation of several facial muscles, with the most prominent being the zygomaticus major and levator labii muscles (**Fig. 1**). Resultant simultaneous elevation of the upper lip and oral commissure, dental display, and periocular wrinkling are described as a positive display of emotion.[42] In attempts to restore the dynamic smile display zones, multivector free gracilis transfers have been developed. In one such approach, two muscle paddles are oriented independently of each other and inserted along two vectors.[43] Successful functional outcomes are the improved oral commissure symmetry and lip excursion in two dimensions. When inserted close to the lateral orbital region, a favorable dynamic periorbital wink is observed, which is characteristic of a genuine (Duchenne) smile.[43]

Most recently, a novel gracilis free tissue transfer approach was described using a trivector approach, including a periocular component to achieve a Duchenne smile (**Fig. 2**). In this technique, three muscle bellies are created from the harvested gracilis, two of which are placed with the intention of creating a natural multivector smile. The third vector is oriented to create a dynamic contraction in the periocular region and is draped from medial to lateral canthus.[44] Marked dynamic reduction in MRD2 (distance from the pupil center to the lower eyelid), as well as a marked improvement in dental displayed, was reported.[44]

Static Techniques

For patients who seek enhancement of existing outcomes, or are poor surgical candidates for dynamic reanimation, static procedures are a great option to restore some facial symmetry. Static procedures are also an acceptable option for temporary facial

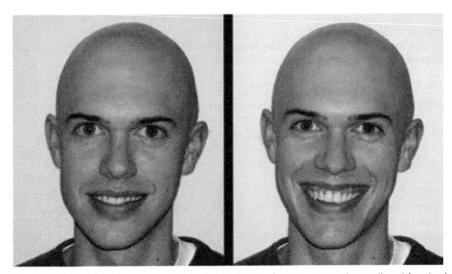

Fig. 1. Left: Non-Duchenne or social smile. Right: Duchenne or genuine smile with raised cheeks raised oral commissure and periocular wrinkling. (Courtesy of Dr. Marianne LaFrance, Ph.D.).

paralysis when nerve recovery is expected. Static techniques can be used for repairing specific cosmetic or functional deficits of the periorbital and perioral regions and to address nasal obstruction due to nasal valve collapse.

MANAGEMENT OF THE UPPER THIRD OF THE FACE
Eye

Lagophthalmos, or incomplete eye closure, is one of the most dangerous consequences of facial paralysis, and can lead to exposure keratopathy, corneal ulcerations, and blindness. Static techniques in treatment of the periorbital deficits are summarized as follows.

Upper eyelid loading with gold or platinum weight placement restores a gravity-assisted eye closure. Thin-profile platinum weights are more discrete and demonstrate decreased incidence of allergy as compared with gold implants. Palpebral spring procedure involves placement of a spring spanning between the superior orbital rim periosteum and the superior aspect of the tarsus. Lateral tarsorrhaphy

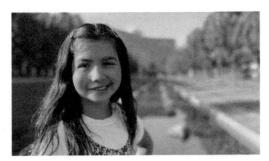

Fig. 2. Patient with a unilateral congenital facial paralysis with a Duchenne smile following a trivector gracilis free tissue transfer for facial reanimation. (Courtesy of Sergio and Carolina Gonzalez.).

involves coaptation of the lateral aspects of the upper and lower lid tarsal plates. Tarsorrhaphies are typically reserved to address exposure keratitis or loss of the corneal sensation.[45]

In treatment of a paralytic lower eyelid ectropion, lateral tarsal strip technique can be used to shorten the horizontal aperture. Alternatively, a medial canthopexy can be performed to address medial paralytic ectropion of the lower eyelid using a precaruncular, transcaruncular or transcutaneous approach.[45,46]

Brow

Brow ptosis can affect cosmesis and visual acuity. Numerous treatment approaches for brow lift have been described and are beyond the scope of this review.[46,47]

MANAGEMENT OF THE MIDFACE AND LOWER FACE
Midface

Static suspension with fascia lata can considerably improve nasal obstruction and also support the midface. Fascia lata can be coapted between the alar base and the zygoma/temporalis fascia to stent open the external nasal valve.[20] Patients with underdefined or overprominent nasolabial folds can undergo a simple suture technique to create or efface the nasolabial fold.[47]

Lip

Static facial slings for increased support and tone are commonly placed from the zygomatic arch/temporalis fascia to the oral commissure. Various materials have been described for use as the sling material including fascia lata, Gore-Tex, and AlloDerm. In addition, multivector suture techniques have also been described for facial suspension.[45]

Interventions for Synkinetic/Hyperkinetic Face

Non-flaccid facial paralysis is defined as involuntary synkinetic or hyperkinetic movement of the facial muscles. Synkinesis is an aberrant regeneration of nerves due to unsuccessful myelination and reorganization of neural networks following injury.[48] Botulinum toxin type A (BTX-A) injections temporarily paralyze muscles by blocking acetylcholine release at the neuromuscular junction, improving synkinesis on the ipsilateral side and reducing hyperkinesis on the contralateral face.[49,50] This can resolve periocular synkinesis, mentalis muscle dimpling, and platysmal hypertonicity.[4] The strategic treatment of the face bilaterally can assist with restoration of facial symmetry and improve functional outcomes.

In addition to serial injections with BTX, injection of local anesthesia, most commonly into the depressor anguli oris muscle followed by selective neurectomy and myectomy are also performed (**Fig. 3**). Contralateral depressor labii inferioris resection can improve smile in patients with unilateral facial nerve paralysis resulting in lower lip asymmetry.[51]

A novel surgical reanimation technique termed "modified selective neurectomy" entails transection of distal facial nerve branches causing unwanted movements of the face.[52] On average, six nerves are transected, and most patients undergo simultaneous procedures such as rhytidectomy, first stage of CFNG, and end-to-side coaptation of transected buccal branch to the zygomatic branch.

Physical Therapy

Physiotherapy may optimize functional outcomes and improve the quality of life and psychological health of patients suffering from facial paralysis. A wide variety of

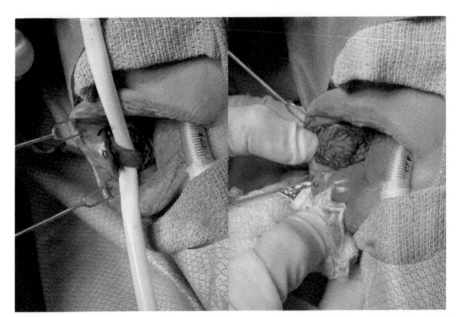

Fig. 3. Selective depressor anguli oris (DAO) myectomy. Left: Isolating and dividing DAO muscle. Right: Confirming a complete division of DAO muscle with visualization of subdermal fat.

physiotherapy techniques exist, including exercise, electric stimulation, biofeedback, and neuromuscular retraining.[53] Neuromuscular rehabilitation aims for selective muscle control to improve muscle discrimination and reduce synkinesis.[54] Muscle rehabilitation via EMG biofeedback and home exercises are shown to be efficacious for muscle reeducation.[27,52–54]

SUMMARY

Facial paralysis is an exceedingly complex and devastating condition that is challenging to manage. Owing to severe emotional consequences and social isolation, patients' quality of life is significantly impacted. Functional, esthetic, and emotive facial reanimation may require nerve transfer, muscle transposition, or free muscle transfer. Nonsurgical treatments serve as an adjunct to further address synkinesis, improve nasal obstruction, and tone to the paralyzed face. Surgical acumen and comfort with several techniques allows the choice of the most appropriate approach for the patient. Further exploration and standardization of objective measures to monitor recovery and compare techniques is needed to define the optimal treatment plan. Given severe emotional and physical consequences of facial paralysis, there is also a need for clinical trials to assess the efficacy of psychological intervention. Promising novel approaches for free tissue transfers, artificial nerve grafts, and conduits in line with innovations in biomedical tissue engineering are being further explored. New technological advancements will continue to advance and alter future practices in facial reanimation.

FINANCIAL DISCLOSURES

None.

CONFLICT OF INTEREST

None.

REFERENCES

1. Dey JK, Ishii LE, Byrne PJ, et al. Seeing is believing: objectively evaluating the impact of facial reanimation surgery on social perception. Laryngoscope 2014; 124:2489–97.
2. Lindsay RW, Bhama P, Hadlock TA. Quality-of-life improvement after free gracilis muscle transfer for smile restoration in patients with facial paralysis. J Am Med Assoc Facial Plast Surg 2014;16:419–24.
3. Dey JK, Ishii M, Boahene KD, et al. Impact of facial defect reconstruction on attractiveness and negative facial perception. Laryngoscope 2015;125:1316–21.
4. Garcia RM, Hadlock TA, Klebuc MJ, et al. Contemporary Solutions for the Treatment of Facial Nerve Paralysis. Plast Reconstr Surg 2015;135:1025e–46e.
5. Secil Y, Aydogdu I, Ertekin C. Peripheral facial palsy and dysfunction of the oropharynx. J Neurol Neurosurg Psychiatry 2002;72:391–3.
6. Boahene K. Reanimating the paralyzed face. F1000Prime Reports 2013;5:49–59.
7. Harris B, Tollefson TT. Facial reanimation. Curr Opin Otolaryngol Head Neck Surg 2015;23:399–406.
8. Bailey BJ, Johnson JT. Acute paralysis of the facial nerve. In: Head and neck surgery – otolaryngology, Vol2. 4th edition. Lippincott Williams and Wilkins; 2006. p. 2138–54 (Chapter 144).
9. Divi V, Deschler DG. Re-animation and rehabilitation of the paralyzed face in head and neck cancer patients. Clin Anatomy 2012;25:99–107.
10. Dvali L, Mackinnon S. Nerve repair, grafting, and nerve transfers. Clin Plast Surg 2003;30:203–21.
11. Matsuyama T, Mackay M, Midha R. Peripheral nerve repair and grafting techniques: a review. Neurol Med -Chir 2000;40:187–99.
12. Kim J. Neural Reanimation Advances and New Technologies. Facial Plast Surg Clin North Am 2016;24(1):71–84. https://doi.org/10.1016/j.fsc.2015.09.006. PMID: 26611703.
13. Harris B, Tollefson T. Facial reanimation: evolving from static procedures to free tissue transfer in head and neck surgery. Curr Opin Otolaryngol Head Neck Surg 2015;23(5):399–406. https://doi.org/10.1097/MOO.0000000000000193.
14. Bedarida V, Qassemyar Q, Temam S, et al. Facial functional outcomes analysis after reconstruction by vascularized thoracodorsal nerve free flap following radical parotidectomy with facial nerve sacrifice. Head Neck 2020;42:994–1003. https://doi.org/10.1002/hed.26076.
15. Albathi M, Oyer S, Ishii LE, et al. Early nerve grafting for facial paralysis after cerebellopontine angle tumor resection with preserved facial nerve continuity. JAMA Facial Plast Surg 2016;18:54–60.
16. Wu P, Chawla A, Spinner RJ, et al. Key changes in denervated muscles and their impact on regeneration and reinnervation. Neural Regen Res 2014;9:1796–809.
17. Conley J. Hypoglossal crossover–122 cases. Trans Sect Otolaryngol Am Acad Ophthalmol Otolaryngol 1977;84:763–8. ORL.
18. Asaoka K, Sawamura Y, Nagashima M, et al. Surgical anatomy for direct hypoglossal-facial nerve side-to-end "anastomosis". J Neurosurg 1999;91:268–75.
19. Ridgway JM, Bhama PK, Kim JH. Rehabilitation of facial paralysis. In: Cummings otolaryngology head and neck surgery, Vol III. 6th edition. Saunders; 2015. p. 2643–61 (Chapter 172).

20. Hadlock TA, Cheney ML, McKenna MJ, et al. Facial reanimation surgery. Surgery of the ear and temporal bone. Philadelphia (PA): Lippincott Williams and Wilkins; 2005. p. 461–72.
21. Dougherty W, Liebman R, Loyo M. Contemporary techniques for nerve transfer in facial reanimation. Plast Aesthet Res 2021;8:6. https://doi.org/10.20517/2347-9264.2020.195.
22. Henstrom DK. Masseteric nerve use in facial reanimation. Curr Opin Otolaryngol Head Neck Surg 2014;22:284–90.
23. Murphey AW, Clinkscales WB, Oyer SL. Masseteric nerve transfer for facial nerve paralysis: a systematic review and meta-analysis. JAMA Facial Plast Surg 2018; 20:104–10.
24. Banks CA, Jowett N, Iacolucci C, et al. Five-year experience with fifth-to-seventh nerve transfer for smile. Plast Reconstr Surg 2019;143. 1060e-71e.
25. Wang W, Yang C, Li Q, et al. Masseter-to-facial nerve transfer: a highly effective technique for facial reanimation after acoustic neuroma resection. Ann Plast Surg 2014;73:S63–9.
26. Tate JR, Tollefson TT. Advances in facial reanimation. Curr Opin Otolaryngol Head Neck Surg 2006;14:1–7.
27. Pinkiewicz M, Dorobisz K, Zatoński T. A Comprehensive Approach to Facial Re-animation: A Systematic Review. J Clin Med 2022;11(10):2890.
28. Aum JH, Kang DH, Oh SA, et al. Orthodromic transfer of the temporalis muscle in incomplete facial nerve palsy. Archives of plastic surgery 2013;40(4):348–52.
29. Balaji S. A modified temporalis transfer in facial reanimation. Int J Oral Maxillofac Surg 2002;31:584–91.
30. Boahene KD. Dynamic muscle transfer in facial reanimation. Facial Plast Surg 2008;24(2):204–10.
31. Byrne PJ, Kim M, Boahene K, et al. Temporalis tendon transfer as part of a comprehensive approach to facial reanimation. Arch Facial Plast Surg 2007; 9(4):234–41.
32. Boahene KD, Farrag TY, Ishii L, et al. Minimally invasive temporalis tendon trans-position. Arch Facial Plast Surg 2011;13:8–13.
33. Harii K, Asato H, Yoshimura K. One stage transfer of the latissimus dorsi muscle for reanimation of a paralyzed face: a new alternative. Plast Reconstr Surg 1998; 102:941–50.
34. Biglioli F, Frigerio A, Rabbiosi D, et al. Single-stage facial reanimation in the sur-gical treatment of unilateral established facial paralysis. Plast Reconstr Surg 2009;124:124–33.
35. Leckenby J, Butler D, Grobbelaar A. The axillary approach to raising the latissi-mus dorsi free flap for facial re-animation: a descriptive surgical technique. Arch Plast Surg 2014;42:73–7.
36. Chuang DC-C, Lu JC-Y, Chang TN-J, et al. Comparison of Functional Results Af-ter Cross-Face Nerve Graft-, Spinal Accessory Nerve-, and Masseter Nerve-Innervated Gracilis for Facial Paralysis Reconstruction. Ann Plast Surg 2018;81: S21–9.
37. Davis M, Greene J. Advances and Future Directions in the Care of Patients with Facial Paralysis. Operat Tech Otolaryngol Head Neck Surg 2022;33. https://doi. org/10.1016/j.otot.2022.02.010.
38. Kumar V, Hassan KM. Cross-Face Nerve Graft with Free-Muscle Transfer for Re-animation of the Paralyzed Face: A Comparative Study of the Single-Stage and Two-Stage Procedures. Plast Reconstr Surg: February 2002;109(2):451–62.

39. Biglioli F, Colombo V, Tarabbia F, et al. Double innervation in free-flap surgery for long-standing facial paralysis. J Plast Reconstr Aesthetic Surg 2012;65(10): 1343–9.

40. Sforza C, Frigerio A, Mapelli A, et al. Double-powered free gracilis muscle transfer for smile reanimation: a longitudinal optoelectronic study. J Plast Reconstr Aesthetic Surg 2015;68(7):930–9.

41. Boonipat T, Robertson CE, Meaike JD, et al. Dual innervation of free gracilis muscle for facial reanimation: What we know so far. J Plast Reconstr Aesthetic Surg 2020;73(12):2196–209.

42. Duchenne B, Cuthbertson RA. The mechanism of human facial expression or an electro-physiological analysis of the expression of the emotions. Cuthberson Trans. Cambridge, England: Cambridge University Press; 1990 (Original work published 1862).

43. Boahene KO, Owusu J, Ishii L, et al. The multivector gracilis free functional muscle flap for facial reanimation. JAMA Facial Plastic Surgery 2018;20(4):300–6.

44. Byrne PJ, Novinger LJ, Genther DJ. Tri-vector gracilis microneurovascular free tissue transfer with periocular component to achieve a Duchenne smile in patients with facial paralysis. Facial Plastic Surgery & Aesthetic Medicine 2022; 24(6):494–6.

45. Mehta RP. Surgical treatment of facial paralysis. Clinical and experimental otorhinolaryngology 2009;2(1):1–5.

46. Chan JY, Byrne PJ. Management of facial paralysis in the 21st century. Facial Plast Surg 2011;27(4):346–57.

47. Hadlock TA, Greenfield LJ, Wernick-Robinson M, et al. Multimodality approach to management of the paralyzed face. Laryngoscope 2006;116(8):1385–9.

48. Hjelm N, Azizzadeh B. Modified selective neurectomy with symmetrical facial repositioning. Facial Plastic Surgery & Aesthetic Medicine 2020;22(1):57–60.

49. Cooper L, Lui M, Nduka C. Botulinum toxin treatment for facial palsy: A systematic review. J Plast Reconstr Aesthetic Surg 2017;70:833–41.

50. De Almeida JR, Al Khabori M, Guyatt GH, et al. Combined Corticosteroid and Antiviral Treatment for Bell Palsy. JAMA 2009;302:985–93.

51. Hussain G, Manktelow RT, Tomat LR. Depressor labii inferioris resection: an effective treatment for marginal mandibular nerve paralysis. Br J Plast Surg 2004; 57(6):502–10.

52. Azizzadeh B, Irvine LE, Diels J, et al. Modified selective neurectomy for the treatment of post–facial paralysis synkinesis. Plast Reconstr Surg 2019;143(5): 1483–96.

53. Novak CB. Rehabilitation Strategies for Facial Nerve Injuries. Semin Plast Surg 2004;18:47–51.

54. Husseman J, Mehta RP. Management of Synkinesis. Facial Plast Surg 2008;24: 242–9.

The Future of Vestibular Schwannoma Management

Lindsay Scott Moore, MD[a,1], Konstantina M. Stankovic, MD, PhD[a,b,*]

KEYWORDS

- Vestibular schwannoma • Neurofibromatosis type 2 (NF2)
- Human induced pluripotent stem cell models (hiPSC) • Biomarkers
- Fluorescence-guided surgery • Immunotherapy • Adoptive cell therapy
- Gene therapy

KEY POINTS

- The ultimate goal for the future of vestibular schwannoma (VS) management is personalized, precision medicine.
- Innovations that will define the future of the diagnosis, prognosis, and monitoring of VS include biomarker identification using liquid biopsy of the blood and inner ear, artificial intelligence algorithms, intracochlear endomicroscopy, advanced targeted imaging strategies, gene editing, next-generation sequencing techniques, and patient-derived cellular models of VS and inner ear.
- Advances that will revolutionize future treatment paradigms of VS include ultra-high dose rate radioterhapy, surgery guided by targeted molecular imaging, novel and repurposed targeted therapeutics, immunotherapies such as checkpoint inhibitors, adoptive T cell therapies, and tumor vaccines, and both in vivo and ex vivo gene therapeutic strategies.

INTRODUCTION

As a critical part of the multidisciplinary teams caring for patients with both sporadic and neurofibromatosis type 2 (NF2)-associated vestibular schwannomas (VSs), which carry potential for significant morbidity,[1] otolaryngologists must strive to improve the management of patients with VS. Fortunately, doing so is more feasible than ever by capitalizing on the exciting era of unprecedented technologic and biomedical advancements that shape the current climate of research and clinical medicine. In this scoping review, we envision the future by highlighting the most promising developments published, ongoing, planned, or harboring potential applications for VS.

a Department of Otolaryngology – Head and Neck Surgery, Stanford University School of Medicine, 801 Welch Road, Palo Alto, CA 94304, USA; b Department of Neurosurgery, Stanford University School of Medicine, 453 Quarry Road, Palto Alto, CA 94304, USA
1 Present address. 801 Welch Rad, Palo Alto, CA, 94304-1611, USA
* Corresponding author. 801 Welch Road, Palo Alto, CA 94304-1611.
E-mail address: kstankovic@stanford.edu

Otolaryngol Clin N Am 56 (2023) 611–622
https://doi.org/10.1016/j.otc.2023.02.018
0030-6665/23/© 2023 Elsevier Inc. All rights reserved.

oto.theclinics.com

DIAGNOSIS, PROGNOSIS, AND MONITORING

Although the treatment paradigms for VS garner greater clinical and public attention, there is an equally important need to improve our management of these patients earlier in the process. Diagnosis occurs only after tumors have caused often irreparable damage, such as sensorineural hearing loss (SNHL), in the majority of cases. Monitoring protocols lack standardization, and both diagnostic and monitoring algorithms are limited only to expensive and burdensome serial MRI. Early screening protocols and accurate prognostics for VS are virtually nonexistent. Fortunately, a flurry of emerging technologies and innovations will reshape the diagnosis, prognosis, and monitoring of VS (**Fig. 1**).

BIOMARKERS
Tumor Tissue-Derived Molecular Biomarkers

Modern oncologic research is focused on identifying unique histologic, cellular, and molecular biomarkers involved in the underlying pathophysiologic signaling pathways. An increasing number of histologic and molecular VS biomarkers have been discovered, as summarized in recent reviews by Zhang and colleagues and Ren and colleagues.[2,3] However, unlike most solid tumors in oncology research, VS location precludes diagnostic biopsy, meaning VS tissue is available only at surgical extirpation, if at all, because the majority of tumors do not undergo surgical resection. As such, although histologic and molecular biomarkers from tumor tissue offer irrefutable value in elucidating the underlying pathophysiology of VS, they are relatively impractical. Therefore, future identification of molecular biomarkers will rely on sampling of more easily and safely accessed patient tissues, such as serum, CSF, or perilymph, as part of an exciting and rapidly progressing approach in oncology known as "liquid biopsy" (LB).

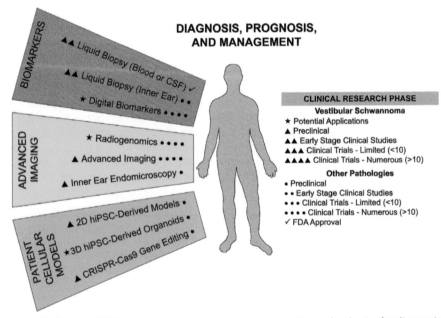

Fig. 1. The future of VS management: Innovations and emerging technologies for diagnosis, prognosis, and monitoring. hiPSC, human induced pluripotent stem cells.

Liquid Biopsy of Circulating Biomarkers

LB, or the detection and analysis of tumor-derived components or other biomarkers of disease from circulating biofluids rather than tumor tissue, is a minimally invasive technique that also allows for critical longitudinal assessments through repeated sampling. Circulating tumor cells, DNA, RNA, proteins, metabolites, extracellular vesicles, miRNA, and novel biomarkers identified in patient plasma, CSF, urine, sweat, saliva, and other fluids have demonstrated efficacy in enabling early detection and screening to improve diagnosis in many cancer types.[4]

VS is poised to benefit from the advantages offered by LB of circulating biomarkers within a patient's serum, perilymph, or CSF. For VS, ideal circulating biomarkers could improve current management paradigms by offering earlier diagnosis, monitoring, or even screening without the need for expensive imaging, enabling selection of targeted therapeutics, detecting drug resistance, assessing for radiosensitivity and detecting changes in tumor biology during the course of radiation, predicting ease of surgical resectability and facial nerve outcomes, and perhaps even guiding resection in real-time.

Vestibular Schwannoma Circulating Biomarkers

Several promising circulating biomarkers have already been identified for VS in blood and CSF (**Table 1**).

Liquid Biopsy of the Inner Ear

Perilymph fluid contains molecules and proteins secreted by cells of the inner ear and by VS and may therefore offer the advantage of harboring the widest variety and highest concentrations of important biomarkers given the relative separation of the inner ear from systemic circulation by the blood-labyrinthine barrier and the proximity of VS to the inner ear. In addition to secreted tumor biomarkers present in perilymph informative of growth, adhesion, and candidacy for targeted therapeutics for VS, LB of the inner ear, likely via the round window, will inform mechanisms of and treatment options for the SNHL associated with VS.

In addition to perilymph biomarkers with diagnostic, prognostic, and surveillance indications, as pharmacologic and genetic options become available for the treatment of VS and associated SNHL, LB of the inner ear will enable assessing therapeutic candidacy, determining inner-ear specific drug levels, monitoring treatment response, and detecting the development of therapy resistance. Looking toward the future, most microneedles for diagnostic LB of perilymph are also being designed with the capability of infusion of therapeutic agents, including pharmacotherapeutics, immunotherapies, and gene therapies directly into the inner ear to optimize target delivery and minimize unwanted off-site effects.[13,14] Pairing of LB tools with otologic microendoscopes will facilitate direct visualization of the round window membrane and precise therapeutic delivery.[13]

Digital Biomarkers

In a time where smart phones are ubiquitous and advances in AI have exploded, digital biomarkers represent the inevitable future of precision medicine. Sensors within connected or wearable hardware and software collect data from users in real time, often continuously, and apply machine learning algorithms to interpret the data in the intended medical context. Digital biomarkers have the potential to enable earlier, more accurate diagnoses, monitor disease progression or treatment response, allow for more personalized care, and offer the advantages of decreased time and travel burden for patients with remote medicine.[15,16] Wearable tech placed in or around the ear is already nearly as abundant as smart phones, with wireless headphones at

Table 1
Circulating biomarkers for vestibular schwannoma

Blood	Candidate Biomarker	Finding
	Vascular endothelial growth factor-D; Stromal cell derived factor 1α	Elevated plasma levels correlated with tumor size reduction in NF2 patients undergoing bevacizumab treatment[5,6]
	Fibroblast growth factor 2	Elevated plasma levels observed in NF2 patients undergoing bevacizumab treatment who experienced an improvement in hearing[6]
	Hepatocyte growth factor	Elevated plasma levels observed in NF2 patients undergoing bevacizumab treatment whose hearing did not improve[6]
	Neutrophil-to-lymphocyte ratio	Elevated levels in VS subjects with growing VS;[7] Elevated NLR is a validated indicator of systemic inflammation and a negative prognostic biomarker in multiple solid tumors[8]
	Matrix metalloprotease 14	Plasma levels and proteolytic activity correlated with degree of VS-induced SNHL and extent of VS surgical resection[9]
CSF		
	Hyaluronan	Levels elevated 17-fold in NF2-related VSs compared with patients without VS;[10] Proliferation rates positively correlated with amount of HA secreted by tumor cells in primary VS culture;[10] Normal HA binding to Schwann cell surface CD44 receptor is disrupted in VS formation and is a tumor suppressor target of merlin[11]
	Kruppel like factor 11; ATP binding cassette subfamily A member 3	Upregulated in CSF proteome analysis in patients with large and growing sporadic VSs[12]
	Brain abundant membrane attached signal protein; Peroxiredoxin 2	Downregulated in CSF proteome analysis in patients with large and growing sporadic VSs[12]

the most basic; the ear is therefore a prime location for sensor devices, furthering the relevance to and potential applications in otologic health.[17]

With the approval of over-the-counter hearing aids and several validated applications capable of audiologic testing already available, it is likely that "hearing health" technology continues to advance, and audiologic screening may become widely available and even encouraged through smartphones and digital health devices, especially as the companies selling these devices come to market with their own amplification products and are further incentivized to capture SNHL. Digital biomarkers could be used for earlier diagnosis of VS by detecting subtle changes in hearing, vestibular function, or facial movement before they are clinically evident; for home-based hearing, vestibular, and facial paralysis rehabilitation programs capable of monitoring progress; and even for surveillance and detection of tumor growth or recurrence.

ADVANCED IMAGING

Although biomarkers have the potential to augment or partially replace cross-sectional imaging for diagnosis and surveillance, imaging will likely always play a role in VS management, especially as advances in imaging technologies expand the capabilities. Recently, whole body MRI was used in patients with NF1 for radiogenomics, in which the relationship between the underlying genomic and proteomic composition of a tumor (obtained through next-generation sequencing) and the imaging phenotype are explored to identify correlations.[18] Although no studies of radiogenomics in NF2 or sporadic VS have been published, this technology promises to provide useful imaging-based biomarkers for personalized predictions of disease prognosis and therapeutic response, as demonstrated in cancer.[19]

Management on the horizon for VS will incorporate targeted imaging agents (including antibodies, nanoparticles, peptides, adaptamers, small molecules, and others) that can be combined with existing routine imaging modalities (such as MRI, computed tomography, and positron emission tomography) or advanced imaging modalities (such as various optical imaging platforms) to predict growth or other tumor characteristics, inform treatment selection, monitor treatment response, improve surveillance protocols, or even offer dual diagnostic and therapeutic applications. For example, optical imaging of near-infrared fluorescent probes conjugated to commercially available antibodies targeting receptors known to be overexpressed in VS are in multiple clinical trials in brain and head and neck cancers.[20,21] Such targeted, dual-functionality, advanced imaging agents and technologies will revolutionize management of and facilitate precision medicine for VS.

PATIENT-SPECIFIC STEM CELL-DERIVED MODELS

Patient-specific stem cell-derived models have the potential to revolutionize preclinical VS work because of their scalability, transformative utility in personalized medicine, and potential for rapid and cost-efficient translation to clinical trials by bypassing the need for animal models, which so commonly fail to accurately reflect outcomes of human studies. Briefly, patient skin or blood cells are reprogrammed into human induced pluripotent stem cell (hiPSC), which can then be differentiated into Schwann cells or various inner ear cell types to allow patient-specific characterization and treatment of their tumor or inner ear. The hiPSC-derived cells can be grown in two-dimensional models or allowed to self-assemble into three-dimensional organoids that model the tissue of interest.[22]

This approach is particularly valuable for the not-readily-accessible inner ear and VS because the cellular models can be used for understanding of disease mechanisms, for functional assays, for testing of promising therapeutics, such as small molecules or gene-editing platforms, and for therapy based on transplantation of wild-type cells or cells with corrected disease-causing mutations.[22,23] Significant strides have recently been made in the utilization of these platforms for SNHL, [22,23] and while less work has been done for VS, emerging preclinical studies are paving the way for this model to change forever the way VS is studied ex vivo and the translatability of knowledge gained in the laboratory.[24,25]

TREATMENT

Although current treatment options for growing VS are limited to radiotherapy and microsurgery, the future of VS management will not only include improvements in these traditional treatment modalities, but will also utilize systemic biological, genetic, and pharmacologic therapies (**Fig. 2**).

THE FUTURE OF RADIATION THERAPY

Continued innovations in computer technology, biomedical engineering, radiobiology, advanced imaging, targeted therapeutics, artificial intelligence, and integrated omics approaches will drive the progress in the development and clinical implementation of stereotactic radiosurgery. The future of dual targeted therapeutics combining pharmacologic and radiation therapy (RT) that act synergistically promises to reduce adverse effects of RT by reducing the required therapeutic dose.[26] Radiomics offers a powerful tool to deliver patient-tailored and tumor-tailored radiation regimens.[26] Proton radiation, which is an emerging area of active investigation in cancer and for VS, has the advantages of superior dose distribution, resulting in decreased toxicity to surrounding normal tissues, as well as 10% greater biological effectiveness.[26]

A cutting-edge development in the field of radiation oncology is ultra-high dose rate radiotherapy, or FLASH-RT (or FLASH) which, when ultimately translated to VS, promises to significantly improve patient outcomes and reduce neurotoxicity and ototoxicity. FLASH manipulates the *rate* of radiation delivery, and ultra-high dose rate therapy constitutes the use of dose rate of 40 Gy/s or greater, which is roughly 1000 times the dose rate of conventional RT.[27] Advantages of FLASH include decreased toxicity with at least equivalent tumor control, significantly decreased time and number of therapies, subsequently decreased interdose and intradose variabilities that affect RT efficacy and accuracy, and the potential for an overall

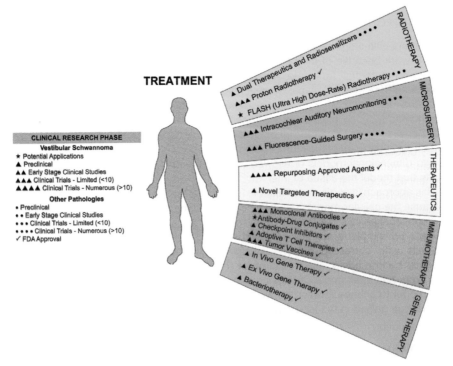

Fig. 2. The future of VS management: Innovations and emerging technologies for treatment.

improvement in RT-related morbidity and mortality.[28,29] To date, only one study has been published on the use of FLASH-RT in humans and demonstrated promising outcomes; as a result, three more clinical trials are now underway.[30]

THE FUTURE OF MICROSURGERY

Ultimately, surgery for VS may be largely replaced by the development of safe and effective targeted pharmaceuticals, biologics, immunotherapies, gene therapies, or a combination of these. However, before clinical implementation of these therapies becomes routine and widespread, the push to improve surgical extirpation and patient outcomes must continue undaunted. Innovations that will truly revolutionize and redefine surgical management paradigms of VS will be those that enhance the surgeon's ability to obtain real-time feedback to guide safer nerve dissection and more complete tumor resection. Intracochlear electrically evoked auditory neuromonitoring to guide cochlear microdissection is one such technology currently in a clinical trial (NCT04241679). Technologies augmenting tissue-specific visualization and providing enhanced, more accurate feedback of nerve location and functionality, especially when designed with dual therapeutic capabilities or combination functionalities, will shape the future of VS surgical management.

Perhaps, the most promising visualization technology is the utilization of optical imaging agents to guide surgery, commonly referred to as "fluorescence-guided surgery" (FGS). In general, FGS uses fluorescence agents (fluorophores) and compatible imaging systems to visually distinguish a tissue of interest based on the difference in the properties of the absorption and emittance of light between the target tissue and other tissues around it.[31,32] Emerging optical agents are based on molecularly-targeted fluorophores created by conjugated fluorescent molecules to antitumor monoclonal antibodies, peptides, or other chemotherapeutic agents.[31,32] Recent success with a nontargeted optical agent to guide VS surgery is promising,[33] and targeted fluorophores will likely offer even more robust success.

THERAPEUTIC AGENTS
Repurposing Approved Therapeutics

Perhaps the fastest pathway of clinical translation and approval of therapeutics is to repurpose Food and Drug Administration (FDA)-approved drugs that may have previously unknown utility to treat VS. Novel therapeutics take an average of 10 years to advance from bench to bedside, and almost 90% of therapeutics in this pipeline fail.[2] Identifying drugs that have already demonstrated safety for human use and obtained FDA approval can save significant amounts of time and money, and has the added benefits of long-term human safety data, affordable pricing given patent expiration and generic options, and an expansion of the population for whom a drug is relevant.

Most FDA-approved drugs that are being considered for repurposing in VS have been recently reviewed and are summarized in tabular format in several recent reviews.[2,34,35] Briefly, of the approved targeted small molecule drugs in clinical trials, only lapatinib, an inhibitor of human epidermal growth factor receptors type 1 (EGFR) and type 2 (HER2/neu), has consistently demonstrated efficacy in Phase I and II trials in patients with NF2, with modest improvements in hearing and tumor volume reduction in ~30% of patients.[36]

Novel Targeted Therapeutics

Antibodies, peptides, small molecules, and other agents that target critical players in pathways underlying VS growth, ototoxicity and neurotoxicity, and adhesion to cranial and central nervous tissues, such as merlin pathway proteins and inflammatory agents, have the potential to offer tumor control, hearing preservation, tumor shrinkage, or even cure. Combinations of different targeted therapeutics should enable decreased dosing, and therefore fewer adverse side effects, of agents used in combination.[2,37] Targeted therapeutics could also play a role in multimodality therapy, which will likely become an option for treatment of VS in the future. "Targeted therapeutics" can be inherently therapeutic or used as a tumor-targeting vessel to deliver a therapeutic agent, including cytotoxic substances, radiotherapy or photoimmunotherapy sensitizers, immune modulators, regulators of apoptosis, and even vectors that affect epigenetic and genetic expression.[2,37]

IMMUNOTHERAPY
Monoclonal Antibodies and Immune Check Point Inhibitors

In addition to monoclonal antibodies, exemplified by bevacizumab as the most successful targeted therapeutic for NF2-VS to date, immune check point inhibitors hold promise for VS. In many cancers, binding of tumor PD-L1 to T cell PD-1 results is a decrease in activated CD8 positive cytotoxic T cells that eliminate tumor cells, and blockade of immune checkpoint proteins with checkpoint inhibitors is thought to have therapeutic effect at least partially due to reactivation of antitumor cytotoxic T cells. Relevantly, histologic studies of VS tissue revealed high PD-L1 expression and the presence of CD8 positive tumor infiltrating lymphocytes, which are both well-established biomarkers predictive of positive response to immune checkpoint inhibitor therapy.[38]

Adoptive Cell Therapies

Adoptive cell therapies, also called T-cell transfer therapies, utilize cytotoxic T cells isolated from a patient's peripheral blood, which are then modified ex vivo in one of several ways to enhance their tumor-killing ability, and then reinfused into the patient to target and destroy tumor cells. The 3 main types of adoptive cell therapies are tumor-infiltrating lymphocyte (TIL) cell therapy, chimeric antigen receptor (CAR) T cell therapy, and engineered T cell receptor (TCR) T cell therapy. In general, a sample of the patient's peripheral blood or tumor tissue is acquired, and naturally occurring cytotoxic T cells that have the potential to target and destroy tumor cells are isolated. These cells are then multiplied and activated outside of the body.[39] In TIL therapy, these cells are then transfused back into the patient's blood. The premise of this therapy is to overcome two of the major barriers prohibiting innate tumor-targeted lymphocytes from successfully controlling tumors: too few activated TILs.[39]

The more involved, advanced strategies of CAR-T and TCR-T cell therapy include additional genetic engineering of the T cells to encode receptors that recognize and target tumor-specific antigens before they are transfused back into the patient. These adoptive cell therapies represent the cutting-edge of personalized tumor therapy, and while only a handful are currently FDA approved (for leukemia and lymphomas only), the explosion of preclinical and clinical trials in every phase of testing reflects the tremendous promise this highly sophisticated technology has to revolutionize oncologic therapy, perhaps including for VS.[39] The first human clinical trial exploring CAR-T cell therapy against tumors in patients with neurofibromatosis and schwannomatosis is ongoing in China (NCT04085159).

Tumor Vaccines

Tumor vaccines can work in a number of ways, but the overall approach is conceptually identical to that of their more familiar application for viral and bacterial diseases:

the immune system is exposed via the vaccine to antigens specific to the target and subsequently stimulated to recognize and mount an attack against these antigens within the body, often using cytotoxic T cells. Thus, tumor vaccines work by activating the body's inherent tumor-targeting lymphocytes in vivo, rather than ex vivo, as described for adoptive cell therapies.[40] Excitingly, a landmark clinical trial demonstrated preliminary efficacy and encouraging safety of a peptide vaccine targeting vascular endothelial growth factor receptor (VEGFR)-derived epitopes for progressive VS in patients with NF2.[40] In the era of molecular therapeutics and mRNA vaccines, as seen for coronavirus disease 2019, and the ongoing developments of biomarker discovery, therapeutic vaccines for VS, which may have the advantage of minimizing toxicity from binding to target antigens in nontumor tissues, may play a role, alone or as combination therapy, in the future of VS management.

GENE THERAPY
In Vivo and Ex Vivo Gene Therapy

Gene therapy involves the introduction of genetic material into cells to modify gene product expression, usually to replace or silence mutated genes. A delivery vector is utilized to carry and deposit the desired genetic material into the cell's nucleus. Regardless of chromosomal integration, the cellular machinery inherent in the nucleus transcribes and/or translates the introduced genetic material to produce the protein or other product of interest. Gene therapy is generally administered using either the in vivo approach, in which gene therapeutics are injected directly into the patient, or the ex vivo approach, in which patients' cells are removed and isolated, the genetic therapeutic agent is applied to the cells outside the patient, and the gene-corrected cells are then expanded and reinfused back into the patient to exhibit their therapeutic effect.[41]

Although gene therapy has been a field of investigation since the 1970s and no genetic therapeutics are currently approved for VS, advances in technologies for cellular and genetic engineering are accelerating progress in gene therapy research. Currently, there are 2 FDA-approved gene therapies in the United States and more than 200 ongoing clinical trials for gene therapy, with an estimated 2,500 in the global pipeline.[41] Several clinical trials for gene therapy in VS are well into planning stages.

Bacteriotherapy

Bacteriotherapy is a unique strategy to treat tumors that serves as a form of both immunotherapy and gene therapy. Bacteria, which can have potent antitumor-effects in isolation, can be genetically engineered with relative ease, penetrate hypoxic areas of tumor resistant to other treatment modalities, can be used as vectors to deliver tumoricidal agents of a variety of sizes and types, and are known to be additionally efficacious in combination with radiotherapy or chemotherapy.[42]

Excitingly, bacteriotherapy has already demonstrated efficacy in preclinical studies for NF2 in which engineered bacteria (live-attenuated *Salmonella typhimurium*) were shown to kill NF2 tumor cells in vitro and reduce tumor volume in human xenograft and mouse syngeneic schwannoma murine models in vivo.[42] A first-in-human clinical trial of bacteriotherapy for NF2 has been licensed, the bacteriotherapeutic agent granted orphan drug designation status in the United States and Europe, and enrollment will reportedly open this year.

SUMMARY

In this scoping review, we have highlighted the critical gaps and challenges in VS management, including the need for improved diagnostic and monitoring strategies and safer, more effective surgical and radiotherapy techniques, as well as the glaring absence of reliable prognostics and systemic therapeutic options. We have illustrated how the development, adoption and integration of powerful emerging technologies in this unparalleled time of biotechnological progress has potential to revolutionize VS management by enabling personalized, precision medicine that will improve patient outcomes and quality of life.

CLINICS CARE POINTS

- There is a paucity of biomarkers for vestibular schwannoma capable of offering clinically actionable information to alter the course of management. Numerous circulating biomarkers sampled through the technique of "liquid biopsy" have been used to facilitate early detection, screening, and personalized treatment regimens for multiple cancer types, and this technology is being increasingly investigated for applications for vestibular schwannoma.

- Advanced imaging techniques, included targeted molecular and fluorescence imaging, have been used to improve both the diagnosis and treatment of many tumors, including those of the head and neck. Early clinical trials using fluorescence to guide microsurgery for vestibular schwannoma have demonstrated preliminary success that is driving further investigations into this technology.

- Ultra-high dose rate radiation therapy is a novel technique in radiation oncology that has demonstrated decreased toxicity to normal tissues surrounding tumors in a multitude of preclinical studies. Clinical trials are needed to validate the so-called "FLASH" effect in humans and optimize parameters of therapeutic regimens before the exciting potential of this technology could be utilized for vestibular schwannoma.

- A number of gene therapy and adoptive cell therapy techniques have gained approval for use for different diseases, with thousands more in various phases of the clinical pipeline. Preclinical work in these fields for applications for vestibular schwannoma has been promising, and a handful of clinical trials are reportedly on the way.

DECLARATION OF INTERESTS

The authors have no financial disclosures for this article.

ACKNOWLEDGMENTS

We gratefully acknowledge support from National Institute on Deafness and Other Communication Disorders grant U24 DC020857 (K.M. Stankovic), Bertarelli Foundation Professorship (K.M. Stankovic), Larry Bowman (K.M. Stankovic), and Tahbazof Scholarship (L.S. Moore).

REFERENCES

1. Slattery WH. Neurofibromatosis type 2. Otolaryngol Clin North Am 2015;48(3): 443–60.
2. Ren Y, Chari DA, Vasilijic S, et al. New developments in neurofibromatosis type 2 and vestibular schwannoma. Neurooncol Adv 2020;3(1):vdaa153.
3. Zhang Y, Long J, Ren J, et al. Potential Molecular Biomarkers of Vestibular Schwannoma Growth: Progress and Prospects. Front Oncol 2021;11:731441.
4. Lone SN, Nisar S, Masoodi T, et al. Liquid biopsy: a step closer to transform diagnosis, prognosis and future of cancer treatments. Mol Cancer 2022;21(1):79.

5. Dilwali S, Roberts D, Stankovic KM. Interplay between VEGF-A and cMET signaling in human vestibular schwannomas and schwann cells. Cancer Biol Ther 2015;16(1):170–5.
6. Blakeley JO, Ye X, Duda DG, et al. Efficacy and Biomarker Study of Bevacizumab for Hearing Loss Resulting From Neurofibromatosis Type 2-Associated Vestibular Schwannomas. J Clin Oncol 2016;34(14):1669–75.
7. Kontorinis G, Crowther JA, Iliodromiti S, et al. Neutrophil to Lymphocyte Ratio as a Predictive Marker of Vestibular Schwannoma Growth. Otol Neurotol 2016;37(5): 580–5.
8. Templeton AJ, McNamara MG, Šeruga B, et al. Prognostic role of neutrophil-to-lymphocyte ratio in solid tumors: a systematic review and meta-analysis. J Natl Cancer Inst 2014;106(6):dju124.
9. Ren Y, Hyakusoku H, Sagers JE, et al. MMP-14 (MT1-MMP) Is a Biomarker of Surgical Outcome and a Potential Mediator of Hearing Loss in Patients With Vestibular Schwannomas. Front Cell Neurosci 2020;14:191.
10. Ariyannur PS, Vikkath N, Pillai AB. Cerebrospinal Fluid Hyaluronan and Neurofibromatosis Type 2. Cancer Microenviron 2018;11(2–3):125–33.
11. Bai Y, Liu YJ, Wang H, et al. Inhibition of the hyaluronan-CD44 interaction by merlin contributes to the tumor-suppressor activity of merlin. Oncogene 2007; 26(6):836–50.
12. Huang X, Xu J, Shen Y, et al. Protein profiling of cerebrospinal fluid from patients undergoing vestibular schwannoma surgery and clinical significance. Biomed Pharmacother 2019;116:108985.
13. Leong S, Aksit A, Feng SJ, et al. Inner Ear Diagnostics and Drug Delivery via Microneedles. J Clin Med 2022;11(18):5474.
14. Early S, Moon IS, Bommakanti K, et al. A novel microneedle device for controlled and reliable liquid biopsy of the human inner ear. Hear Res 2019;381:107761.
15. Motahari-Nezhad H, Fgaier M, Mahdi Abid M, et al. Digital Biomarker-Based Studies: Scoping Review of Systematic Reviews. JMIR Mhealth Uhealth 2022; 10(10):e35722.
16. Jeong H, Jeong YW, Park Y, et al. Applications of deep learning methods in digital biomarker research using noninvasive sensing data. Digit Health 2022;8. 20552076221136642.
17. Choi JY, Jeon S, Kim H, et al. Health-Related Indicators Measured Using Earable Devices: Systematic Review. JMIR Mhealth Uhealth 2022;10(11):e36696.
18. Liu Y, Jordan JT, Bredella MA, et al. Correlation between NF1 genotype and imaging phenotype on whole-body MRI: NF1 radiogenomics. Neurology 2020; 94(24):e2521–31.
19. Aerts HJ, Velazquez ER, Leijenaar RT, et al. Decoding tumour phenotype by noninvasive imaging using a quantitative radiomics approach. Nat Commun 2014;5:4006, published correction appears in Nat Commun. 2014;5:4644]. Cavalho, Sara.
20. Zhou Q, van den Berg NS, Rosenthal EL, et al. EGFR-targeted intraoperative fluorescence imaging detects high-grade glioma with panitumumab-IRDye800 in a phase 1 clinical trial. Theranostics 2021;11(15):7130–43.
21. Lee YJ, Krishnan G, Nishio N, et al. Intraoperative Fluorescence-Guided Surgery in Head and Neck Squamous Cell Carcinoma. Laryngoscope 2021;131(3): 529–34.
22. Stojkovic M, Han D, Jeong M, et al. Human induced pluripotent stem cells and CRISPR/Cas-mediated targeted genome editing: Platforms to tackle sensorineural hearing loss. Stem Cell 2021;39(6):673–96.

23. Zine A, Messat Y, Fritzsch B. A human induced pluripotent stem cell-based modular platform to challenge sensorineural hearing loss. Stem Cell 2021; 39(6):697–706.

24. Nourbakhsh A, Gosstola NC, Fernandez-Valle C, et al. Characterization of UMi031-A-2 inducible pluripotent stem cell line with a neurofibromatosis type 2-associated mutation. Stem Cell Res 2021;55:102474.

25. Ishi Y, Era T, Yuzawa S, et al. Analysis of induced pluripotent stem cell clones derived from a patient with mosaic neurofibromatosis type 2. Am J Med Genet 2022;188(6):1863–7.

26. Malicki J, Piotrowski T, Guedea F, et al. Treatment-integrated imaging, radiomics, and personalised radiotherapy: the future is at hand. Rep Pract Oncol Radiother 2022;27(4):734–43.

27. Gao Y, Liu R, Chang CW, et al. A potential revolution in cancer treatment: A topical review of FLASH radiotherapy. J Appl Clin Med Phys 2022;23(10):e13790.

28. Harrington KJ. Ultrahigh Dose-rate Radiotherapy: Next Steps for FLASH-RT. Clin Cancer Res 2019;25(1):3–5.

29. Schüler E, Acharya M, Montay-Gruel P, et al. Ultra-high dose rate electron beams and the FLASH effect: From preclinical evidence to a new radiotherapy paradigm. Med Phys 2022;49(3):2082–95.

30. Bourhis J, Sozzi WJ, Jorge PG, et al. Treatment of a first patient with FLASH-radiotherapy. Radiother Oncol 2019;139:18–22.

31. Nagaya T, Nakamura YA, Choyke PL, et al. Fluorescence-Guided Surgery. Front Oncol 2017;7:314.

32. Crawford KL, Pacheco FV, Lee YJ, et al. A Scoping Review of Ongoing Fluorescence-Guided Surgery Clinical Trials in Otolaryngology. Laryngoscope 2022;132(1):36–44.

33. Szczupak M, Peña SA, Bracho O, et al. Fluorescent Detection of Vestibular Schwannoma Using Intravenous Sodium Fluorescein In Vivo. Otol Neurotol 2021;42(4):e503–11.

34. Long J, Zhang Y, Huang X, et al. A Review of Drug Therapy in Vestibular Schwannoma. Drug Des Devel Ther 2021;15:75–85.

35. Tamura R, Toda M. A Critical Overview of Targeted Therapies for Vestibular Schwannoma. Int J Mol Sci 2022;23(10):5462.

36. Karajannis MA, Legault G, Hagiwara M, et al. Phase II trial of lapatinib in adult and pediatric patients with neurofibromatosis type 2 and progressive vestibular schwannomas. Neuro Oncol 2012;14(9):1163–70.

37. Ren Y, Sagers JE, Landegger LD, et al. Tumor-Penetrating Delivery of siRNA against TNFα to Human Vestibular Schwannomas. Sci Rep 2017;7(1):12922.

38. Wang S, Liechty B, Patel S, et al. Programmed death ligand 1 expression and tumor infiltrating lymphocytes in neurofibromatosis type 1 and 2 associated tumors. J Neuro Oncol 2018 May;138(1):183–90.

39. Zhao L, Cao YJ. Engineered T Cell Therapy for Cancer in the Clinic. Front Immunol 2019;10:2250.

40. Tamura R, Fujioka M, Morimoto Y, et al. A VEGF receptor vaccine demonstrates preliminary efficacy in neurofibromatosis type 2. Nat Commun 2019;10(1):5758.

41. Sinclair A, Islam S, Jones S. Gene therapy: an Overview of approved and pipeline technologies. In: CADTH Issues in emerging health technologies. Ottawa (ON): Canadian Agency for Drugs and Technologies in Health; 2018. p. 1–23.

42. Ahmed SG, Oliva G, Shao M, et al. Intratumoral injection of schwannoma with attenuated Salmonella typhimurium induces antitumor immunity and controls tumor growth. Proc Natl Acad Sci U S A 2022;119(24). e2202719119.

Moving?

Make sure your subscription moves with you!

To notify us of your new address, find your **Clinics Account Number** (located on your mailing label above your name), and contact customer service at:

Email: journalscustomerservice-usa@elsevier.com

800-654-2452 (subscribers in the U.S. & Canada)
314-447-8871 (subscribers outside of the U.S. & Canada)

Fax number: 314-447-8029

Elsevier Health Sciences Division
Subscription Customer Service
3251 Riverport Lane
Maryland Heights, MO 63043

*To ensure uninterrupted delivery of your subscription, please notify us at least 4 weeks in advance of move.

Printed and bound by CPI Group (UK) Ltd, Croydon, CR0 4YY

03/10/2024

01040468-0003